*Air*Veda

Ancient & New Medical Wisdom Digestion & Gas

Joseph B. Weiss, MD, FACP, FACG, AGAF
Clinical Professor of Medicine,
Gastroenterology
University of California, San Diego

© 2016 Joseph B. Weiss, M.D.
     SmartAsk Books
     Rancho Santa Fe, California, USA
     www.smartaskbooks.com

ISBN-13: 978-1-943760-18-3 (Volume One)
ISBN-13: 978-1-943760-19-0 (Volume Two)
ISBN-13: 978-1-943760-10-7 (Combined Volumes)

Cover photo: © Byheaven87 | Dreamstime.com license

Last digit is the print number: 9 8 7 6 5 4 3

Dedication

This volume is dedicated to clearing the air of the misperception that intestinal gas is anything other than a normal physiologic process common to all humanity. Nature and natural processes should be universally accepted as one of the cherished principles of fundamental human rights. The pursuit of health and happiness, and the accessible knowledge and resources of how to do so, should be available to all.

I am indebted to my loved ones Nancy, Danielle, Jeremy, Courie, Lizzy, & Indy. They have offered their insights, suggestions, comments, and unwavering support throughout the long process of having this project finally come to pass. You will always be the mighty wind beneath my wings.

Table of Contents

Preface

This is a very unusual book, both in content and intent. Dealing with matters of health and wellness the goal is to be factually correct and accurate, as well as to be informatively entertaining. With time, science and medicine will progress and no doubt a portion of the content will become outdated. In my chosen field of specialization, internal medicine, and especially in my field of sub-specialization gastroenterology, the advances have been dramatic and rapid.

As is to be expected, life, health, wellness, and disease are very complicated and complex subjects. The life sciences such as physiology, genomics, microbiology, etc. are interdependent with the basic sciences of chemistry, biology, physics, mathematics, and others. The applied sciences of engineering, pharmacology, epidemiology, and the myriad others add to the resources for deeper understanding and discovery.

The greatest age of discovery is still ahead of us, and the excitement and challenges in the fields are palpable. The history of medicine and science offer important lessons that are all too often forgotten as time progresses. Some of the most repeated and avoidable errors in health care is that business and profit opportunities from premature marketing of presumed medical and health advances are often later discredited, all too often with serious health consequences and not just financial losses.

This volume, and the others in the series, cover a wealth of topics related to the health and wellness of the digestive process, with an emphasis on intestinal gas and feces as examples of common health concerns that are intimately associated with normal daily health yet are rarely discussed. As a gastroenterologist who has seen tens of thousands of patients from all over the world, and all walks of life, I can unequivocally confirm that they are common concerns across the spectrum of humanity. The humorous references in this volume attempt to be tasteful and light, to compensate for some of the more technical and scientific content provided for those who wish to delve deeper into the subject.

As the book can be read as random short separate entries, or from cover to cover, the reader can choose how they wish to explore the wealth of information contained within these pages. Other volumes in the series provide additional resources for exploring what the author believes to be a fascinating and important subject, although it has been unfortunately suppressed by the embarrassment of cultural and societal norms.

It is ironic and humbling that often times in medicine, it is ancient wisdom that is rediscovered and appreciated anew. As you read these pages the amazing new wisdom and discoveries related to the gut microbiome, genomics, and the brain-gut-microbiome-diet axis were often already reflected in the insights and wisdom of the ancients.

*Air*Veda: Ancient & New Medical Wisdom

Introduction

Human health and longevity have always been dependent on adequate nutrition, shelter, and avoidance of mortal threats. The average life expectancy was limited to the early reproductive years because of high infant mortality and the lack of effective treatment for most injuries, infections, and illnesses. As communities and social structure evolved, the healing arts developed, often in association with religious beliefs and practices. The oldest known system of the healing arts and medicine was established in Ancient India over five thousand years ago and is known as Ayurveda. The word Ayurveda is derived from the Sanskrit terms Ayu meaning life and Veda meaning knowledge, wisdom, and learning. A major focus of this health system approach, which remains in active practice today, is the vital role of digestion and diet in health and disease.

Ancient Egyptian civilization also developed a system of medicine where digestion and the bowels were a focus of concern and attention. The chief physician of the supreme leader, known as the Pharaoh, was given the honorific title of Keeper of the Royal Rectum. The term physician is a reference back to the priority focus on the digestive organs as the source of health and illness, as the term physic was applied to purgatives and laxatives. A physician was a health professional trained in the use of prescribed physics. Even in more recent Western societies such as the realm of King Henry the Eighth of England the bowel function of the head of state was a closely guarded state secret. The Keeper of the Stool was the given title of the first member of the King's Privy Council, the private closed inner circle of the King's most trusted advisors. The term privy is still in use today as a euphemism for the water closet (WC) or toilet.

Digestive disorders, nutrition, and diet are the most common of health concerns, and justifiably so, since virtually all health matters are ultimately influenced by this basic function and source of vitality. The Greek and Latin term Gastro referring to the stomach, and Entero referring to the intestines, have been added to the suffix -ology meaning knowledge, to arrive at the present name Gastroenterology. Often shortened to the acronym GI for gastrointestinal, it is the name of the internal medicine subspecialty dealing with the digestive organs, health, and disease. Western medicine, most often referred to by the misnomer Allopathic Medicine, tends to focus on disease states and their treatment to allow a return to health. Other healing approaches, especially those taking a more holistic perspective, have gained greater appreciation over recent years. Initially described as Alternative or Complementary Medicine, they are now more often identified as Integrative Medicine. Whatever the name, most practitioners would agree that if the approach provides health and healing benefits, they should be a welcomed addition to the armamentarium of modern medicine.

*Air*Veda: Ancient & New Medical Wisdom

My own background is based on the Western Allopathic model. My cultural background and early education included Judaic studies of the original ancient Hebrew texts, as well as the original Aramaic texts of the Babylonian Talmud. One of my personal heroes was the compassionate and brilliant Middle Ages Royal Court physician and scholar Maimonides. My interest in medical history has been a lifelong fascination, and I have a profound appreciation for the challenges facing each generation of healers and physicians. It is always the case that we are dealing with a primitive state of medical knowledge, and limited therapeutics, compared to what we know will be the advances to come just over the horizon of time. My cultural and ethnic background exposed me to the common Yiddish exclamation of desperation, Oy Vey! With self-deprecating humor, I would consider the allopathic medicine focus on disease to be a form of OyVeydic Medicine!

Although I pursued a traditional Western medical education in the U.S., I maintained my international and multicultural perspective with postgraduate studies in medicine in Europe, Africa, and Latin America. I completed specialty training in Internal Medicine and Gastroenterology with further interests in tropical medicine, microbiology, nutrition, and metabolism. Maintaining an active clinical practice along with research, teaching, and administrative responsibilities allowed continuous advancement of an extensive experience and education in health matters. Serving in a volunteer capacity for over thirty-five years at the Veterans Administration Medical Center and on the clinical faculty of a major teaching and research university has been extremely rewarding and fulfilling. One of the many significant lessons I learned over and over during my decades of practice in medicine, and being honored with the care entrusted to me by my patients, has been the healing power of empathy and caring. The ability to see the humor that is ever present in the human condition is also a gift worth nurturing. Since I consider myself an amateur humorist, I like to share the philosophy stated in the phrase 'Laughter is the Best Medicine'.

As the culmination of my professional knowledge as a gastroenterologist, my passion for education as a clinical professor at a prestigious university medical school, and my avocation as a humorist and entertainer, I have written a series of books for the lay public. The books are purposefully focused on subjects that are rarely discussed, but that I know from discussions with tens of thousands of patients over the years are of great public interest. Since I have a longstanding interest in medical history, and some knowledge of Ayurveda Medicine, I feel comfortable describing my specialty knowledge (in Sanskrit described as Veda) on digestion and intestinal gas as the founding of the new discipline of AirVeda Medicine.

*Air*Veda: Ancient & New Medical Wisdom

Since I enjoy sharing what I believe to be valuable and entertaining information, I have published a number of volumes. My books to date include:
AirVeda: Ancient & New Medical Wisdom, Digestion & Gas
The Scoop on Poop! Flush with Knowledge
You Don't Know Sh*t! Until You Read This Book (same content as Scoop)
To 'Air' is Human: Everything You Ever Wanted to Know About Intestinal Gas
Artsy Fartsy, Cultural History of the Fart
How Do You Doo? Everybody Pees & Poops!
The Quest for Immortality: Advances in Vitality & Longevity

Now after introducing the reader to my humorous tongue-in-cheek creations of OyVeda and AirVeda, let's return to the original and authentic healing system of Ayurveda. One of the most remarkable aspects of Ayurveda, beyond its ancient history and longevity, is that only recent advances in science and technology have provided a deeper understanding of its properties and benefits. The current research advances in the microbiome, immunology, genomics, epigenetics, diet, nutrition, meditation, herbal remedies, nutraceuticals, and the life sciences in general are opening new appreciation for this ancient and venerable body of knowledge. Ayurveda is the world's oldest health discipline in that it originated in Ancient India over five thousand years ago. It is a holistic approach to body, mind, and spirit which defines disease as the absence of vibrant health. This is a different approach than taken by traditional Western Allopathic Medicine, which typically defines health as the absence of disease. Ayurveda surgical techniques and medical therapies were the basis of many advances adopted by Western medicine. Other aspects are still considered alternative or complimentary medicine, with newer advances in research technology capabilities encouraging their reassessment and adaptation by what we consider Modern Medicine.

In Ayurveda the presence of disease is believed to be attributable to either physical imbalance, emotional turbulence, or spiritual disconnection. Treatment modalities include diet, herbs, massage, meditation, yoga, detoxification, emotional regulation, breath management, and proper sensory input. The balance of Mind, Body, and Spirit are characterized as the three doshas representing various combinations of Akasha (space/potential), Vayu (air/movement), Agni (fire/transformation), Jala (water/protection), and Prithivi (earth/structure). Vata is the combination of space and air, Pitta is the combination of fire and water, and Kapha is the combination of water and earth. Each dosha has a primary site in the body, Kapha is the stomach, chest, and head, Pitta is the small intestine, liver, and blood, and Vata is the colon. Each person has different proportions of each dosha comprising their constitution, and imbalance of the doshas can result in health issues. The Ayurveda approach to treatment is to return the doshas to the proper balance for the individual.

Digestion and nutrition play a vital role in both the Ayurveda and Allopathic Medicine. In Ayurveda health is ascribed to the potency of digestive Agni, defined as the powerful digestive fire. A strong Agni allows the body access to Ojas, the subtle nourishment and nutrition present in food. A weak Agni is unable to properly process and digest intake which allows the accumulation of Ama, the toxic residue and waste of the incomplete digestive and absorptive process. The beneficial Ojas or toxic Ama then enter the Srota, the circulatory channels, and are distributed to the body. The Dhatus are the tissues of the body and are classified as Rasap (plasma), Rakta (blood), Mamsa (muscles), Meda (fat), Asthi (bone), Majja (nerves and bone marrow), and Shukra (reproduction). The waste products are called Mutra (urine), Purisha and Mala (feces), and Sweda (sweat).

The qualities of the Vata Dosha are dry, light, cold, rough, quick, mobile, changeable, irregular, and subtle. Its functions are transportation, movement, and communication. The qualities of the Pitta Dosha are light, hot, sharp, slightly oily, intense, penetrating, acidic, moist, flowing, liquid, and pungent. Its functions are metabolism, digestion, and transformation. The qualities of the Kapha Dosha are oily, heavy, cool, slow, stable, sticky, solid, smooth, steady, enduring, and dull. Its functions are structure, cohesion, and lubrication. In most people, one or two doshas predominate. Although determined at conception and called Prakruti, experience and choice influence an individual's current balance of doshas, called Vikruti.

Ayurveda doshas Shutterstock/GL Sonts

Ayurveda describes six tastes: Madhura (sweet), Amla (sour), Lavana (salty), Katu (pungent), Tikta (bitter), and Kashaya astringent. Sweet is considered the taste of energy which builds tissues. Included in this category are grains, pasta, bread, nuts, dairy, oils, sweet fruits, starchy vegetables, animal products, and sugar. The sour taste includes organic acids which promote appetite and digestion. This includes citrus fruits, berries, tomatoes, sour fruits, yogurt, cheese, vinegar, pickles, fermented foods, and alcohol. The taste of salt promotes digestion and includes table salt, fish, meat, seaweed, soy sauce, processed foods, condiments, and sauces. Pungent taste is found in essential oils and is believed to stimulate digestion and assist in detoxification. Examples include pepper, cayenne, ginger, garlic, onions, leeks, chilies, radish, horseradish, salsa, basil, thyme, cloves, and mustard. Bitter taste is considered to be the taste of information and includes anti-inflammatory and detoxifying properties. It is found in green and yellow squash, broccoli, greens, spinach, kale, and Brussels sprouts. The astringent taste is the taste of dryness and lightness and is believed to have healing and compacting properties. It is found in beans, legumes, peas, lentils, tea, cranberries, pomegranate, apples, and dark leafy greens.

In Ayurveda the six stages of disease are Sanchaya (accumulation), Prakopa (aggravation), Prasara (spread), Sthana-samshraya (localization), Vyakti (manifestation), and Bheda (differentiation). The Ayurveda evaluative techniques include Roga Pariksha the examination of the disease and Rogi Pariksha the examination of the patient. Dravya Guna Karma Shastra is the Ayurveda science of pharmacology. The term Dravya describes substances, herbs, and drugs. Guna is the term for their properties and qualities, and Karma is the term for their action and effect. Shastra is the term for science, Veerya means potency, Prabhava is a unique property, and Vipaka is a post-digestive effect. The Ayurveda term Soma is the cooling essence of physiology, Sattva is defined as purity, clarity, and evolution. Additional terms include Rajas meaning dynamism, movement, and energy, and Tamas meaning inertia, darkness, and ignorance.

Pancha Karma is the Ayurveda purification therapy that includes Shodhana and Shamana the terms for detoxification and rejuvenation. The methodology of Pancha Karma detoxification includes Vamana the inducement of vomiting (emesis), especially for the Kapha Dosha. For the Pita Dosha Virechana, the inducement of purgation with laxatives and cathartics, is often prescribed. Nasya, the nasal passage cleansing, using a netti pot and saline solution is often prescribed for the Kapha and Vata Doshas. Basti are colonic enemas that are either Anuvasana (oil based) or Niruha (water based) and often used on the Vata Dosha. Raka Moksha is bloodletting and was used for the Pitta Dosha. Swedena is the use of heat to induce sweating (diaphoresis). Snehana is oleation, the use of oils both internally and externally. Rasayana is the process of rejuvenation utilizing nutrition, rest, exercise, meditation, herbs, and other modalities.

Ayurveda, still predominantly found in India, is taught and practiced around the world. The herb turmeric, often found in curry, is a natural anti-inflammatory product that is just as potent as the strongest prescription pharmaceuticals. Western Allopathic medicine has traditionally taken a reductionist approach, looking for a single key feature or chemical which offers a specific mechanism of action. A limited number of diseases are fully explained and successfully approached with this methodology. Ayurveda takes a more holistic systems biology approach, where multiple compounds in a natural product may require synergy to provide a full benefit. The life sciences are providing more evidence that the systems biology approach is necessary for the vast majority of illnesses and therapeutics. The nearly infinite variability of the human genome, combined with the complexity and interaction of human microbiome diversity, emphasizes the importance of the systems biology approach.

Air is critical for life, and has played a major part in the long history of medicine from the focus on the air nature of the Vata Dosha of Ayurveda to the airborne transmission of communicable diseases and environmental pollutants. The entire specialty of pulmonary medicine deals with the respiratory organs and the absorption and elimination of the various gases that comprise the air we breathe and body metabolism. The gastrointestinal tract also deals with air issues, including the air we swallow, known as aerophagia, the gasses produced by our digestive process, and finally the gasses produced by the microbiome, the community of microbes residing within our body. The purpose of this volume is to offer insight and knowledge about this common concern, which has been all too often been an unnecessary source of confusion and embarrassment.

Many people incorrectly believe the age of discovery and exploration was in the past. The rapid advances in technology over the past century occurred at a dizzying pace. Remarkably the age of flight from the Wright brothers at Kitty Hawk progressed to supersonic jets and man traveling and returning to the moon in less than a hundred years. The first telegraph wire to wireless communication of smart computing phones with video conferencing capabilities to anywhere in the world took place in a blink of evolutionary time. The understanding of a hidden microbial world continues to astound with entirely new life forms identified in only the last few decades. One of these, Archaea, was hiding in plain sight and has the remarkable ability to survive and thrive in places once thought impossible, such as within rocks miles underground, and in extreme temperatures. The recognition that the human microbiome is intimately involved with human health and disease will without doubt revolutionize medicine. Other discoveries of similar or greater magnitude are likely over the years to come, so it remains humbling how little we know.

Air in the gastrointestinal tract is normal. The presence of air, especially if found in excess, can have three or more results. The first is the release of air as an eructation, more commonly known as a burp or belch. The second is distention, also known as bloat. The third result is flatulence, more commonly known as the passage of gas as flatus or as a fart. The word fart is the correct word to use in the English language, and indeed is one of its oldest words. The alternative terms used, such as flatus and flatulence are not original English words as they have been borrowed from the Latin. There is controversy as to the derivation of the word fart. It is thought to have Indo-European roots in the Germanic language word farzen. One thought is that it originated as an onomatopoeia, a word that phonetically imitates the sound of the event it describes. Another thought is that it was related to the term for partridge, as the bird makes a similar sound when it is disturbed in its natural habitat and takes flight.

Farts are ubiquitous, all living creatures generate gas from cellular metabolism and respiration, and humans are no exception. The bacteria of your colonic flora, part of the microbiome of living organisms that lives on and within humans, generate gas which collect in the bowel. They are joined with the air swallowed throughout the day and night, particularly at meals. Aerophagia is universal and we swallow on average three to five cubic centimeters (one teaspoonful) of air with every swallow. Additional gasses are produced during the enzymatic digestive processes as well as the neutralization of gastric hydrochloric acid by pancreatic and duodenal bicarbonate. The result is a significant volume of gasses within and transiting the bowel.

Fortunately, the vast majority of the gasses produced are absorbed by the gut, then into the bloodstream through diffusion and finally exhaled when they each the alveoli of the lungs. The component gasses have very different properties of diffusion through the bowel wall and into the bloodstream. Carbon dioxide readily diffuses and enters solution and is exhaled promptly. Although it is the largest volume of gas generated, and temporarily contributes to distension and postprandial (after meal) discomfort, it is the easiest to eliminate from the bowel and is only a minor contributor to flatulence.

The volume of gasses in the gastrointestinal tract is dependent on the quantity and nature of foods ingested, the body's ability to produce enzymes for the various food types, the microbiome and gut flora, and gastrointestinal transit time. The often quoted figure of twelve farts per day is a reasonable average number of farts passed but there is a very wide range of what is considered normal. The fact is that air is critical for our survival, as well as ubiquitous in nature and in our digestive tract. It is my hope that this book and its companion volumes will serve to inform and entertain the public. The knowledge gained with progress in medicine and the life sciences will hopefully enhance health and vitality as well as extend the human lifespan. Perhaps there is more than a little truth to the phrase Life is a Gas.

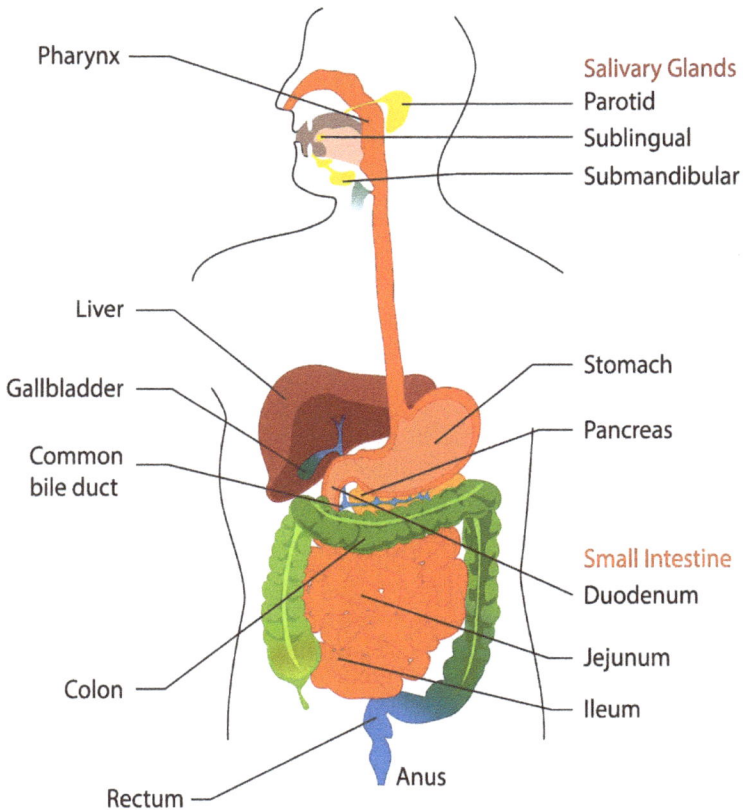

Pharynx

Salivary Glands
Parotid
Sublingual
Submandibular

Liver

Stomach

Gallbladder

Pancreas

Common
bile duct

Small Intestine
Duodenum

Jejunum

Colon

Ileum

Anus

Rectum

Shutterstock/yaruna

This book is organized in an alphabetical order of subjects, much like an encyclopedia. This allows one the luxury to skip around to read entries of interest, and to spend as little or as much time as one wishes reading at one sitting. The image of the digestive tract on this page is a useful reference to its anatomy and terminology. Reading the entry on digestion is also a very good place to start to give an overview of this fascinating subject vital to good health, as well as understanding the passage of air in the digestive tract.

Activated Charcoal

Commercially available products to trap and contain the dispersion of noxious gasses and toxins have been available for some time. Adapting these properties to address the aroma of a fart have also been marketed with some success. They rely on the adsorptive properties of activated carbon also known as activated charcoal, activated coal, or carbo activatus. Activated charcoal is a form of carbon processed to increase the surface area available for adsorption or chemical reactions.

Activated charcoal, microscopic view increased surface area. Creative Commons License

The term adsorption and absorption are frequently confused. Absorption allows another material to be integrated into the volume of the absorptive matter. Adsorption is when the material being incorporated adheres to the surface of the material, and is not absorbed into its interior. An example of the difference between the two terms would be the drinking of water leads to its absorption that is it becomes internalized within your bodily tissues. Water that coats your skin in the shower or after spilling it on yourself is adsorbed, that is it is only on the outer surface of your body, and it is not absorbed.

Its very large surface area is a key concept to understanding the effectiveness of activated charcoal. A single cube of charcoal has a much smaller surface area for adsorption to take place, than an identical volume cube that has been subdivided into many smaller cubes. The following illustration helps to visualize how the surface area can be dramatically increased with the same volume of material.

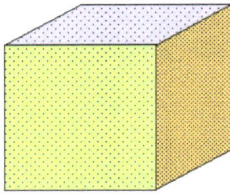

a one-meter cube has 6 square meters of suface area

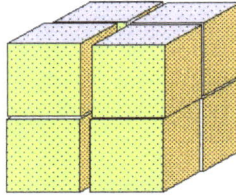

pieces half the original size have twice the surface area

pieces one quarter of the original size have 4 times the surface area

pieces one-eighth of the original size have 8 times the surface area.

a cubic meter of fine sediment can have millions of square meters of surface area

Increase in surface area illustrated. Phil Stoffer, Ph.D. Geology Cafe geologycafe.com Creative Commons License

Activated carbon is used in the purification, decaffeination, metal extraction, water purification, and sewage treatment processes. It is also used in the air filters in masks and respirators, filters in compressed air, and to filter vodka and whiskey to remove impurities that would affect taste. In cases of the ingestion of toxins or poisons it has been used orally to bind to the toxin to prevent its absorption into the victim.

It is also effective in adsorbing offensive smelling gasses in flatus. Due to its porosity a single gram of activated carbon can have a surface area in excess of five hundred meters squared, with one thousand five hundred meters squared being possible with further refining. Its adsorption ability varies amongst gasses and liquids and it is known to be a poor adsorbent of carbon monoxide, which is toxic and odorless. It is particularly effective in adsorbing most of the volatile odoriferous gasses.

The key to the success or failure of the product is the degree to which the fart can escape without having passed through the activated charcoal. The tighter the seal, the less likely for odiferous gasses to escape. The sitting pad was least effective trapping about twenty percent of gasses. Underwear pads ranged from fifty to seventy-five percent effectiveness, while the tight fitting entirely lined with activated charcoal underwear were the most effective, but also the most expensive.

Flat-D activated carbon technology provides a thin barrier with sponge-like surface area for blocking the release of odor molecules.

ODOR ABSORBING TECHNOLOGY

Activated charcoal pad products. Flat-D Innovations, Inc. Used with permission

Activated carbon is used to treat oral poisonings by binding to and preventing the poison from being absorbed by the gastrointestinal tract. The home remedy of eating burnt toast for food poisoning was based on the adsorptive properties of activated charcoal. Charcoal biscuits were marketed in the early 19th century as an antidote to flatulence, and are still sold today for diarrhea, indigestion, flatulence, and as a pet care product. Unfortunately, orally ingested charcoal pills are not effective in appreciably reducing intestinal gas. This may be because the adsorptive capacity of the activated charcoal is fully utilized before it finally gets to the colon where its gas adsorbing properties are needed. Fortunately, bismuth products do provide a significant advantage by binding to the sulfur compounds and eliminating them without producing offensive gas.

Aerogel

Aerogel was developed by Samuel Kistler (1900-1975) at the College of the Pacific in Stockton, California in 1931. It was a silica material with a chemical structure similar to glass with gas in its pores rather than liquid. It is an open celled material that is ninety-five percent air, with pores less than one ten-thousandth of the diameter of a human hair. Further refinements allowed the air to be replaced by a vacuum, and the silica to be replaced by other materials. Kistler developed aerogels made of alumina, tungsten oxide, ferric oxide, tin oxide, nickel tartarate, cellulose, cellulose nitrate, gelatin, agar, egg albumen, and rubber. Further advancements and refinements in production have led to greater commercial applications.

The pore diameter being measured in nanometers gives it a nanoporous nature leading to the lowest thermal conductivity of any known solid. It has an extremely high surface area to mass ration with just two grams of aerogel having a surface area of a square kilometer (one thousand meters squared)

Aerogel. Stardust.jpl.nasa.gov Public Domain

Aerogel is made from a wet gel that is dried. The substance has been described as feeling like volcanic glass pumice; a very fine, dry sponge; and extremely lightweight Styrofoam. NASA Public Domain

Though with a ghostly appearance like a hologram, aerogel is very solid. It feels like hard Styrofoam to the touch. Aerogel. Stardust.jpl.nasa.gov Public Domain

It is so lightweight that it has unmatched utility as an insulating material and has been utilized by NASA for the space shuttle and space exploration. The development of this product has allowed exploration of extreme environments such as outer space and deep sea exploration, where humans are exposed to the high and low extremes of atmospheric pressure that dramatically effect intestinal gas pressure and volume

Crayons placed on top of a piece of silica aerogel will not melt from the heat of a flame. Certain types of aerogel provide thirty-nine times more insulation than fiberglass. NASA Public Domain

Aerogel. Stardust.jpl.nasa.gov Public Domain

Aerogel eetd.lbl.gov Public Domain

Aerogel. A five-pound (two and one-half kilogram) brick is supported on top of a piece of aerogel weighing only two grams. Stardust.jpl.nasa.gov Public Domain

Aerophagia (Air Swallowing)

Air swallowing is a universal event in humans and is also known as aerophagia. We do it with every one of the on average two thousand swallows we take every day, ingesting approximately five milliliters (one teaspoonful) of air with every swallow. Air is seventy-eight percent nitrogen, which is a poorly absorbed gas. If it is not released in a burp, it will contribute to bloating and distension. The volume of air swallowed is impressive, but is only a small percentage of what the digestive process can generate in terms of gas production.

Aerophagia is the swallowing of air, allowing it to enter the digestive tract, and it occurs naturally and without thinking in every individual. There is a variation of aerophagia in which the behavior becomes a purposeful, and at times obsessive-compulsive, behavior. More often, when excessive spontaneous aerophagia is occurring it is a subconscious or unconscious behavior, much like a nervous tic. The volume of air swallowed in these conditions can be impressive and a plain x-ray of the abdomen may demonstrate that the entire digestive tract is filled with air from esophagus to rectum.

Various studies have estimated the volume of each swallow as approximately twenty milliliters or four teaspoons. Many people swallow larger gulps of food on purpose and some even go to extremes in demonstrating their swallowing abilities. Sword swallowing is just one example where swallowing has been taken to a level of competition or entertainment.

Air swallowing (aerophagia) is universal and occurs with every single swallow including swallows of food, food, saliva, etc. Shutterstock/yuris

At the other extreme, some people take very small swallows and may sip foods at a teaspoon or less per swallow. They may be surprised to learn that sipping smaller volumes may actually increase the total amount of air they swallow. In general, the larger the total number of swallows, the larger the volume of air consumed.

If we took twenty milliliters as the volume of a normal average swallow, and the individual only took in small five milliliters sip of soup, each twenty milliliters swallow would include an additional fifteen milliliters of air. This is why hard candy and chewing gums, which generates small volumes of saliva and frequent swallows that mainly consist of air, lead to excessive aerophagia.

Baby bottles are a common source of aerophagia in infants. If the milk or formula does not completely cover the nipple of the bottle the baby will suck in and swallow air. Shutterstock/Nicolesa

Since the digestive tract of the newborn is sterile, there are no microorganisms generating gas through cellular metabolism. All of the gas the newborn infant begins to pass is swallowed air. If an infant is bottle-fed rather than breast-fed they are much more likely to swallow even more air.

The first exposure to microorganisms that will be swallowed and begin to colonize the infant digestive tract are from the birth mother if the delivery is vaginal. The microorganisms that colonize the infant become its microbiome and play a major role in its ongoing health and wellness. The gut flora is one aspect of the microbiome, with skin, ears, mouth, genitourinary, and every surface of the body exposed to the external environment developing its own unique microbiome. Infants born by Caesarean section have exposure to different organisms, which establish a microbiome that is not believed to be as beneficial as via a natural vaginal delivery.

Baby bottles are a common cause of aerophagia in infants as they suck in and swallow air if the formula does not always cover the nipple. Burping the baby after a feeding is the means of allowing the swallowed air to escape, otherwise it will cause distension and discomfort. Some bottles are designed to use an internal plastic sleeve to prevent air from reaching the nipple, when the formula is depleted the sleeve forms a vacuum so the infant is not sucking in air.

The air swallowed is the same as the air in the atmosphere, about seventy-eight percent nitrogen, twenty-one percent oxygen, one percent argon, and other gasses. Included in the other gasses that make up one percent of air is argon, comprising the vast majority at zero point nine three percent. In spite of global warming carbon dioxide makes up only a fraction of one percent of air, with the remainder including trace amounts of neon, helium, methane, krypton, and hydrogen. Seventy-eight percent of air is nitrogen and the gastrointestinal tract poorly absorbs this gas compared to oxygen and carbon dioxide.

Once the nitrogen is swallowed it has only two ways to get out of the digestive tract. Coming up as a burp or belch is its closest exit, but it has to overcome the lower esophageal sphincter, the upper esophageal sphincter and the oncoming rush with peristalsis and gravity of more food, fluid, drink, saliva, and yes even more air being swallowed. With every single swallow about five milliliters, or one teaspoonful, of air is swallowed whether you are eating, drinking, or just resting between meals. You swallow approximately every thirty seconds while awake, and about every five minutes while asleep.

The average person swallows about two thousand times a day, but many swallow much more than that. Foods that are extremely hot or cold tend to be swallowed in smaller quantities, resulting in more swallows being necessary to eat or drink the same volume at a moderate temperature. If you chew gum, use a lozenge or sucking candy, or use any product that is a sialagogue, i.e. generates saliva, you will be doing a lot more swallowing. Don't forget that with each swallow you are taking in much more air than saliva.

Aerophagia and Belching / Supragastric Belching

Belching is swallowed air returning to the mouth. This is usually the result of reflex LOS relaxation to vent excess gastric air after eating; however it is possible to voluntarily induce belching. This is achieved by swallowing air (aerophagia) and abdominal contraction to force gastric air across the LOS (the same mechanism as rumination).

Supragastric belching is the result of swallowing air immediately followed by abdominal *and* diaphragmatic contraction. This increases abdominal pressure and closes the LOS by closure of the diaphragmatic hiatus thus forcing air back.

Similar to rumination, aerophagia with belching and / or supragastric belching may be subconscious, maladaptive behaviour. Affected patients present with 'uncontrollable, persistent burping'. Investigation is with concurrent manometry and impedance. Treatment is with biofeedback techniques.

Supragastric Belching

UOS relaxes in response to oesophageal distention

Simultaneous rise in pressure (and impedance)

Air forced back at unopened LOS

Abdominal wall Contracts to increase gastric pressure. Diaphragm contracts to close LOS

www.bmj.com

The same is true of chewing tobacco and even smoking tobacco whether as cigar, pipe, cigarette, or electronic smokeless cigarette. Do you want to hold a conversation while you are eating? Go ahead but it will cause even more air swallowing, as will drinking from a straw or tilting your head back to drink from a bottle or can. Rush through your meals, and you swallow more air than food or drink.

Talking while eating leads to excess air swallowing. Shutterstock/R.legosyn

Tobacco smoked as a cigarette, pipe, or cigar, or even chewed contributes to aerophagia
Shutterstock/branislavpudar

If you are a baby, just lean back and drink from your baby bottle, even those designed to keep the amount of air swallowed to a minimum. Well, the good news for babies is that most caregivers know how to get them to burp up the air swallowed after a feeding. Then again, the associated spit ups could best be avoided by changing the posture at feeding times to reduce air swallowing.

Chewing and bubble gum, as well as use of sucking candy and throat lozenges can lead to excessive air swallowing. Shutterstock/billionphotos

Other conditions recognized to increase air swallowing include poor fitting dentures, not chewing food well, drinking from a straw or bottle, talking while eating, and racing through a meal. In another category is the notorious adolescent male who loves to swallow air on purpose so he can generate belches and burps worthy of a dinosaur. Although he may be proud of his newfound talent, it will take many years to achieve the maturity to recognize the sounds generated are an ineffective mating call to attract the female of the species.

Aerophagia air swallowing is the most common source of excess intestinal gas. Ill-fitting dentures will contribute to more air being swallowed. Shutterstock/stocksnapper

Some individuals also develop a rumination syndrome, where they subconsciously regurgitate and re-swallow food mixed in with even more air. Fortunately, it is unusual to see a different form of purposeful aerophagia since the development of the artificial larynx or voice box. Years ago, individuals who unfortunately developed cancer of the vocal cords or throat and lost their voice box, used to be taught to swallow air and generate esophageal speech. Esophageal speech was primarily air swallowing followed by controlled belching to create a modified vocalization.

Going back to the average of two thousand swallows a day we are talking about ten liters of air swallowed every single day. Even incorrectly assuming that one hundred percent of the oxygen in the swallowed air was absorbed, we are looking at about eight liters of nitrogen that has been taken in and now needs to get out. That is a lot of nitrogen, and the most direct exit, the shortest distance to travel, and the fastest way to get relief, is to burp or belch.

Sometimes the social situation or environment discourages and suppresses the natural inclination to release the swallowed air. Even if you could burp at will that is an awful lot of gas swallowed throughout the day and night. It is much more than the most frequent and dedicated burpers and belchers are able to release through eructation. The retained nitrogen will contribute to bloating and distension, before it eventually makes its way out of the other end of the intestinal tract as flatus, more commonly known as a fart.

Meals with a high fat content trigger the release of hormones that slow down gut motility. As the food spends more time in the digestive tract, continued bacterial fermentation produces increasing quantities of gas. In addition, foods that are extremely hot or cold tend to be swallowed in smaller quantities, resulting in more swallows being necessary to eat or drink the same volume at a moderate temperature. As each swallow contributes an additional quantity of air entering the esophagus and digestive tract, more swallows results in more air ingestion. Foods or snacks that require excess chewing with resultant excess swallowing of saliva, such as chewing or bubble gum, also contribute to excess air ingestion.

Drinking directly from a bottle or can, or using a straw, can lead to excess aerophagia.
Shutterstock/AnnaJurkovska

A hidden source of swallowed air is the air content present within many foods. Fruits contain a great deal more air than you might have imagined. If you compress an apple and add the volume of the juice and the pressed fruit together you will find that it was only sixty percent of the volume of the original fruit. In other words, of the entire fruit that you swallowed forty percent was air.

We have been in love with ice cream for thousands of years. All ice creams are not prepared in an identical manner. There is another important factor that leads to differences besides the ingredients such as cream or milk fat content, flavorings, sweeteners, stabilizers, emulsifiers, lactose, whey, casein, etcetera. It may be surprising to learn that the two largest ingredients in ice cream by volume are water (between fifty-five percent and sixty-four percent) and air (between three percent and fifty percent).

The other ingredients are measured as a percentage by weight. These include milk fat (minimum ten percent) or in premium ice creams, butter fat (up to nineteen percent). Other ingredients include sweeteners (twelve percent to sixteen percent), milk solids including proteins like casein and whey, and carbohydrates like lactose (between nine percent to twelve percent). Additional ingredients include stabilizers and emulsifiers like agar-agar or carrageenan extracted from seaweed that prevent the fat and water contents from separating (between zero point two percent to zero point five percent). Although air is a large percent by volume, it has virtually zero weight.

The finest ice creams have the lowest percentage of air, but the air is a necessary ingredient to provide a smooth, silky, creamy texture. Without the added air the ice cream would be denser, harder, and feel colder to the tongue. The size of the air bubbles is important as the smallest bubbles provide the smoothest texture. The industry term for air added to foods such as ice cream is 'overrun'. If one liter of ice cream is aerated to double the volume of the mixture to two liters, the overrun is one hundred percent. Most commercial ice creams aim for an overrun of seventy-five percent to one hundred percent, with super-premium ice creams achieving overruns of approximately twenty percent.

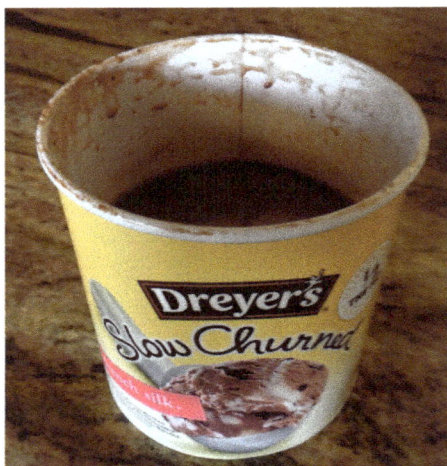

Overrun is the term used to describe air that is added into the finished food product to expand its volume as well as for texture. Air content of ice cream ranges from three percent to fifty percent and has a significant influence on texture, taste, and the value of the product purchased since ice cream is typically sold by volume, not weight. Photo by Lizabeth Weiss.

Have you ever noticed that the volume of ice cream decreases as it melts? If you have accidently left a full container of ice cream out of the freezer and it melted, you would find that it would only be about sixty percent full. You can quickly tell the difference in air content by lifting up equivalent size containers of super-premium ice creams and lower priced competitors. The super-premiums weigh much more, but also contain a lot more content, calories, and fat grams. If half of the volume of ice cream you eat is simply hidden air, you have just been spared half the calories and get the bonus of having swallowed more air to entertain your family and friends.

One of the advantages of a higher overrun, besides higher profits by selling a volume of air at the price of ice cream, is the fact that the air cells as bubbles may prevent ice crystals from forming. If you have ever had ice cream with ice crystals, you know that the raspy cutting feeling on the tongue quickly ruins a pleasurable experience. The Food and Drug Administration has standardized the weight of ice cream to not fall below four and one-half pounds to the gallon. This weight standard has limited the amount of air that can be added to the ice cream to approximately fifty percent by volume.

The research team that developed the concept of aeration of ice cream included Baroness Margaret Thatcher, the former Prime Minister of Great Britain and contemporary of US President Ronald Reagan. Perhaps there is a kernel of truth that it was a right-wing conservative conspiracy to allow the addition of air allowing ice cream companies to double their profit by selling half a container of air at the full price of ice cream!

Gelato and ice cream are not identical and have a different composition and nutritional value. In the U.S. ice cream is required to have at least ten percent milkfat, with most medium to high end brands actually containing between fourteen percent to seventeen percent milkfat. Ice cream is churned at a high speed to incorporate air into the mixture to create a smooth and fluffy texture. Ice cream typically contains more than fifty percent air after the churning process both for enhanced mouth feel as well as profitability since it is sold by volume not weight. By contrast, gelato contains between three percent and eight percent milkfat, and twenty -five percent to thirty percent air.

Gelato is denser than ice cream due to its lower air content. A scoop of gelato weighs more than the same size scoop of vanilla ice cream. Since the nutritional comparison is based on ounces of weight and not volume, a scoop of gelato that is the same size as a scoop of ice cream may have more total calories, fat and sugar than ice cream. On average, a three and one-half ounce serving of vanilla gelato contains ninety calories, three grams of fat and ten grams of sugar. A typical three and one-half ounce serving of vanilla ice cream contains one hundred and twenty-five calories, seven grams of fat and fourteen grams of sugar. The fat in content coats the taste buds of the tongue, preventing them from completely experiencing the flavors. Because gelato has a lower fat content the taste buds experience flavors more intensely, and gelato does not need as much added sugar as ice cream for sweetness

The same proposition is true for bread and most baked goods. The baking process often uses baking powder or yeast. When the dough rises you are seeing the additional volume of gasses such as carbon dioxide being produced by the yeast fermentation process. Many foods are whipped with air to increase their volume, which adds to the smoothness and creaminess of the product. It also adds to the bottom line of profitability to the manufacturer, as you are paying for a product typically sold by volume. As long as they don't push it to the detriment of flavor and texture the more air added to a product increases its volume and profitability.

Carbonated beverages are very popular worldwide. In the United States sales of carbonated beverages exceed twenty billion dollars per year, four times the sales volume of dairy products. The majority consumed today already comes carbonated with large amounts of carbon dioxide forced into solution under high pressure. As the pressure seal of the can or bottle is released the carbon dioxide forms bubbles and comes out of the solution, giving a pleasant tickling sensation on the palate, and a full at times bloated feeling in the stomach and gut.

Many soft drinks have high concentrations of simple carbohydrates such as glucose, fructose, and sucrose. Oral bacteria ferment these carbohydrates and produce acidic products, which can erode the tooth enamel beginning the dental decay process. A large number of soft drinks are already acidic and have phosphoric acid added in the manufacturing process bringing their pH level to three or lower. To put this value in perspective, neutral water has a pH of seven and gastric hydrochloric acid has a pH of two. Many dentists advocate avoid the brushing of teeth shortly after an acidic beverage because the tooth enamel is more vulnerable to abrasions after being softened by acid.

Carbonated champagne uncorking photographed with a high-speed air-gap flash.
Shutterstock/lightwork

Mineral water cures were very popular in the middle ages and beyond. Going to the source of mineral springs and the drinking of its contents was referred to as 'taking the waters'. The waters had a variety of mineral content depending on source locale and included various salts and sulfur contents. The sites of such resources became well known as spas, baths, and wells and developed into destinations for the ill and infirm, as well as those who wished to preserve their good health. The term Seltzer water was originally a trademarked name for the German town of Selter that had a famous mineral spring.

The bottling of mineral waters became a profitable enterprise by offering people the opportunity to partake of the presumed beneficial waters in their own locales. An attempt to imitate the effervescent effect of the mineral waters was made by Joseph Priestley in 1767. Some fans of carbonated beverages believe this should be his claim to fame rather than his discovery of oxygen. J. J. Schweppes of Switzerland commercialized the process in 1783, moving his factory and enterprise to England in 1783.

Have you ever wondered how much carbon dioxide gas is released from a soft drink or carbonated beverage? You have already gotten a visual demonstration if the bottle or can was dropped or shaken before being opened. This agitation accelerates the release of the carbon dioxide, and it can form a jet stream of gassy bubbles to be sprayed on everyone within a dozen feet of the demonstration. This social activity is very popular amongst preadolescent boys. The quantification of how much carbon dioxide is in a one-liter bottle of a carbonated soft drink is calculated using a formula known as Henry's Law.

The gas content in a one-liter bottle is a surprising two point eight liters. In other words, there is nearly three times the volume of the original container in excess gas under pressure hidden in those tiny bubbles. Do not forget another important law of the physics of gasses, Charles' Law. This law defines the activity of gasses expanding as the temperature increases. If you drink a cold carbonated beverage, and after swallowing it is warmed up to body temperature, it will exhibit another substantial increase in the volume of gasses released. The burping and belching that occurs after drinking a cold carbonated beverage may seem out of proportion to the small amount consumed. Just remember that whatever the volume of liquid carbonated beverage swallowed, there is nearly three times that volume of dissolved gas waiting to be released.

Diet Coke and Mentos Geyser by Michael Murphy Creative Commons License.

If you want further visual proof that Henry's Law is accurate take a look at the photographic evidence of another popular activity. The harmless addition of a Mentos brand mint candy tablet to a liter bottle of a carbonated beverage, such as Diet Coke, sounds like such an innocent activity. This demonstration is repeated in countless elementary school science classes. The *Guinness Book of World Records* described one thousand three hundred and sixty students in the historic university town of Leuven, Belgium creating simultaneous Mentos with Diet Coke geysers. See the entry on carbonation for more details about this process and phenomenon.

In some beverages the carbon dioxide would interfere with the taste and flavor by reacting with the ingredients, giving it an acid taste from carbonic acid. An alternative is to use nitrogen as the gas of choice as it is a neutral gas and would not interact with the beverage. The most popular example is Guinness, which uses nitrogen, or a combination of nitrogen and carbon dioxide, under pressure in kegs.

Shutterstock/JoshuaResnick

The nitrogen provides smaller firmer bubbles with a smoother longer lasting head, and other companies have followed their lead. Guinness also pioneered the use of a widget, an irregularity at the base of the container to serve as the nucleation focus for gas bubbles to form at the base of cans and bottles rather than the surface.

Nitrogenated   Carbonated

Creative Commons License

Nitrogen is poorly soluble in liquids, and the high density of bubbles contributes to a smooth creamy mouth feel. Most beers are saturated with a combination of thirty percent carbon dioxide and seventy percent nitrogen. The head serves both an aesthetic purpose, as well as accomplishing the dispersal of the beer aroma. You can get an idea of how high the nitrogen content is by looking at the size of the head created. A significant percentage of the volume of your drink is the head, and a friendly bartender will discard some of the head to give you more drink for your money, as well as to encourage a larger gratuity.

Beer drinkers are famous for the burping and belching generated. The added nitrogen gives them an edge up in competitive burping and belching contests since it is not as rapidly absorbed and eliminated via the lungs, as is carbon dioxide. Nitrogen is also used in iced coffee beverages, providing a head of bubbles very similar to that of beer.

Aerospace

Intestinal gas, like gasses everywhere, must comply with the laws of physics and the laws of nature. Boyle's law states that at a constant temperature, the product of the volume and pressure of a gas must remain constant. This requires that they maintain an inverse relationship, if one increases the other has to decrease. As such, an increase in pressure will result in the decrease of the volume of the gas, and vice versa. The atmospheric pressure on earth is defined as a standard of one atmosphere at sea level. As you go deeper down into the earth, such as happens in a mineshaft, or diving deeper into the oceans, the atmospheric pressure increases. As you go higher in elevation, whether climbing flights of stairs, ascending a mountain, or in a hot air balloon, the atmospheric pressure decreases. The atmospheric pressure is also not uniform, constantly changing along with the weather.

www.wpclipart.com NOAA Public Domain

The changes in atmospheric pressure in aerospace are even more dramatic than in mountain climbers, both in intensity and rapidity. During World War II, flight surgeons found that at altitudes thirty thousand feet or more above sea level, aviators suffered painful abdominal distension. At that altitude, the atmospheric pressure was a fraction of that at sea level, allowing intestinal gas to balloon to nearly four times its original volume. Painful distension of the abdomen was the result of the dramatic volume expansion of trapped intestinal gas. Because the trapped gas was not near the rectum, it could not be readily released as flatus.

Popularly referred to in the military by its abbreviated acronym, High-altitude flatus expulsion (HAFE) is a common gastrointestinal syndrome seen in pilots and passengers of aircraft. It involves the uncontrollable passage of large quantities of intestinal gasses at high altitudes. As the atmospheric pressure decreases with an increase in altitude, the volume of gas in the intestine increases consistent with the principles of physics (Boyle's Law). Military pilots and astronauts have repeatedly verified the existence of HAFE, with its sensation of distension, and the need to expel the expanding intestinal gasses. With commercial aircraft commonly flying at over thirty thousand feet in elevation, the atmospheric pressure outside of the plane is a fraction of atmospheric pressure at sea level. The pressure loss at that altitude would not be tolerable to passengers, so the aircraft is pressurized to simulate what the atmospheric pressure would be at approximately eight thousand feet above sea level.

The retained pockets of air in your gut will expand quickly, and want to be released even if it comes at the expense of your embarrassment. Airlines, pilots, and flight attendants are well aware of this effect, but they rarely offer the passenger any warning or explanation. They assume that you will not comment on the natural discomfort you are experiencing, or the subsequent release of intestinal gas, either your own or of the person sitting directly in front of you. In fact, it is to be expected that there is much more air turbulence inside an aircraft than outside.

Pressure — Number of moles — Temperature

$$PV = nRT$$

Volume — Gas constant

A visual example of the differences in atmospheric pressure between beings on the ground closer to sea level, and at an atmospheric pressure equivalent to an altitude of eight thousand feet is often served to you by a flight attendant. Take a close look at what happens to carbonated beverages served at high altitude. Have you ever noticed that the release of the bubbles of carbon dioxide from a carbonated beverage is much more dramatic when flying? Flight attendants have to spend more time while pouring the carbonated beverages, pausing to let the bubbles release themselves as they fill your glass. If they did not pause to let the gasses be released, you would be handed a container of fizz and foam instead of the beverage you wanted.

$$PV = FaRT$$
(Ideal gas law)

rlv.zcache.com

Aerospace has another concern that increases the volume and frequency of farts within the tight confines of a space capsule or space station. In an environment without gravity, the weightlessness leads to muscle weakness and atrophy. As the abdominal muscles weaken, the intestinal gasses expand further distending the gut and results in an increase in fart volume and frequency. While traveling in space, even in a pressurized space capsule, there is a very significant reduction in pressure, which means that gasses must exhibit a proportional increase in volume.

NASA Public Domain

For those involved in space travel, including the growing population of space tourists, the pressure changes are unparalleled. Many people are knowledgeable about the dangers of scuba and deep-sea divers, especially if surfacing from the depths too quickly. The nitrogen gas in the air that is breathed in at higher pressures dissolves in the bloodstream and body fats. When returning to the surface too quickly, the diver is subjected to a rapid drop in atmospheric pressure. The nitrogen gas comes out of solution, and forms bubbles of gas in the circulation. Decompression sickness, caisson disease, or 'the bends' is a risk for the space traveler as well.

The air and space traveler would likewise experience a rapid decrease in atmospheric pressure if not for the ability to pressurize the aircraft or spacecraft. The ambient atmospheric pressure within a spacecraft is typically maintained at fourteen point seven pounds per square inch (psi), or one hundred and one kilopascals (kPa). The most dramatic exposure to a rapid decrease in atmospheric pressure occurs when space travelers leave the pressurized spacecraft for spacewalks, more formally known as extravehicular activity.

Without the pressurized spacesuit, known more formally as extravehicular mobility units, the rapid reduction in atmospheric pressure may be life threatening. The spacesuit is typically pressurized to four point three pounds per square inch (thirty kPa). Without the spacesuit, decompression sickness also known as caisson sickness or the bends can develop in astronauts just as it does in deep-sea divers. As the atmospheric pressure is rapidly reduced the nitrogen gas that was previously in solution forms bubbles. These form in the bloodstream, nerves, joints and can cause pain, as well as circulatory collapse

Because the reductions in atmospheric pressure remain significant and put them at risk of life-threatening decompression sickness, the space travelers are given pure oxygen to breathe for several hours prior to the spacewalk. Breathing pure oxygen for several hours reduces the nitrogen dissolved in their circulation and fat stores, and further reduces the risk of nitrogen bubbles forming in their bloodstream leading to decompression sickness.

The early pioneers of space travel were appropriately heralded as heroes known for 'the right stuff'. They balanced the dangers and unknowns with a mixture of bravado and humor. As space travelers are at the extreme of reduced atmospheric pressure, they have a carte blanche to blame Boyle's Law for any and all gas bubbles they may wish to release. Alan Shepard, Jr. (1923–1998) was an American naval aviator, test pilot, and NASA astronaut. In 1961 Shepard became the first American, and second person after Soviet Cosmonaut Yuri Gargarin, to travel into space. When reporters asked Shepard what he was thinking about as he sat atop the potentially explosive Redstone rocket waiting for liftoff he replied "The fact that every part of this ship was built by the low bidder!" Ten years later, Alan Shepard was at the command of the Apollo 14 mission to the moon. Despite thick gloves and a stiff spacesuit Shepard struck two golf balls on the lunar surface driving the second golf ball "miles and miles and miles."

Benjamin Franklin was quoted as saying "Instead of cursing the darkness, light a candle." Alan Shepard created another memorable quote while waiting for the end of the interminable delays to launch. NASA engineers had delayed his first flight so many times that the Soviets were able to send the first man into orbit. On the day of his successful voyage, Shepard sat on the launch pad, waiting inside his rocket for over four hours while engineers corrected one challenging problem after another. The wait was longer than expected, and Shepard exceeded his bladder capacity. He ended up having to urinate inside his spacesuit. They had to turn off his monitoring equipment so that he did not create a short circuit. When one more problem cropped up, Shepard exclaimed, "Why don't you fix your little problem and light this candle!" The quote became the title of his biography, *Light This Candle.*

The U.S. space program was concerned about intestinal gas during space flight. After liftoff, while experiencing weightlessness, Shepard also experienced this other anticipated consequence of virtually zero atmospheric pressure. His internal gas bubbles expanded with the production of near continuous farting, which he graphically described over the radio communications with mission control. If you listen closely to the recording of the conversations, not all of the background noise was static!

As director of the astronaut program, Shepard received the following memorandum from astronaut John Young. "RE: Safety Issues. No less than six times have I had to listen to Borman complain about his lactose intolerance when someone stole his weird not-milk milk stuff. Additionally, when Borman drinks regular milk, he gets the farts. That's all I'm going to say about that." In the microgravity environment of space, farting results in the body being propelled when the 'digestive gas thruster is fired'. On the U.S.S.R. and Russian space station Mir, restraining devices were installed on the toilet seat, so the user would not be thrust off the seat with a fart.

Bathroom on the space shuttle. NASA Public Domain

Gus Grissom was scheduled to go into space two months after Shepard's inaugural flight on Friendship Seven. He insisted that the 'potty' problem had to be solved, and a naval flight surgeon was assigned to the task. He sent one of the nurses into town to buy a women's panty girdle, which was layered with absorbent pads. Grissom was the first astronaut to go into space wearing women's lingerie. Astronauts, cosmonauts, and taikonauts have to deal with bodily functions in space, and modifications have been required. The Hamilton Standard Company was the maker of the U.S. astronaut spacesuits, and male astronauts used a condom catheter under the spacesuits for spacewalks and moonwalks. Ingenuity was required to come up with a comparable solution for female astronauts.

When the Gemini program began, the astronauts graduated to urine and fecal bags and special diapers for spacewalks. Urine waste was disposed of by an overboard dump valve. The solid waste was handled differently with a germicide placed in the storage bag, which was sealed in a locker. Since the lunar model itself was not designed with an overboard dump valve or storage cabinet, astronauts left very personal mementos of their visits behind. More than the national flag of the United States of America was deposited on the moon surface and remains there to this day. At the time the waste was left behind science believed than none of the microbes present in the feces could survive in the hostile environment of outer space or the moon. The remarkable discoveries since then of extremophiles (see Microbiome, Archaea) raises the possibilities that the material left behind still has viable and living microbes that could be the basis of a science fiction thriller with a scatological theme. When the Space Shuttle program was being engineered, a specially designed space toilet called the "Waste Collection Facility" or WCF for short was developed. It was budgeted to cost three million dollars to develop, but with cost over-runs it ended up being the world most expensive toilet by far costing more than thirty million dollars.

For those living in high altitude communities such as Mexico City at over seven thousand feet above sea level, the atmospheric pressure is much lower than at sea level. Commercial aircraft are pressurized to an equivalent of eight thousand feet above sea level. With the atmospheric pressure at just over two-thirds of sea level, the gas volume expands by about forty percent. That is more than enough to cause a person to notice a significant increase in their flatulence, and an increase in the flatulence of everyone else as well.

Air Enema

An air enema is often used during a barium enema study, when the air is inflated into the colon via the enema tube to provide air as a contrast to the barium. This type of barium study is called an air contrast or double-contrast barium enema. Air may also be inflated into the colon as the self-practice of the air enema that is described in the ancient yoga literature. The advanced yogi may develop anal sphincter control, and control of the abdominal muscles to create an abdominal suction effect to vacuum air into the lower intestine.

*Air*Veda: Ancient & New Medical Wisdom

Shale Basti, also called Vat Basti, Air Basti, is an air enema used as an advanced Hatha yoga technique and is best learned from an expert teacher. There are a number of different approaches and techniques, but mastery of voluntary control of the anal sphincter is a challenging practice. See the entry on yoga for more details, as well as entry on Le Pétomane a stage performer who mastered this technique to great critical acclaim and commercial success.

www.flickr.com Creative Commons License

Air Fart

The ability to air fart is the common term for the ability to control the anus and muscles of the abdomen and respiration, including the diaphragm, to cause air to be aspirated into the colon and then released voluntarily as a fart. It is also known colloquially as the ability to butt breathe. The air fart and butt breathe technique is known in more enlightened society as an air enema and has been practiced as a part of yoga colon hygiene for thousands of years. Although usually considered under involuntary control these muscles can be trained, and yogis attain remarkable proficiency. At the turn of the twentieth century, the performer Joseph Pujol, under the stage name Le Pétomane, became an international sensation by demonstrating his prowess at butt breathing. This ability is not limited to trained yogi and stage performers. According to the results of an internet-based survey on farting performed in 2001, with over one thousand three hundred participants, over fifteen percent of respondents were able to accomplish this with the benefit of being able to fart on command.

Fart survey question for men: Can you fart on command also called "Butt Breathe"?

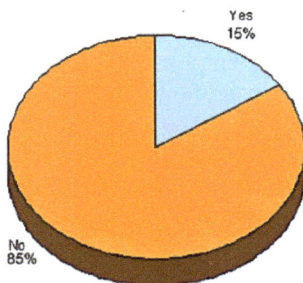

Yes
15%

No
85%

Only fifteen percent of the men surveyed can fart voluntarily by suctioning air into the colon. One-third of all men did not even know that this is possible!

Fart survey question for women: Can you fart on command also called "Butt Breathe"?

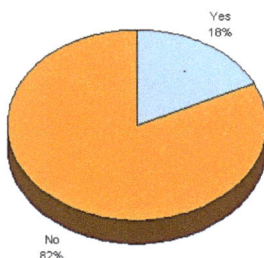

Yes
18%

No
82%

Eighteen percent of the women surveyed can fart voluntarily by suctioning air into the colon. This is either a remarkably high or low number, depending on the perspective.

Air, Gas Composition

If the entire abdomen is distended with air-filled loops of the intestine, a bowel obstruction may be its cause. Marked distension of the stomach can occur with gastroparesis, a neuropathy that delays stomach emptying seen most often in diabetics or when the pyloric channel or upper small bowel is obstructed. Iatrogenic is a fancy way of saying a physician was the cause. Iatrogenic air in the gastrointestinal tract is common after endoscopic procedures such as upper gastrointestinal endoscopy (esophagoscopy, gastroscopy, esophagogastro-duodenoscopy, EGD), endoscopic retrograde cholangiopancreatography (ERCP), or colonoscopy (proctoscopy, sigmoidoscopy, colonoscopy, ileoscopy, enteroscopy). The official name of the endoscopic procedure undertaken is defined by the anatomy of the organs examined.

The coming advances including capsule endoscopy will replace many of these multi-syllable, expensive, and invasive diagnostic tests. Developed initially by Given Imaging, a high-tech company based in Israel, a swallowed capsule travels through the digestive tract like a spying submarine. With remarkable visual clarity, it examines the lining of the bowel for abnormalities. Further development will allow it to obtain tissue samples and even therapeutic lasers bringing the science fiction movie *Fantastic Voyage* one step closer to reality. Other technology companies are pursuing this and other nanotechnology marvels that will travel through the body for diagnostic and therapeutic purposes.

Air is the typical gas inflated, and it may be several hours to up to a day for the excess gas to be eliminated. As described below carbon dioxide is the preferred gas for inflation since it is so readily absorbed and eliminated, but for either ease of access or because of the low cost, air continues to be used by most endoscopists. The radiologist also uses air insufflation with radiographic studies such as the barium enema. When the study is enhanced by air insufflation it is called an air-contrast or double-contrast barium enema.

Barium studies are not performed as often today, but they can provide valuable diagnostic information. A number of years ago I had a patient who was scheduled to have a barium enema to examine the colon, to be followed a few days later by a barium swallow to examine the esophagus. In about twenty percent of patients undergoing barium enema, the contrast material passes through the ileocecal valve and into the small bowel. This can be useful in providing additional diagnostic information about the distal small bowel, such as the presence of inflammatory bowel disease. In this individual, the barium entered the small intestine, but before the radiologist could reduce the pressure of the barium flow it refluxed all the way into his stomach and esophagus and the patient vomited up the barium. With disgust, the patient told the radiologist to cancel the barium swallow. When asked why, the patient told him he would never be able to drink the barium because it tasted like shit!

Iatrogenic (physician caused) distension with gas is routine in the performance of laparoscopy where tube-like visual instruments are used to examine the abdomen and pelvis. The gas used to inflate the abdominal cavity, creating a pneumoperitoneum, is carbon dioxide. The carbon dioxide gas is rapidly absorbed by the body and eliminated via exhalation through the lungs. If air were used the less than one percent component of carbon dioxide would be rapidly absorbed. The twenty-one percent portion of the air comprised of oxygen would be slowly absorbed over a few days. The remaining seventy-eight percent majority consisting of nitrogen is poorly absorbed. The nitrogen gas would remain within the peritoneal cavity for an extended period of time, being slowly absorbed over a period of several days to weeks.

Air, Iatrogenic

Iatrogenic is a fancy way of saying a physician was the cause. Iatrogenic air in the gastrointestinal tract is common after endoscopic procedures such as upper gastrointestinal endoscopy (esophagogastroduodenoscopy, EGD, esophagoscopy, gastroscopy), endoscopic retrograde cholangiopancreatography (ERCP), or colonoscopy (proctoscopy, sigmoidoscopy, colonoscopy, ileoscopy, enteroscopy). The official name of the endoscopic procedure undertaken is defined by the anatomy of the organs examined.

Shutterstock/CedricCrucke

Air is the typical gas inflated, and it may be several hours to up to a day for the excess gas to be eliminated. As described below carbon dioxide is the preferred gas for inflation since it is so readily absorbed and eliminated, but for either ease of access or costs air continues to be used by most endoscopists. The radiologist also uses air insufflation with radiographic studies such as the barium enema. When the study is enhanced by air insufflation it is called an air-contrast or double-contrast barium enema. Iatrogenic (physician caused) distension with gas is routine in the performance of laparoscopy where tube-like visual instruments are used to examine the abdomen and pelvis. The gas used to inflate the abdominal cavity, creating a pneumoperitoneum, is carbon dioxide.

Argon < 1%

Carbon Dioxide .04%

Other Gases < 1%

Oxygen 21%

Nitrogen 78%

The carbon dioxide gas is rapidly absorbed by the body and eliminated via exhalation through the lungs. If air were used the less than one percent component of carbon dioxide would be rapidly absorbed. The twenty-one percent portion of the air comprised of oxygen would be slowly absorbed over a few days. The remaining seventy-eight percent majority consisting of nitrogen is poorly absorbed. The nitrogen gas would remain within the peritoneal cavity for an extended period of time, being slowly absorbed over a period of several days to weeks.

Allopathic Medicine (Western Medicine)

Allopathic medicine (Greek ἄλλος, állos, other + πάθος, páthos, suffering) is a description commonly used by homeopaths and advocates of other forms of alternative medicine to refer to mainstream Western or modern medicine. The term was created in 1810 by the founder of homeopathy, Samuel Hahnemann (1755–1843). Allopathic medicine uses pharmacologically active agents or physical interventions to treat the causes and symptoms of diseases or conditions.

Hahnemann used the term allopathic medicine to contrast it from his homeopathic (Greek homeo similar) medicine philosophy of using diluted substances that would cause symptoms similar to the illness being treated. Early in its use, allopathic medicine was considered an offensive term and was not accepted by Western Medicine. Although it is literally incorrect it is now a commonly accepted term to describe Western or modern medicine.

Alpha Galactosidase

Beano, Bean-Zyme, Say Yes To Beans, and competing products are an enzyme-based dietary supplement that is used to reduce the intestinal production of gas from dietary oligosaccharides such as raffinose, stachyose, and verbascose from legumes. Beano contains the enzymes alpha-galactosidase and invertase, which are derived from the fungus *Aspergillus Niger. Aspergillus Niger* and its fermentation products are 'generally recognized as safe' (GRAS) by the United States Food and Drug Administration (FDA). Because pets, such as dogs and cats, also release intestinal gas, the identical product was released to be marketed for pets under the brand name Curtail. Although it may be effective, it reduced the ability of guilty humans to blame a fart on the dog or cat and is no longer on the market as that brand name.

Refueling station and restaurant. Cindy Cornett Seigle www.flickr.com Creative Commons License

The alpha-galactosidase is effective but must be taken with the first bite of food. Because heating inactivates it, it cannot be used in the cooking process, and must be taken when eating the food. It does not have any effect on lactose or other enzyme deficiencies. Additional doses of alpha-galactosidase will be needed if large quantities of legumes are consumed, or a substantial period has passed since the dose was taken.

Another approach is to soak the beans for several hours and discard the fluid, which leaches out some of the complex sugars. Allowing the seeds to germinate allows the bean plant itself to begin to produce alpha-galactosidase. Within twenty-four hours of germination the internally generated enzyme breaks down most of the complex sugars. Using the herb asafetida can also reduce flatulence although the herb itself has an aroma that may be worse than the farts you are trying to prevent. The name of the herb itself may give you a clue as fetida has the same root as the word fetid. These words are derived from the Latin word foetidus and *foetēre* meaning 'to stink'

Certain beans are being developed that have lower concentrations of the challenging complex sugars. The enzyme hydrolyses the polysaccharides and oligosaccharides of the raffinose family including stachyose, verbascose, and galactinol found in foods such as the legumes beans and peanuts, and the cruciferous vegetables cauliflower, broccoli, cabbage, and Brussels sprouts. Beano was marketed by Alan Kligerman of AkPharma, Inc. in 1990. Originally in the dairy farm business, he was the developer of the commercially successful lactase (lactose milk sugar enzyme) supplement Lactaid. Beano received a US patent in 1995, which is estimated to expire in 2015. There are more than fifty competing products on the market. It should be noted that the use of these products enhances the digestibility of certain foods and increases the nutrients and calories absorbed.

www.flickr.com Creative Commons License

The intellectual concept for a product to reduce or mask the aroma of intestinal gas was proposed in the 1780's by Benjamin Franklin. He submitted an essay "A Letter To A Royal Academy" suggesting that an award be given to the inventor of a food additive that would make the aroma of flatus attractive instead of offensive. Benjamin Franklin was known as for his sense of humor, and although some thought his proposal was serious, it was written tongue in cheek.

Simple sugars are produced in the malting process of barley to brew beer. The complex sugars that are not hydrolyzed or fermented and consumed by the beer drinker may contribute to its well-recognized ability to increase flatulence. Some home brewers have added Beano to the mash in an attempt to reduce this occurrence. The use of the prescription drug Acarbose or Miglitol used in the treatment of diabetes mellitus will cause a dramatic increase in flatulence because of its enzyme inhibitor activity. These drugs are used to treat type 2 diabetes mellitus by inhibiting the glycoside hydrolases, the alpha-galactosidae family of enzymes necessary for the digestion of many starches. It specifically inhibits alpha-glucosidase enzymes in the brush border of the villi of the small intestines, pancreatic alpha-amylase, maltase, isomaltase, glucoamylase, sucrose, and invertase.

Alpha-glucosidase inhibitors are the competitive, reversible inhibitors of pancreatic alpha amylase and membrane bound intestinal alpha glucosidase hydrolase enzymes. Use of these drugs leads to a blockade of the the enzymatic degradation of complex carbohydrates in the small intestine, decreasing the amount and delaying the absorption of these sugars. Acarbose, which is not absorbed by the body, has the following preferred affinity for blocking the alpha glucosidase enzymes: glycoamylase > sucrase > maltase > dextranase and has no affinity for the alpha glucosidase enzymes, such as lactase. Miglitol is a more potent inhibitor of sucrase and maltase than acarbose and has no effect on alpha amylase.

Pancreatic alpha amylase hydrolyzes complex starches to oligosaccharides in the chyme being digested in the lumen of the small intestine. The intestinal alpha-glycosidase further hydrolyzes oligosaccharides, trisaccharides, and disaccharides to glucose and other monosaccharides at the brush border of the villi in the small intestine. Inhibition of these enzyme systems reduces the rate of digestion of complex carbohydrates and decreases the amount of glucose available for absorption. It should be taken at the start of a meal, and as more complex carbohydrates pass to the colon undigested, increased bacterial fermentation will result. Increased flatulence is reported in the vast majority of patients, and approximately fifteen percent develop diarrhea. The gastrointestinal side effects may diminish with continued use over time. Adverse side effects may also include elevation of liver function tests, which usually resolves with discontinuation of the medicine.

There has been a significant increase in average size and stature of adults in a wide diversity of countries around the world over a span of only one or two generations. The obvious explanation is the improvement in access to not only additional calories but also the critical nutrition role played by vitamins, dietary minerals, and trace elements. The full role of diet, nutrition, hormones, enzymes, the gut flora and microbiome, genetics, epigenetics, and other factors is still in the process of being elucidated.

NEW FOOD PYRAMID

outlined by the authors distinguishes between healthy and unhealthy types of fat and carbohydrates. Fruits and vegetables are still recommended, but the consumption of dairy products should be limited.

Public Domain

Certain types of vegetables and fruits contain carbohydrates with substantial quantities of sugars and starches that may be poorly digested by people but happily fermented by bacteria comprising the gut flora. The starches, including potatoes, corn, noodles, and wheat are the source of the majority of gasses generated by the gut microbial flora. Rice is the one starch exception and rarely contributes to intestinal gas production. Wheat has the other 'distinction' of having the protein glutamate, which contains the nitrogen base product that contributes to the generation of ammonia-like aromatic compounds. The most common food intolerance is for the milk sugar, lactose when an individual has decreased quantities and activity of the necessary enzyme for its digestion, lactase.

Amino Acid

Aromatic amino acids are a category of amino acids that include the chemical structure of an aromatic ring. Examples include the essential amino acids

49

phenylalanine, tryptophan, histidine, and the semi-essential amino acid tyrosine. Essential amino acids are those that humans or other animals cannot synthesize for themselves and must be obtained from the diet.

Tyrosine is semi-essential in that it can be synthesized, but only if phenylalanine is ingested. The disorder phenylketonuria occurs when there is an absence of the enzyme phenylalanine hydroxylase, which is required for tyrosine synthesis.

Essential	Conditionally Non-Essential	Non-Essential
Histidine	Arginine	Alanine
Isoleucine	Asparagine	Asparatate
Leucine	Glutamine	Cysteine
Methionine	Glycine	Glutamate
Phenylalanine	Proline	
Threonine	Serine	
Tryptophan	Tyrosine	
Valine		
Lysine		

The twenty standard amino acids, divided into essential, conditionally non-essential and non-essential categories; Non-essential amino acids are synthesized in the body, while essential amino acids must be obtained from food. All plants and microorganisms synthesize their aromatic amino acids, unlike animals, which obtain them through their diet. Animals have lost these energy intensive metabolic pathways, since they obtain aromatic amino acids through their diet. Herbicides and antibiotics inhibiting enzymes involved in aromatic acid synthesis are toxic to plants and microorganisms dependent on this pathway, but not to animals which do not utilize these enzymes.

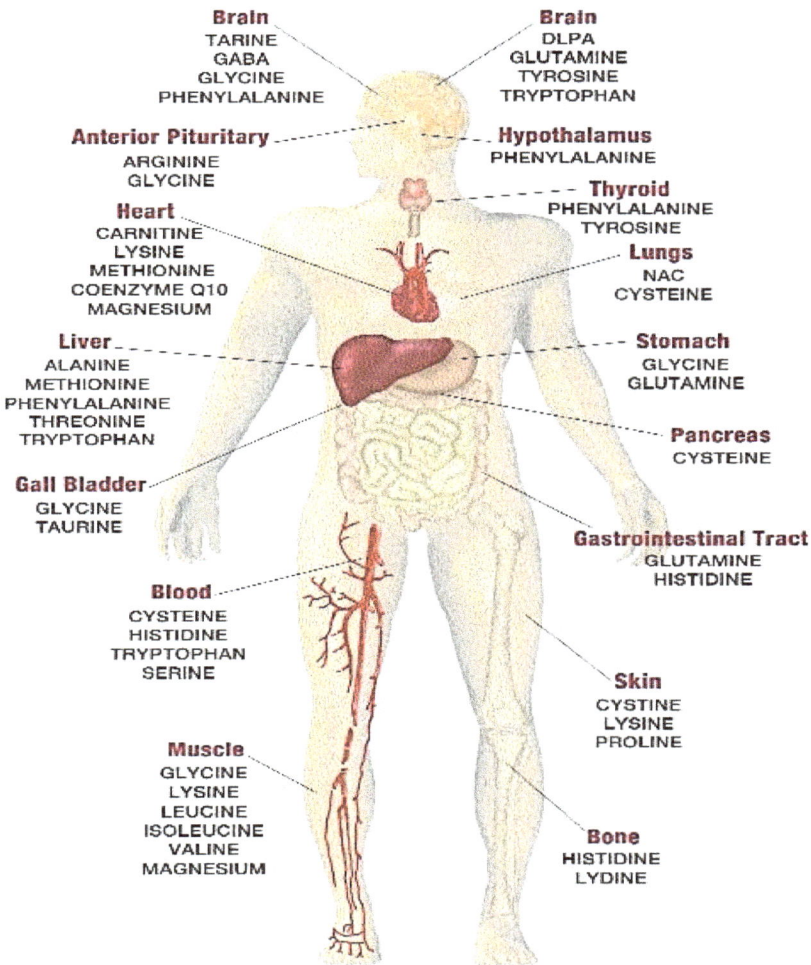

Brain
TARINE
GABA
GLYCINE
PHENYLALANINE

Brain
DLPA
GLUTAMINE
TYROSINE
TRYPTOPHAN

Anterior Pituritary
ARGININE
GLYCINE

Hypothalamus
PHENYLALANINE

Heart
CARNITINE
LYSINE
METHIONINE
COENZYME Q10
MAGNESIUM

Thyroid
PHENYLALANINE
TYROSINE

Lungs
NAC
CYSTEINE

Liver
ALANINE
METHIONINE
PHENYLALANINE
THREONINE
TRYPTOPHAN

Stomach
GLYCINE
GLUTAMINE

Pancreas
CYSTEINE

Gall Bladder
GLYCINE
TAURINE

Gastrointestinal Tract
GLUTAMINE
HISTIDINE

Blood
CYSTEINE
HISTIDINE
TRYPTOPHAN
SERINE

Skin
CYSTINE
LYSINE
PROLINE

Muscle
GLYCINE
LYSINE
LEUCINE
ISOLEUCINE
VALINE
MAGNESIUM

Bone
HISTIDINE
LYDINE

Amino Acid needs by body location.

L-Tyrosine

L-Tryptophan

L-Phenylalanine

Aromatic amino acids.

The aromatic amino acids are precursors for important neurotransmitters. The same enzyme, L-aromatic amino acid decarboxylase is required for the synthesis of the monoamines serotonin and dopamine. If the amino acid precursors of one system dominate the enzyme in monoamine synthesis it could lead to an unbalance and depletion of the other monoamine.

The same enzyme, L-aromatic amino acid decarboxylase (AAAD), is responsible for synthesis of the monoamines serotonin and dopamine.

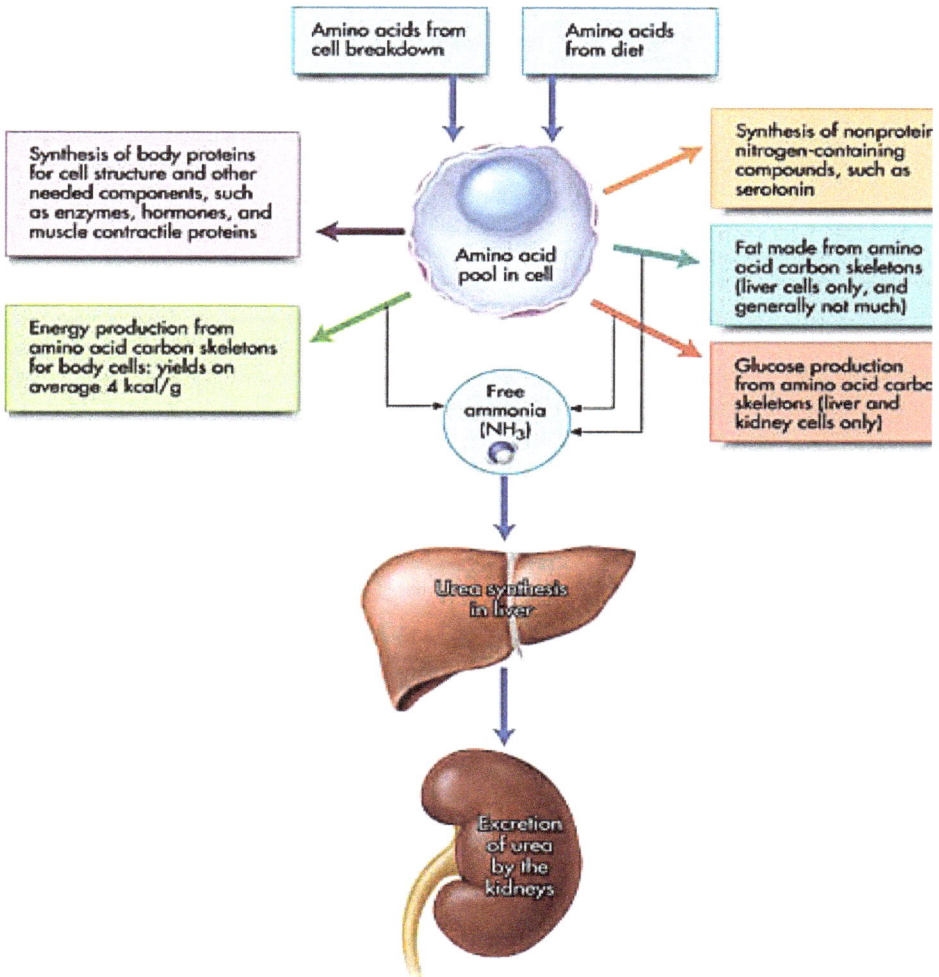

Amino acids from cell breakdown

Amino acids from diet

Synthesis of body proteins for cell structure and other needed components, such as enzymes, hormones, and muscle contractile proteins

Synthesis of nonprotein nitrogen-containing compounds, such as serotonin

Amino acid pool in cell

Fat made from amino acid carbon skeletons (liver cells only, and generally not much)

Energy production from amino acid carbon skeletons for body cells: yields on average 4 kcal/g

Glucose production from amino acid carbon skeletons (liver and kidney cells only)

Free ammonia (NH_3)

Urea synthesis in liver

Excretion of urea by the kidneys

Amylase

Amylase is an enzyme that catalyzes the degradation of starches into sugars. Erhard Friedrich Leuchs (1800–1837) documented that starch was hydrolyzed and the active enzyme identified in the saliva was named amylase. You can see the effect of amylase in saliva by chewing on starchy food like potatoes for a few minutes. The salivary amylase breaks the starches down to glucose and the chewed starch begins to taste sweeter as the glucose is produced.

In addition to the salivary glands, the pancreas also produces amylase. The amylase enters the duodenum from the pancreatic duct via the Ampulla of Vater. It hydrolyzes the dietary starch into disaccharides and trisaccharides. These are further digested by other enzymes in the small intestine converting them to monosaccharides such as glucose, which can be more readily absorbed.

Plants, yeast, and some bacteria also produce amylase. Amylase also plays an important role in converting starches to sugars in the processing of bread and beer. For wheat, alpha-gliadins are seed-storage proteins, but also act as inhibitors of alpha-amylase activity.

Anus

The anal canal is the distal and terminal portion of the large intestine of the gastrointestinal tract, with the anus being the outlet for digestive waste. In the long tube like structure of the gastrointestinal tract, the term proximal means closest to the mouth, and distal means closest to the anus. In the intestines the term terminal means the end of the tube like structure. It is not used as the term for the end of life like the phrase terminal illness, it is more like the use of the word as in train terminal, where the travel line ends.

The proximal portion of the anal canal begins at the superior aspect of the pelvic diaphragm, where the rectal ampulla narrows. This is at the level of the U-shaped sling formed by the puborectalis muscle. The canal is approximately one and one-half inches (three and one-half centimeters) long. The distal aspect of the anal canal ends at the anus itself, the terminal outlet of the alimentary canal.

Rectum

Internal hemorrhoid tissue

Levator ani muscle

Internal anal sphincter

External anal sphincter

External hemorrhoid tissue

Anus

Shutterstock.com/AlilaMedicalMedia

Fecal continence is a function of the coordinated activity of the involuntary internal and voluntary external anal sphincters. The sympathetic nervous system maintains the tone of the involuntary internal sphincter. This tone allows it to remain closed, except during filling of the rectal ampulla. The rectoanal inhibitory reflex is the involuntary internal anal sphincter relaxation in response to rectal distention. This reflex is one reason why an enema can be promptly effective in stimulating a bowel movement. The loss of the tone of the internal anal sphincter leading to fecal incontinence with capital punishment is known to the executioner, but is rarely known to those who commit suicide by this means. Perhaps this knowledge would deter this form of suicide by those who believe they are selecting a very sanitary way of leaving the world behind. The greatest deterrent might be if they were aware of how much grief and pain they leave behind for their loved ones, and how a tragic suicide is all too often a permanent 'solution' for a temporary problem.

The anal sphincter tone may also be relaxed and inhibited during parasympathetic stimulation inducing contraction of the rectum. During these events, the closure must be maintained by voluntary contraction and heightened tone of the puborectalis and external anal sphincter, to prevent defecation before it is socially appropriate.

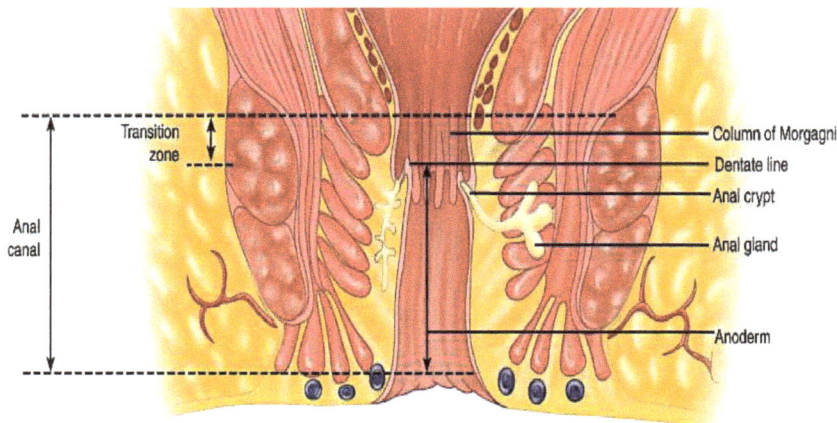

www.knowyourbody.net/wp- Creative Commons License

Internally the pectinate line is a visible landmark that demarcates the transition from visceral to somatic innervation and vascular supply. The canal is surrounded by superficial and deep venous plexuses, which normally have a varicose appearance. The hemorrhoidal vascular plexus contributes to the maintenance of fecal continence.

The external anal sphincter is usually under voluntary control. The sphincter is a large muscle forming a broad band across both sides of the lower two-thirds of the anal canal. The external anal sphincter is supplied through the inferior rectal nerve, which also serves the levator ani and puborectalis. They contract simultaneously to preserve continence when the internal sphincter is inhibited or relaxed, except during defecation. Internally the superior half of the anal canal has a series of longitudinal ridges called anal columns. Within these columns are the terminal vessels of the superior rectal artery and vein. The anorectal junction is demarcated by the proximal ends of the anal columns. It is at this point that the wide rectal ampulla narrows as it traverses the pelvic diaphragm.

The distal ends of the anal columns are bridged by anal valves. Proximal to the valves are small indentations called the anal sinuses. When compressed by feces the anal sinuses exude mucus, which aids in lubrication and the evacuation of feces from the anal canal. The distal limit of the anal valves forms an irregular line called the pectinate line. This line demarcates the junction of the superior and inferior portions of the anal canal.

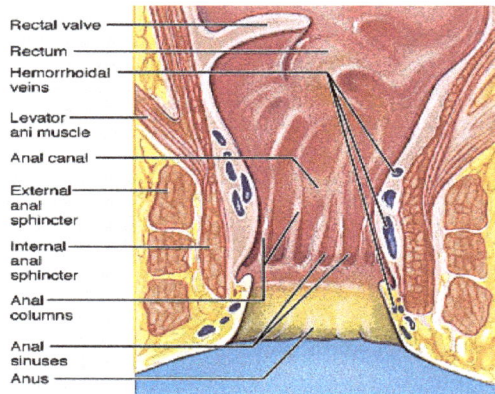

Anal canal anatomy http://www.webdicine.com Creative Commons License

The anal canal proximal to the pectinate line has significant differences from the part that is distal to this landmark. The pectinate line is the anatomical landmark that separates the arterial supply, innervation, venous circulation, and lymphatic drainage of the proximal and distal portions. These differences are the result of the separate embryological origins of the proximal and distal parts of the anal canal. The proximal portion is visceral and derived from the embryonic hindgut. The distal portion is somatic and is derived from the embryonic proctodeum.

Proximal to the pectinate line, the anal canal cannot sense pain, touch or temperature. The proximal anal canal is sensitive only to stretching, which evokes sensations at both the conscious and the unconscious reflex levels. For example, distension of the rectal ampulla inhibits and relaxes the tone of the internal anal sphincter. Distal to the pectinate line, the sensory nerves of the anal canal have somatic innervation. As somatic sensory nerves they are able to sense pain, touch, and temperature. This is why internal hemorrhoids that occur above the pectinate line are painless. External hemorrhoids that occur distal to the pectinate line can be excruciatingly painful. Efferent fibers of the somatic nerves cause contraction of the voluntary external anal sphincter when stimulated.

Based on the histology of cellular tissue the anal canal may be divided into three parts. The zona columnaris is the proximal portion of the anal canal and is lined by simple columnar epithelium. The distal half of the anal canal, below the pectinate line, is further divided into two zones separated by Hilton's white line. The two parts are the zona hemorrhagica lined by stratified squamous non-keratinized epithelium and the zona cutanea, lined by stratified squamous keratinized epithelium.

The anal glands or sacs are sebaceous glands located in the anal canal of many mammals including dogs and cats that secrete a liquid used in the marking of territory. The anal glands are emptied passively with the passage of solid feces. With soft or loose stools the glands may not be sufficiently emptied and impaction can develop. Humans have anal glands as well, and can identify the scent of their own feces and flatus.

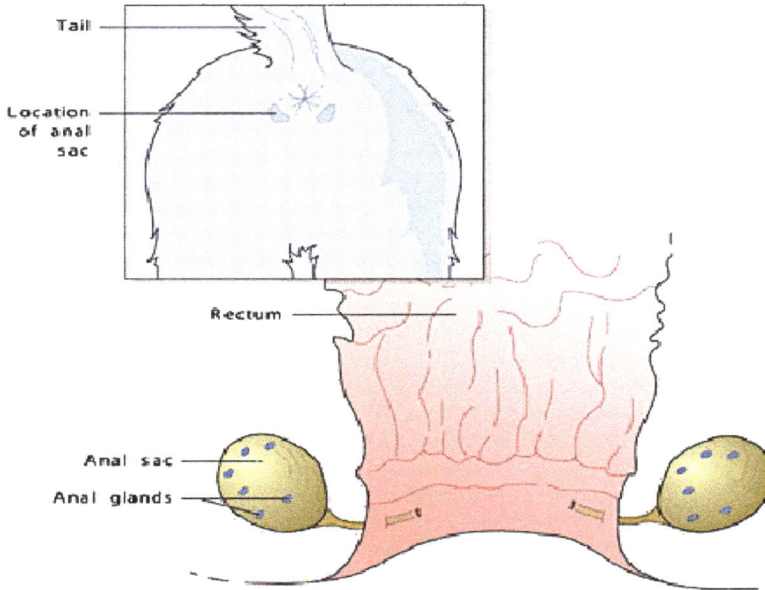

Anal glands. www.michigananimalhospital.com

Irritation or impaction of the glands can lead to pruritus ani (anal itching), perianal pain, and abscess formation. Perirectal abscess is a very painful and potentially dangerous condition that responds to antibiotics after surgical incision and drainage. Perirectal fistula may also develop and are often associated with an inflammatory bowel condition such as Crohn disease. Perianal disease such as abscess, fistula, and fissures are best treated early for pain relief and healing.

In dogs, these glands may be referred to as 'scent glands', and butt sniffing is a means of identification of territorial markers. If the anal glands are impacted it can lead to scooting its bottom on the ground or floor, tail chasing, or licking and biting the anus. Dog groomers often perform anal sac expression for the hygiene and comfort of the animal. In cats impacted glands can cause defecation outside of the litter box. Skunks anal glands generate the foul smelling spray they utilize as a defense mechanism.

Some humans find the scent of the anal glands attractive, and many people are surprised that they find the scent of their own farts particularly appealing. Perhaps even more unexpected is how many find the aroma of farts of others attractive. Musk (Sanskrit muskies - testicle) is a class of aromatic substances used in perfumery. It is also used in Ayurveda, the traditional medical healing system developed in ancient India, where it is considered a life-saving drug in cardiac, mental, and neurological disorders. Musk was obtained from a gland of the now endangered male musk deer. By weight it is has three times the value of gold. The organic compound responsible for the musk odor is mascon. Nearly all musk used in perfumes today is synthetic.

Deer Musk (Moschidae) Author: F. Spangenberg Creative Commons License

Throughout history high quality musk was stored in special containers and vessels made of gold, silver or brass. These were often placed in the royal palace for its intoxicating fragrance. Musk is produced in a special gland found in a hairy sac midway between the stomach and the genitals of the musk deer *Moschus moschiferus*. The name musk is derived from the Sanskrit term muska, which means testicle. This is actually a misnomer as the musk gland is not the testicle and the hairy sac in which it is anatomically located is not the scrotum.

The musk deer is a shy and nocturnal animal that is about three feet in length and one and a half feet tall. Hunters have historically resorted to entrapment to capture the musk deer. Its natural habitat is in the Himalaya Mountains, highlands, and forests of Tibet, as well as Siberia, and northwest China. Somewhat ironically for a product named after the testicle, the female of the musk deer species is the primary producer of black musk. This premier product is a high quality perfume additive.

Musk sniffffffff.blogspot.com Creative Commons License

Historically, hunters would unnecessarily kill the deer for the musk sac, which is then dried under direct sunlight, or dipped in very hot oil. Musk can actually be harvested in the proper season without killing the animal. The musk deer whose life has been spared may be available for future musk harvesting. Musk comes from several countries including China, Tibet, Nepal, and Siberia in Russia.

Shutterstock/jcfmorata

Skunks (also called polecats) are mammals related to the ferret, which spray a liquid with a strong offensive odor from their anal glands as a defense mechanism. The skunk can aim the spray, which contains sulfur containing thiols and mercaptans, accurately over a distance of over ten feet (three meters). They are generally reluctant to release their spray, as it takes them up to two weeks to replenish the supply once dispensed.

Shutterstock/JamesColeman

Anal cleansing after defecation was historically accomplished with sticks, leaves, stones, clay, corncobs, water, or literally whatever was available at hand. The ancient Greeks used clay and stone. Romans used a water soaked sponge on a stick. Toilet paper has been used for the cleaning of the anus and urethra after elimination for well over one thousand years. The first recorded use of toilet paper was in China in the sixth century.

Toilets in ancient Rome had sophisticated sewer lines with running water to remove waste. Remarkably many countries around the world have more primitive systems in place today than the Romans had over two thousand years ago. shutterstock/AbelFeyman

*Air*Veda: Ancient & New Medical Wisdom

Toilet is derived from the French word toilette meaning the act of washing, dressing, and preparing oneself. In Western society human feces waste management is usually a matter of a toilet with indoor plumbing, and a sewer or septic system. Anal cleansing after defecation was historically accomplished with sticks, leaves, stones, clay, corncobs, water, or literally whatever was available at hand. In many parts of the world only the left hand was used for wiping and cleansing after defecation. That may have contributed to the use of the right hand for social greetings and shaking hands. The Hongwu Emperor was the first ruler of the Ming dynasty (1368-1644). Chinese imperial court documents show that fifteen thousand sheets of 'thick but soft' perfumed toilet paper were ordered in 1393. The royal family was recorded as using 720,000 sheets of toilet paper a year. The large sheets of two feet by three feet were for general use at the court, but smaller and even better quality sheets that were three inches square were designed for the exclusive use of the imperial family.

In the United States toilet paper was often simply pages torn out of the Farmer's Almanac, or the catalog of merchants such as Sears, Roebuck. & Company. They often came with a pre-punched hole in the catalog for ease of hanging by wire in the bathroom or outhouse. A humorous spinoff on the Sears Roebuck catalog was the 'Rears and Sorebutt' catalog. New York entrepreneur Joseph Gayetty invented aloe-infused sheets of Manila hemp in 1857 that he claimed prevented hemorrhoids. The product was sold in 500 sheet packages and marketed as Gayetty's Medicated Paper. The name Gayetty was imprinted on each sheet of the patented paper, and he was happy to see his name so besmirched as his fortune increased every time his customers wiped. In 1872 John Kimberly, Charles Clark , and other investors started a paper manufacturing company in Wisconsin. In 1874 the brothers Thomas, Clarence, and E. Irvin Scott created a competing paper company and in 1890 popularized toilet paper on a roll. Scott advertised that "over 65% of middle-aged men and women suffered from some sort of rectal disease". The Scott brothers claimed that inferior toilet paper was responsible and that "harsh toilet tissue may cause serious injury". The advertisement went on to say "ScotTissue, Sani-tissue and Waldorf are famous bathroom tissues specifically processed to satisfy the three requirements doctors say toilet tissue must have to be safe: absorbency-softness-chemical purity".

In 1901 the Northern Paper Mills in Green Bay Wisconsin developed a toilet paper that was not made from hardwood pulp, but from softer pulp. They advertised it as the first toilet tissue that guaranteed you would not get wood splinters on wiping. The appeal of not getting wood splinters on wiping with toilet paper not surprisingly led to immediate market success. Competitors soon joined in the rush to market splinter free toilet paper. By 1925 the Scott brothers were the largest toilet paper manufacturers in the world. Acquired by Kimberly-Clark in 1995 for just under ten billion US dollars, the Scott brand name of toilet paper remains very popular. Twenty-six billion rolls of toilet paper are sold annually in the United States. Americans use an average of twenty-three and a half rolls per capita a year.

Toilet Paper was medicated, perforated, perfumed, and considered the state the art of anal hygiene in the mid-nineteenth century. Creative Commons License

One tree produces about one hundred pounds (forty-five kilograms) of toilet paper, and global production consumes twenty-seven thousand trees daily. Perforated toilet paper for ease of tearing off sheets was patented in 1871 by New York businessman Seth Wheeler. He established the Albany Perforated Wrapping Paper Company, and toilet paper in those days was more politely referred to as wrapping paper. The patent application specified that the end of the roll of toilet paper was to be on the outside or in the 'over' position. Although the subject of ongoing debate, controversy, and arguments within a household, the official patented invention specifies 'over', and seventy percent of the public dutifully complies. The toilet paper business in the United States is an enormous enterprise. The industry is innovative in finding ways to increase profit margins. According to the financial newspaper The Wall Street Journal in 2013 the Kimberley-Clark Corporation announced that it improved its toilet paper product by making it fifteen percent bulkier, but at the same time reduced the number of sheets by thirteen percent, a process the industry terms desheeting. Desheeting while making bulkier tissue is a money saver as Kimberly-Clark says it doesn't need additional material to make its sheets fluffier. Kimberly Clark is the largest manufacturer of toilet paper in the world with products sold in over 150 countries.

According to Kimberly-Clark's research, Americans use on average forty-six sheets of toilet paper a day over five bathroom trips. Over eighty-three million rolls of toilet paper are manufactured in the United States each day. In 2012 companies sold over ten billion dollars of tissue and toilet paper, a two percent increase over the previous year. Seven billion rolls of toilet paper are sold each year in the United States. In the U.S. more than fifty miles of toilet paper are produced every second. A roll of toilet paper will last five days in the average U.S. household. The average American uses one hundred rolls of toilet paper (twenty thousand sheets) per year, and will require the processing of 384 trees during their lifetime to create the toilet paper they will use. Most of the world has embraced the use of water cleansing for hygienic purposes wherever available. Approximately four billion people around the world do not use toilet paper. The use of only paper products for anal hygiene is counterintuitive, and is surprisingly still the procedure of choice in the United States and many Western countries. The last figures for toilet paper consumption by country were published over twenty years ago. The US led the world with 730 pounds of toilet paper consumption per resident each year. Other countries on the list with pounds of consumption per year for each resident included Finland 669, Belgium 565, Japan 526, Canada 505, Singapore 502, Taiwan 492, Switzerland 476, Denmark 471, New Zealand 468, Brazil 77, China 48, Indonesia 31, and Russia 28. Since the list was published Japan has moved into second place and China a rapidly rising third place.

Designer toiler papers are very popular. They come in various colors, but white remain the most popular followed by beige, and peach. Some come with embossed patterns, and others with writings, poetry, and images. The most exclusive designer toilet paper comes from Japan, where the Hanebisho Company creates handcrafted toilet paper that sells for nearly $20 per roll. It is created from the highest quality wood fiber pulp from Canada, and treated with the purest water fin Japan from the Nyodo River. The special drying process is constantly adjusted for humidity and temperature. The paper is then decorated by highly trained artisans and carefully wrapped and packaged in special decorative boxes. The product has been delivered to the residence of the Emperor of Japan for years. If you were to take toilet paper in your bare hands to wipe your pet or child's behind after a bowel movement, you would probably instantly recognize the unhygienic nature of the activity and wash your hands thoroughly. If you did not know it before now you do, toilet paper has to be at least ten sheets thick to prevent bacteria from easily transiting through the porous paper. Even double and triple folding of toilet paper allows fecal bacteria to be in direct contact with the hands. After wiping the person touches the handle to flush. It should not come as any surprise that the toilet faucet or handle has four hundred times the number of bacteria per square inch than the toilet seat.

In the United States and Western society many people wipe after a bowel movement with only porous toilet tissue paper between their fingers and fecal material. These same fingers are then often used to prepare food or pick up finger food that is often shared with others. In the United States health department codes require that restaurant and food preparation employees wash their hands after using the bathroom. The best approach is to practice regular hand washing with an anti-microbial soap and water. The lack of hand washing after using the bathroom is commonplace, as is the lack of basic hand washing skills. The use of an ultraviolet backlight below demonstrates how the hands harbor pockets of potential sources of infection. The touching of a toilet handle and door knob on leaving the bathroom can allow the further transmission of infectious microbes.

OUTFOXprevention.com. Used with Permission.

*Air*Veda: Ancient & New Medical Wisdom

The United States Center for Disease Control publishes the following guidelines for proper hand washing. Wet the hands with clean, running water (warm or cold), turn off the tap, and apply soap. Lather the hands by rubbing them together with the soap. Lather the backs of hands, between fingers, and under the nails. Scrub the hands for at least twenty seconds. Rinse the hands well under clean, running water. Dry the hands using a clean towel or air-dry them. The U.S. CDC advocates washing hands before, during, and after preparing food, before eating food, before and after caring for someone who is sick, before and after treating a cut or wound, after using the toilet, and after changing diapers or cleaning up a child who has used the toilet. Hand washing is also recommended after nose blowing, coughing, or sneezing, after touching an animal, animal feed, or animal waste, after handling pet food or pet treats, and after touching garbage. Alcohol based hand sanitizers that contain at least sixty percent ethanol is also effective in reducing the transmission of contaminants and infective agents. Hopefully, the advent of high technology toilets incorporating automatic water washing features, as well as warm air blow-drying, obviating the need for toilet paper and touching the anogenital area will be more readily embraced by Western and other cultures.

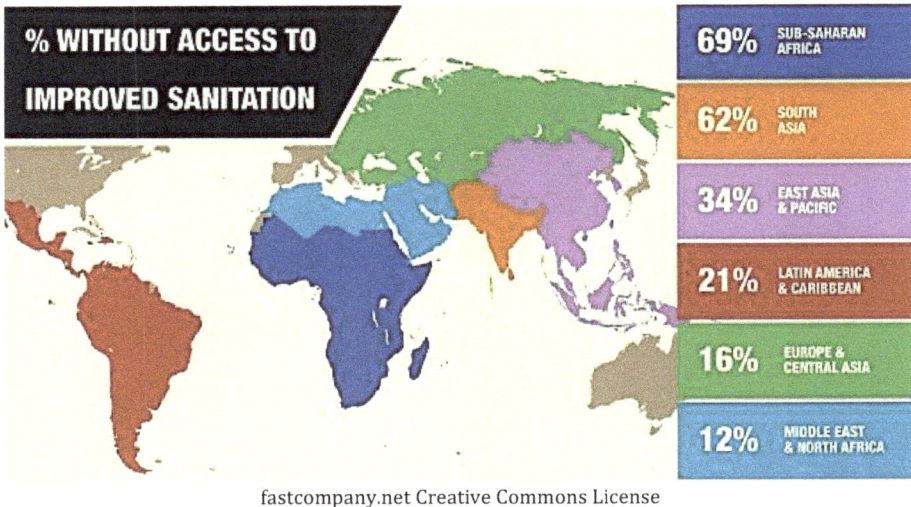

% WITHOUT ACCESS TO IMPROVED SANITATION
69% SUB-SAHARAN AFRICA
62% SOUTH ASIA
34% EAST ASIA & PACIFIC
21% LATIN AMERICA & CARIBBEAN
16% EUROPE & CENTRAL ASIA
12% MIDDLE EAST & NORTH AFRICA

fastcompany.net Creative Commons License

Contrary to popular belief Thomas Crapper did not invent the indoor flush toilet. It had been developed hundreds of years before he established his manufacturing company in Victorian England. Credit for the flushing toilet is usually attributed to Sir John Harrington, a godson of Queen Elizabeth I. One rumor is that his first name is the source of the nickname 'john' for a toilet. Thomas Crapper had a successful plumbing business and the inventor Albert Giblin was an employee of his. Giblin patented a silent siphon valve and Crapper bought the patent and marketed the improved toilet from 1861-1904 at great profit and name recognition. The average person goes to the toilet 2,500 times per year, and spends a total of three years of their lifetime sitting on the toilet. For those musically inclined most toilets flush in the key of E flat. Other trivia of note, one third of Americans flush the toilet while still sitting on it, and there are 40,000 injuries a year while sitting on the toilet seat.

Countries with most open defecation and worst access to sanitation[3]

uwcm-geog.wikispaces.com/Food+Aid Creative Commons License

In France the invention of the bidet in the early eighteenth century made water cleansing popular. The word bidet means pony in French, and using the bidet required that one straddle the bowl of the bidet as if riding a pony. A bidet spray or health faucet is a hand held hose and nozzle that utilizes a water spray for perianal and genitourinary cleansing after defecation and urination. The bidet is commonplace in many countries including Spain (thirty percent), Portugal (seventy percent), Greece (eighty percent), Italy (ninety-five percent), and Japan (fifty percent). In Japan automated and high technology toilets incorporate water washing as well as air blow drying and other features. The water bidet is also very popular in the Middle East, and growing in popularity in the United States.

Although popular in Europe and elsewhere around the world, the United States has been very slow to adopt the preferable water based approach to anal hygiene. In addition to its increased efficacy it has environmental benefits in reducing forest product consumption and sewage disposal of paper waste products. The reluctance of Americans to adopt the use of the bidet may be related to a misconception on the part of American and British troops during World War I. When they were first exposed to the bidet in France they assumed its purpose was purely for the washing of the genitals after sexual intercourse. The bidet incorrectly became associated as a product developed to accommodate French sexual immorality.

*Air*Veda: Ancient & New Medical Wisdom

Although popular in Europe and elsewhere around the world, the United States has been very slow to adopt the preferable water based approach to anal hygiene. In addition to its increased efficacy it has environmental benefits in reducing forest product consumption and sewage disposal of paper waste products. Creative Commons License

Although there are some very expensive models of toilets combined with bidets, the cost of an aftermarket addition of a washlet feature to a toilet is very economical. Many bidet equivalent washlets cost less than one hundred dollars, and with the savings by reduced toilet paper usage the device rapidly pays for itself. On the Indian subcontinent, in spite of the lack of bidets, over ninety-five percent of the population use water for anal cleansing. Many also use soap with water for cleansing after defecating. Use of paper is rare in this region, and hand washing after cleansing is critically important to prevent illness. In Japan the technological innovation of combining the bidet and toilet into a single product was introduced and advanced. Rapid innovations included a heated seat, automatic deodorizing, automatic lid raising and closing, directed water jets for female and male anatomy, music playing during use, vacuum fan ventilation, and warm air blow drying to obviate the need for wiping or use of toilet paper.

Genital and anal infections do not come in contact with the toilet seat in normal use. The intact skin of your buttocks is an efficient barrier against most disease organisms. Most transmission of pathogens is via the fecal to oral route is usually accomplished by way of the hands. The flush handle, sink handles, and door knob are much more likely to be a source of contamination since they are much likely to have been touched by someone whose hands had just been used to wipe their bottoms with a thin piece of toilet paper. It would be a good precaution to use toilet paper or paper towels to prevent your hands from touching the flush, faucet, and doorknobs or handles.

*Air*Veda: Ancient & New Medical Wisdom

Most transmission of pathogens is via the fecal to oral route is usually accomplished by way of the hands. The average human stool contains three trillion microorganisms. Wiping with toilet paper nearly guarantees that the hands will come into contact with fecal microorganisms. After wiping it is not uncommon to find brown streaks on underwear because of inadequate anal hygiene. The average man's underwear contains one-tenth of a gram of feces at laundering. Another infection risk from the toilet is the splashing and aerosol formation that can occur during flushing, particularly when someone with diarrhea has used that toilet. Surprisingly one-third of Americans remain seated on the toilet when they flush, and perhaps mistakenly find the misting of their anogenital region refreshing and hygienic. If they put paper toilet seat covers down before they sit on a public toilet seat for hygienic purposes, they should definitely get off the toilet seat before they flush.

The typical toilet flush creates a mist of contaminated water droplets that can travel up to twenty feet in all directions. It includes fecal matter and pathogens that settle on any exposed surface in the flush zone, including toothbrushes, drinking cups, bath toys, handles and doorknobs. The mist can stay airborne for up to two hours and be easily inhaled. The microbial pathogens can live on surfaces for up to a week. Before you flush, lower the lid to keep the aerosolization and spread to a minimum. Worldwide there are approximately two million fatalities every year due to diarrhea. The majority of these are in children under five years of age. Simple routine hand washing with soap and water could reduce the incidence of diarrhea by approximately fifty percent, and respiratory infections by about twenty-five percent. Hand washing also reduces the incidence of skin diseases, eye infections, and intestinal worms and parasites.

In most cultures and faiths food is not stored, prepared, or consumed in the vicinity of a toilet area. Both Islam and Judaism have a brief prayer of thanksgiving to be offered after the body functions of eliminating waste and the washing of hands. With the risk to health and wellness from exposure to human waste, religious customs and practices often offered practical guidance and hygiene to avoid disease. Istinja (Arabic: استنجاء), a component of Islamic hygiene practices, is the cleansing away of any residue and impurities (najasat) that remain after being passed from the urethra or anus. Istinja requires the use of water if available, and may be utilized with water alone or in combination with toilet paper. If water is not available stones, soil, or other natural material (other than bone or dung) may be utilized in the process known as 'istijmar'. The passage of intestinal gas alone does not require Istinja

Xylospongium replica

*Air*Veda: Ancient & New Medical Wisdom

Xylospongium, also known as *sponge on a stick*, is a device used to clean the perianal area after a bowel movement. It consists of a wooden stick (Greek: ξύλον, *Xylon*) with a sponge (Greek: Σπόγγος, *Spongos*) fixed at one end. In the *baths of the seven sages* in Ostia, a fresco from the 2nd century contains the Inscription *(u)taris xylosphongio* which is the first known mention of the term. Also in the early second century a papyrus letter of Claudius Terentianus to his father Claudius Tiberianus uses the term *xylospongium* in a phrase.

Shit stick is a thin stake or stick used for cleaning the perianal area after a bowel movement. It is used when water or toilet paper was not available for this purpose. The term has also been used in Chinese Buddhism and Japanese Buddhism. A well-known example is *gānshǐjué/kanshiketsu* (乾屎橛 "dry shit stick") from the Chan/Zen *gōng'àn/kōan* in which a monk asked "What is Buddha?" and Master Yunmen/Unmon answered "A dry shit stick". The presumed logic for such language was that most of the great masters of these schools did not directly state what they wished to convey. They often used a shout, or strike with a rod, or striking phrase as above to place their student in a state between comprehensibility and incomprehensibility. According to this logic it somehow promoted their development of enlightenment." Another explanation was that Zen Buddhist masters used the image of a dry shit stick to neutralize and balance of our image of a true person as sine thing other than pure or noble.
Ancient Roman latrines in Ostia Antica

Gaki zōshi 餓鬼草紙 "Scroll of Hungry Ghosts", a *gaki* condemned to shit-eating watches a child wearing *geta* and holding a *chūgi*, c. 12th century. People have used many different materials in the long history of anal cleansing, including leaves, rags, paper, water, sponges, corncobs, earthenware, pottery, and sticks. In ancient times, instruments made from bamboo, possibly in the form of spatulas ([*cèchóu*] 廁籌, [*cèbì*] 廁箆, or [*cèjiǎn*] 廁簡), may have been used with water for cleansing after a bowel movement. the assistance of water in cleaning the body after defecation. Japanese *chūgi* from the Nara period(710-784), shown with modern toilet paper for size comparison. When monks and missionaries introduced Buddhism into China and Japan, they also brought the Indian custom of using a *śalākā, a* small stake, stick, or rod for wiping away fecal residue after a bowel movement. Translators rendered this Sanskrit word into a number of different terms based on the words of *chóu* or *chū* 籌 "small stake or stick", or *jué* or *ketsu* 橛 "short stake or stick". Such terns included the Chinese *cèchóu* 廁籌 and Japanese *chūgi* 籌木. The custom of using shit sticks became popular and had the advantages of being inexpensive, washable, and reusable.

The Chinese invented paper around the 2nd century BCE, and toilet paper no later than the 6th century CE, when Yan Zhitui noted, "Paper on which there are quotations or commentaries from the Five Classics or the names of sages, I dare not use for toilet purposes". The earliest Japanese flush toilets date from the Nara period (710–784), when a drainage system was constructed in the capital at Nara. It was designed as squat toilets built over 4 - 6 inch (10–15 cm) wide wooden conduits that users would straddle. Archaeological excavations in Nara have also found numerous *chūgi* wooden sticks that were used for fecal cleansing. Ming Dynasty Xuande Emperorplaying *touhu*, 15th century. Chinese *Chóu* 籌 and chóumù or Japanese chū 籌 or *chūgi* 籌木 (with 木 "tree; wood") and *cèchóu* 廁籌 (with 廁 "toilet") "small stake; stick" are used as the equivalent terms meaning "shit stick". The Buddhist Sanskrit term *śalāka* or *śalākā* (Pali *salākā*) is its equivalent and may be a small stake, stick, rod, or twig. In Indian Buddhist contexts, *śalākā* can also represent a stick used for purposes other than anal hygiene. particularly meant "a piece of wood or bamboo used for counting or voting". *Salaka-Grahapaka* was the wood or bamboo sticks used in counting votes in general assembly. The Jain term *salakapurusa* "illustrious or worthy person" compounds *salaka* "stick used for voting" and *purusa* "person". *Chou* 籌 originally meant "arrow used in *tóuhú* (an ancient game wth competition on the number of arrows thrown into a pot)" or "tally stick (used in counting)". *Chóu* 籌 "shit stick" was first described in writing around the 3rd century CE. The Jin dynasty (265-420) *Yulin* 語林 by Pei Qi 裴啟 has stories about the ostentatious bathrooms of wealthy merchant Shi Chong 石崇 (249-300) who mocked the politician Liu Shi 劉寔 (220-310) for not being familiar with the perfumed shit sticks offered by two female bathroom attendants.

Chinese *jué* or Japanese *ketsu* 橛 "short wooden stake; stick; peg; post" is compounded with *shi* or *shĭ* 屎 (written with 尸 "body" and 米 "rice") "shit; excrement; dung" into Japanese *shiketsu* or Chinese *shĭjué* 屎橛 "shit stick". The famous term *gānshĭjué* or *kanshiketsu* 乾屎橛 "dry shit stick", modified with *gān* or *kan* 乾 "dry, dried; hollow". Kan-shiketsu 乾屎橛 Excrement-wiping spatula. A Zen word of abuse for a person who clings to things. Kan-shiketsu Japanese, literally a "dry shit stick"; a Zen expression designating a person who is attached to the world of appearance. Chinese *bì* 篦 "fine-tooth comb; spatula" or Japanese *hera* 篦 "spatula; scoop" is compounded into Chinese *cèbì* 廁篦 "toilet spatula" and Japanese *kusobera* 糞篦 "shit spatula" or *kusokakibera* 糞搔く篦 "shit scratching spatula". While most Japanese "shit stick" words have Sino-Japanese roots such as *chūgi* from *chóumù* 籌木, both *kuso* 糞 "shit; crap" and *hera* 篦 "spatula; scoop" are native Japanese terms. Chinese *cèjiăn* 廁簡 or 厕简 "toilet stick" is a synonym of *cèchóu* 廁籌 using the word *jiăn* 簡 "bamboo and wooden slips". During the time of Queen Zhou the Elder (r. 961-964), a monk used a sharpened toilet stick to remove a tumor.

The English language has some *shit(e) stick* parallels in its lexicography parallel to these Asian language terms. The *Oxford English Dictionary* (shyte, shite, shit) quotes two early *shit-stick* examples: "a hard chuffe, a shite-sticks" (1598) and "a shite-sticks, a shite-rags, that is to say, a miserable pinch-pennie" (1659); and defines poop-stick as "a fool, ineffectual person", with the earliest usage in 1930.

The microscopic mist that emanates with each flush of the toilet bowl distributes contaminated water droplets up to twenty feet in reach direction. Creative Commons License

Microbiological surveillance studies of *Escherichia coli* and other fecal bacteria have been performed in typical American household kitchens and bathrooms. The surprising finding was that toilet seats were one of the cleanest areas in the house with a very low microbe count. Faucets and refrigerator handles were more heavily contaminated. The highest concentration of microbes, more than two hundred times that of the toilet seat, were found on kitchen cutting boards. It was theorized this was from poultry, which often has fecal microbe contaminants in processing. Public toilet seats were also surveyed and less than two percent had any *Escherichia coli* or fecal contaminants. Even this small percentage was thought to represent contamination from the water mist that is generated by flushing. The best use of the toilet seat paper protector dispensed would be to use it instead of your bare hands to touch the faucets and door handles in the bathroom. In other public places some of the highest concentrations of fecal bacteria are found on sanitary napkin dispensers, hotel TV remote control units, vending machine buttons, and drinking water fountain controls.

The following twenty-five locations were surveyed in the United States for fecal contaminants with some surprising findings. Fast food restaurants in the US serve ice that had more bacteria than the toilet water in seventy percent of locations surveyed. Public restrooms have about two million bacteria per square inch, while the average toilet seat has only fifty per square inch. The average office desk has four hundred times more bacteria than a toilet. Keyboards can have up to two hundred times more bacteria than a toilet seat. Cell phones and mobile electronic devices can have ten times more bacteria than a toilet seat, and they are frequently in close contact with the fingers, face, and mouth. There are on average one hundred times more bacteria on restaurant menus than on restroom toilet seat. Raw meat carries a very high level of fecal bacteria, so food-chopping boards harbor more fecal contaminants than toilet seats. When the toilet is flushed the plume of toilet water with fecal contaminants often end up on toothbrushes left exposed. With two hundred thousand bacteria per square inch, carpets are four thousand times dirtier than a toilet seat. Humans shed one and one-half million skin cells every hour that helps feed the bacteria carpeting the carpets.

Most refrigerators test positive for the fecal contaminant *Escherichia coli* because thorough cleaning and disinfecting is an infrequent undertaking. Reusable shopping bags have more fecal matter than underwear and are rarely washed. In many households the television remote control is one of the most contaminated items handled. Hands are one of the dirtiest parts of the body, and they are frequently used to grasp and hold doorknobs, which are a reservoir of contaminants. Light switches can have up to two hundred and seventeen bacteria per square inch. The kitchen sink is usually dirtier than the bathroom and is often overlooked when cleaning. The bathtub, although thought of as a place to get clean, typically harbors nearly twenty thousand bacteria per square inch around the drain. Dead skins cells, dust mites, fungal spores, pollens, and other body secretions build up on the pillow, the place the head usually rests at night. After ten years a mattress will nearly double in weight thanks to the number of dust mites and dust mite feces that it has collected. The inside rim of a pet bowl alone contains over two thousand bacteria per square inch.

Currency bank notes can harbor up to two hundred thousand bacteria. It's a good idea to wash the hands after directly handling cash and currency. It brings new meaning to those having lots of money being known as 'filthy rich'. Draperies collect pet fur, mold, dander, debris, dust mites, and dust mite feces. The warm, dark, and moist insides of showerheads are popular breeding grounds for bacteria. Handbags contain cell phone, money, hairbrush, lipstick, cosmetics, and other items teeming with contaminants. Handbags are rarely cleaned and are a notorious source of potential contaminants. The kitchen sponge is nearly always the most heavily contaminated item in the house. With ten million bacteria per square inch the kitchen sponge is nearly a quarter of a million times dirtier than a toilet seat. The toilet seat is usually very clean, and the reason is really pretty simple, it gets cleaned often. A swimming pool visited by one hundred children can have over two pounds of feces floating around. Little kids can carry as much as ten grams of leftover feces around their anus after wiping their rear ends which just rinses off into the pool. Fecal contamination also occurs from adults with less than stellar anal hygiene. The U.S. Center for Disease Control (CDC) found that more than half of swimming pools in the U.S. test positive for the fecal bacteria *Escherichia coli*, which can cause gastroenteritis. Your best line of defense is to try not to swallow any water.

Restaurant menus have over one hundred times more bacteria than a toilet seat. They are held and fingered touched by dozens of people but only wiped down once a day, if that, and usually with a used rag. Instead of washing your hands before you sit down at the restaurant you may want to scrub up and use a hand sanitizer after you order. Be careful to never lay your silverware on top of the menu. Do you like a squeeze of lemon wedge with your water or beverage of choice? Researchers found that nearly seventy percent of the lemons had disease-causing microbes, including fecal contaminants such as *Escherichia coli*. Drinking fountains, especially public water fountains, have high bacteria counts, particularly on the faucet or push button. Ironically, the handles and push buttons on public restroom soap pumps are a breeding ground for bacteria, too. So scrub your hands for at least twenty seconds or better yet, carry your own personal hand sanitizer. And before you reach for that door handle leaving the restroom, think about how many people don't wash after going to the bathroom. The Center for Disease Control says only thirty-one percent of men and sixty-five percent of women do. Kitchen employees are supposed to always wash their hands after using the bathroom, and one can only hope that they do comply with this basic hygiene measure

Shopping cart handles can be swarming with millions of microorganisms, including ones from raw meat from a previous shopper, or fecal bacteria if a diapered child was sitting in the cart earlier in the day. A lot of grocery stores have antibacterial wipes handy, so use them, or put your items directly into paper or plastic bags or boxes. Many people are careful not to touch heavily contaminated door handles, including refrigerator and freezer handles, but are not as wary as they should be of push buttons on elevators, remote controls, computer or bank ATM keypads, etc. In hotel rooms the television remote control is the dirtiest object there and could use a disinfectant wipe before you channel surf. Other potential microbial hotspots include the bedside lamp switch, bedspread, hair dryer, telephone, and unwrapped drinking glasses.

If you take children to a playground, remember it is also a playground for microbes. Playgrounds are rarely cleaned and kids are continuously handling railings, handles, swings, slides. Your child would actually be in less contact with microbes if they were playing with public restroom toilet seats, which are at least cleaned frequently. The worse spot in the playground is the sandbox, with thirty-six times more germs than a restaurant tray. One organism found all too often in the sandbox is the parasitic protist *Toxoplasma gondii*. The U.S. Humane Society estimates that the wild feral cat population in the US exceeds fifty million, and the vast majority carry this dangerous and easily transmissible parasite. They look upon a playground sandbox as nothing more than a giant litter box and frequently defecate in them and mix their feces in with the sand.

Worldwide there are approximately two million fatalities every year due to diarrhea. The majority of these are in children under five years of age. Simple routine hand washing with soap and water could reduce the incidence of diarrhea by approximately fifty percent, and respiratory infections by about twenty-five percent. Hand washing also reduces the incidence of skin diseases, eye infections, and intestinal worms and parasites. In most cultures and faiths food is not stored, prepared, or consumed in the vicinity of a toilet area. Both Islam and Judaism have a brief prayer of thanksgiving to be offered after the body functions of eliminating waste and the washing of hands. With the risk to health and wellness from exposure to human waste, religious customs and practices often offered practical guidance and hygiene to avoid disease.

It is obvious that the transmission of contaminants from the feces of one person to the mouth of another is exceedingly common. Even taking great precautions and frequent hand washing the exposure possibilities are nearly limitless. Did your food preparer was their hands thoroughly after using the bathroom? How about after they touched the kitchen sink faucet or refrigerator door handle? Did you wash your hands after touching a drinking fountain knob, or after shaking someone's hands? Did you hold onto a stairway railing, open a door by turning a knob or touching a handle? Did you handle currency, share a pen, hold a child's hand, touch a computer keyboard, use a remote control, hold a restaurant menu?

Welcome to the world of overwhelming microbial presence. The number of bacteria and Archaea organisms on earth are estimated at five million trillion trillion (called a nonillion in short scale for English speaking countries and quintillion in long scale for non-English speaking countries). For those who prefer numbers in numerical form it is the number five followed by thirty zeroes written as 5,000,000,000,000,000,000,000,000,000,000. Over one half of the world's biomass are bacteria and Archaea, and they outnumber each human by many trillions of organisms. There are approximately ten trillion human cells in the body. The human gut microbiome alone, just the microbes living within the human intestinal tract is over one hundred trillion organisms, and outnumbers all human cells by more than ten to one. Adding in the quadrillions of viruses, prions, protist, fungi, parasites, and other life forms that have yet to be discovered humans are an extremely small minority.

The exposure to human and animal waste is nearly ubiquitous, in spite of our best efforts. Part of the challenge is the sheer quantity of waste generated by the human and animal. There are nearly one and a half billion cattle in the world today, each one producing an average of twenty-seven kilograms (sixty pounds) of feces a day. Fortunately, twenty-four kilograms is water, but that still leaves three kilograms (over six and one half pounds of feces by dry weight). Cows alone generate nearly one hundred billion pounds of feces per day. The world sheep population is one point two billion, each of which produces on average fifteen kilograms (thirty-three pounds) of feces, adding another forty billion pounds of feces a day to the waste challenge.

The world pig population is one billion, each producing seven kilograms (fifteen pounds) of manure a day. The world bird population is estimated at three hundred billion, horse population is sixty million, dog population is three hundred million, cat population is five hundred million. There are hundreds of billions of additional animals, ranging from the enormous blue whale and elephant to the diminutive mouse and termite adding trillions of pounds of feces into the environment every day. Of course, we should not forget our own contribution, with a world human population of over seven point three billion people ewe contribute over a billion pounds of feces per day. Fecal contaminants are commonly in the food and water supply around the world.

Atmospheric Pressure (Barometric Pressure)

Intestinal gas, like gasses everywhere, must comply with the laws of physics and the laws of nature. Boyle's law states that at a constant temperature, the product of the volume and pressure of a gas must remain constant. This requires that they maintain an inverse relationship, if one increases the other has to decrease. As such, an increase in pressure will result in the decrease of the volume of the gas, and vice versa.

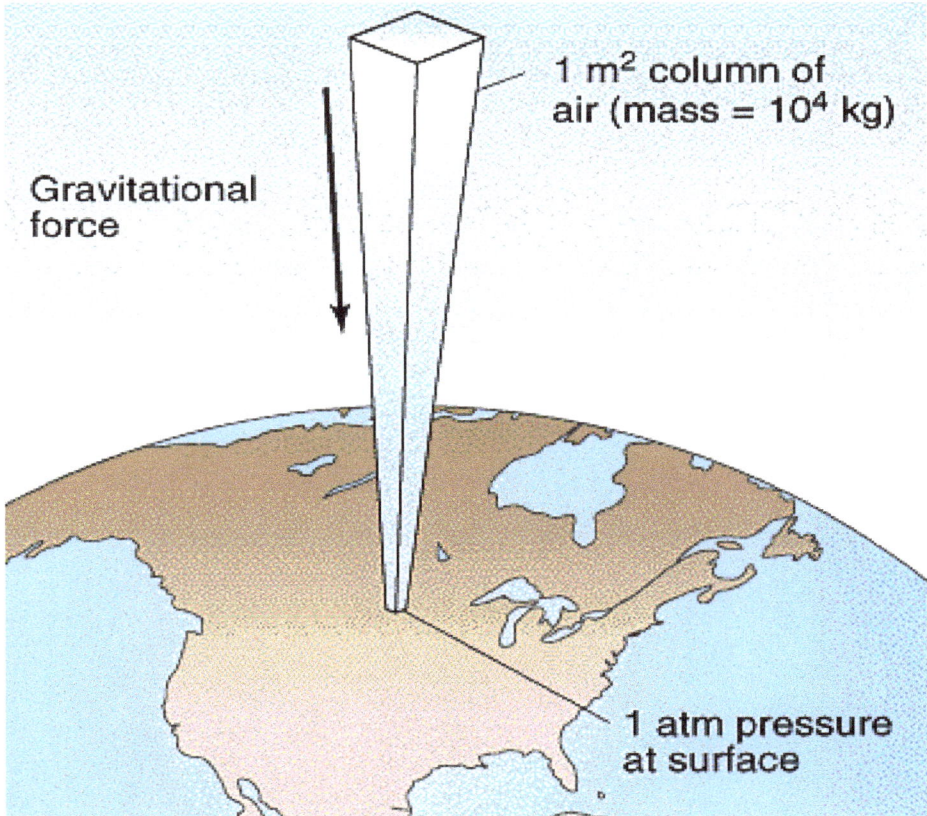

Atmospheric pressure hendrix2.uoregon.edu Creative Commons License

The atmospheric pressure on earth is defined as a standard of one atmosphere at sea level. As you go deeper down into the earth, such as happens in a mineshaft, or diving deeper into the oceans, the atmospheric pressure increases. As you go higher in elevation, whether climbing flights of stairs, ascending a mountain, or in a hot air balloon, the atmospheric pressure decreases. The atmospheric pressure is also not uniform, constantly changing along with the weather.

Atmospheric pressure and the weather are always changing. Shutterstock/polarpx

Using Boyle's law, you can calculate how much the volume will compress as you go deeper underground or underwater and atmospheric pressure increases. You can likewise calculate how much a gas will expand, as you go higher in altitude and the atmospheric pressure decreases. If you have ever gone diving into a swimming pool or scuba diving, you can feel the increasing atmospheric pressure on your eardrums.

Visual depiction of the principle of Boyle's Law, as the pressure increases the volume decreases, and vice versa. Creative Commons License

AirVeda: Ancient & New Medical Wisdom

-10 C

250 C

Visual depiction of the principle of Charles' Law, as the temperature increases the volume increases, and vice versa. Creative Commons License

COOKING TIMES (approximate)

	Whole chicken	Brown rice	Black beans
Regular:	60 min.	50 min.	60 min.
Cooker:	15 min.	20 min.	15 min.

—250° Pressure cooker temp.
—212° Normal boiling point

Pressure regulator

Lock

STEAM

Sealing ring

1 Higher temperatures
The tight-fitting lid prevents steam from escaping. Pressure builds, allowing inside temperatures to rise above normal boiling point of 212°F.

2 Direct contact
The steam's heat is transferred directly to the surface of the food.

IMPROVED SAFETY

■ **Locking handle** cannot be opened when under pressure.

■ **Multiple valves** release pressure.

A pressure cooker is one example of the practical application of the laws of physics. As the pressure within the cooker increases the water can achieve a temperature higher than its boiling point. Creative Commons License

77

Aerospace

Intestinal gas, like gasses everywhere, must comply with the laws of physics and the laws of nature. Boyle's law states that at a constant temperature, the product of the volume and pressure of a gas must remain constant. This requires that they maintain an inverse relationship, if one increases the other has to decrease. As such, an increase in pressure will result in the decrease of the volume of the gas, and vice versa. See earlier entry on aerospace for more details.

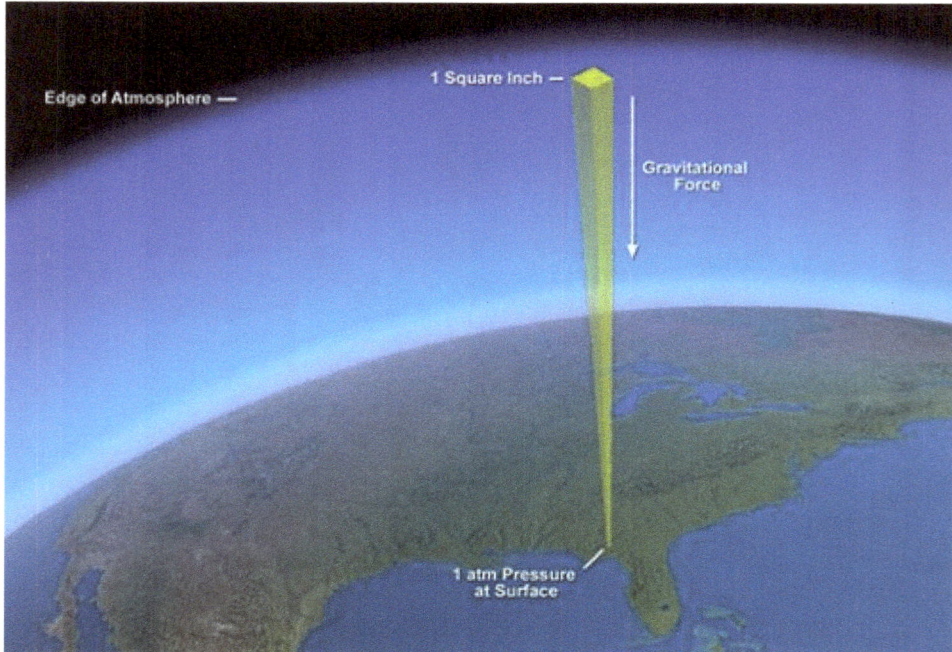

farm7.static.flickr.com Creative Commons License

Elevators

The sensation of the increasing volume of intestinal gas is most noticeable with the rapid decrease in atmospheric pressure experienced in airplane or space travel. A high-speed elevator comes close, and you may first sense the change in air pressure by the inequality of the pressure applied to the eardrums. You may have an ear 'popping' effect from a rapid ascent in the elevator. As you rapidly ascend by the elevator in a high-rise building, driving up a mountain road, or flying in an airplane, you may feel or hear your ears 'pop' as they adjust to the decreasing atmospheric pressure. If they do not 'pop' on their own, you may feel the discomfort of the unequal pressure as the eardrum begins to bulge. Since you are not underwater you can use the more comfortable maneuver of yawning, instead of the Valsalva maneuver (see page 432).

www.flickr.com Kevin Trotman Creative Commons License

Unfortunately, with the elevator's rapid ascent comes the equally rapid expansion of intestinal gasses. This may lead to an increase in the passage of intestinal gasses in the confined space of the elevator. If the elevator is crowded there are lots of people to glare at to take the suspicion off of you. Fortunately, the same risk does not occur as the elevator descends. On the descent the increasing atmospheric pressure causes the volume of intestinal gas to decrease., and the risk of being subjected to your own or someone else's fart in the confined elevator decreases.

High Altitude Community

The majority of the world's population lives close to the seashore and have the standard atmospheric pressure of one atmosphere found at sea level. A significant percentage of the world's population lives at higher altitudes with atmospheric pressures less than one atmosphere. The higher above sea level you are, the lower is the atmospheric pressure you are subjected to. As a consequence, although the number of molecules of gas produced is identical, it will require a larger volume of space to contain it.

If you live in Denver Colorado, the mile-high city with an elevation of five-thousand one-hundred and eighty-three feet (one-thousand six-hundred and nine meters) feet above sea level, the volume will be larger than residing in Los Angeles or New York City. It is all relative as residing in Mexico City, which is at seven-thousand three-hundred and fifty feet (two-thousand two-hundred and forty meters), will produce a much larger volume than Denver.

Manizales, Colombia is at an altitude of six thousand six hundred and ninety feet (2,021 meters) above sea level. Shutterstock/fotos593

For those flying at even higher altitudes the cabin pressure in commercial aircraft limits the reduction in atmospheric pressured to the equivalent of approximately eight-thousand feet above sea level high, much as if you were in Mexico City. With the atmospheric pressure at this altitude just over two-thirds of sea level, the gas volume expands by about forty percent. That is more than enough to cause a person to notice a significant increase in their flatulence and an increase in the flatulence of everyone else as well.

Atmospheric pressure arises from the weight of the air sitting above the observer. The mass of air in the column above the head of the observer is pulled down by the gravity of the Earth and exerts a pressure force on the observer. At the surface of the Earth at sea level the pressure is 14.7 pounds per square inch. This is also described in other measurement units as one atmosphere, 101,000 Pascals, 1kPa (kilopascal), or one bar. At higher altitudes, less air sits above an observer, so there is a lesser amount of atmospheric pressure. hendrix2.uoregon.edu Creative Commons License

High Rise Building

If you work or reside on the higher floors of an office building or residence tower, or if your place of work or residence is at a higher elevation in a mountain community the difference in atmospheric pressure may be significant. Whatever the reason for the change in altitude the resulting changes in atmospheric pressure affects intestinal gasses. They are subject to the same consequences of Boyle's Law as any other gas.

The heights of the tallest skyscrapers continue to reach new world records. Even coastal cities that are nearly at sea level will have buildings in which the changes in atmospheric pressure between those at the ground floor and those at the higher levels will be significant. This is most readily demonstrated by taking a high-speed elevator in a high-rise building. The rapid decrease in atmospheric pressure traveling from the lower to the higher floors often results in pressure changes on the eardrum (tympanic membrane). The equalization of pressure on both sides of the tympanic membrane may give rise to an ear popping sensation.

Burj Khalifa, Dubai, Tallest building in the world. Skyline is depicted above fog level.
Shuttertstock/NaufalMQ

Mountain Climbing

In rock or mountain climbing, the higher the altitude, the lower the atmospheric pressure. Although the number of molecules remain unchanged gastrointestinal gasses will expand by virtue of the laws of physics. The increasing volume of gas will lead to discomfort and ultimately will find a way to exit your digestive tract. Air in the stomach may be released, as a burp or belch, but the larger quantity of gasses in the colon will come out as flatus, commonly called a fart. The higher in altitude you go, the lower the atmospheric pressure, and the more flatus you will be passing.

As you go up the elevator in a high-rise building, or drive up a mountain road, or fly in an airplane you may feel or hear your ears 'pop' as they adjust to the decreasing atmospheric pressure. To relieve the discomfort, you need to equalize pressure on both sides of the eardrum. As these pressure changes occur while not underwater, a simple yawn is easier and more comfortable the Valsalva maneuver to equalize the pressure difference.

Mountain climber. Shutterstock/MyGoodImages

<u>Scuba Diving</u>

Using Boyle's law, you can calculate how much the gas volume will compress as you go deeper underground or underwater and atmospheric pressure increases. You can likewise calculate how much a gas will expand, as you go higher in altitude and the atmospheric pressure decreases. If you have ever gone diving into a swimming pool or scuba diving, you can feel the increasing atmospheric pressure on your eardrums., also known as the tympanic membrane. If you go deep enough, the atmospheric pressure increases to such a degree that it may become painful.

To relieve the discomfort, you have to equalize the pressure on both sides of your eardrums. This equalization of air pressure is usually accomplished by performing the Valsalva maneuver. This procedure can be initiated by attempting to exhale against a closed epiglottis, much like straining during a bowel movement. The open Eustachian tube from the pharynx allows equalization of the atmospheric pressure on both sides of the eardrum.

If unrelieved, or if pressure is increased further, it may exceed the ability of the tissue to withstand it resulting in rupture or perforation. A perforated eardrum is very painful and is more likely to occur if the Eustachian tubes that must be open to equalize the pressure on both sides of the eardrum are swollen shut by infection, inflammation, or other conditions. For this reason, activities, which rapidly or excessively apply pressure on the eardrums, should be avoided if the individual has an upper respiratory or nasal congestion, such as sinusitis, head cold, ear infection, etcetera. The use of a nasal and sinus decongestant may be helpful but caution is still required. Scuba diving, flying, mountain climbing, and other activities require awareness of their potential effects on human health.

*Air*Veda: Ancient & New Medical Wisdom

Shutterstock/timsimages

Other effects of pressure changes on the gasses within human tissue are less frequent but of even greater concern. Scuba divers know better than to eat a gas producing meal, such as chili with beans and carbonated beverages, before a dive. The gas bubbles generated within the gut while at a one-hundred-foot dive depth are compressed into a relatively small volume by the high atmospheric pressure. Upon returning to the surface at the conclusion of the dive that small gas bubble will rapidly expand to a much larger volume as the high atmospheric pressure is reduced back to normal at the surface. As the gas bubble expands the pressure on the intestinal tract wall dramatically increases and can lead to a rupture as the result of barotrauma. Unlike a perforated eardrum, a perforation and rupture of the gut is life threatening and may lead to peritonitis and death if the perforation is not sealed or corrected surgically.

Another gas pressure related condition has to do with nitrogen dissolved in the blood under high pressure, leaving solution and forming actual physical bubbles circulating in the bloodstream. The bubbles can lead to catastrophic effects if they prevent circulation of oxygen carrying blood to vital organs as an air or gas embolism. This condition was first recognized in deep sea divers and is known as caisson disease, decompression sickness, as well as 'the bends' because it often lead to a doubling over because of joint pain within hours of returning to the surface after prolonged dives. The limitation of dive length is calculated by dive tables or computers, and is typically based on the depth of the dive and the composition of the air or inhaled gasses in the dive tanks.

Nitrox was developed to reduce the incidence of nitrogen narcosis, which can lead to dangerous changes in mental awareness because of the buildup of dissolved nitrogen gas in the bloodstream. The term narcosis has the same Greek word root as the word for narcotic. The Greek word αρκωσις (narcosis) is derived from *narke*, which means a decline or loss of senses and movement. Nitrogen narcosis has also been called 'raptures of the deep', inert gas narcosis, and the 'Martini effect'.

During ascent all gases increase in volume as the atmospheric pressure decreases. As the gases in the gastrointestinal tract increases in volume they may produce symptoms including cramping colicky abdominal pain, distension, belching, flatulence, and vomiting. Rare cases of rupture of the stomach and other portions of the gastrointestinal tract have occurred. Severe stomach pains have been reported during chamber dives after the divers drank carbonated beverages while under high atmospheric pressure.

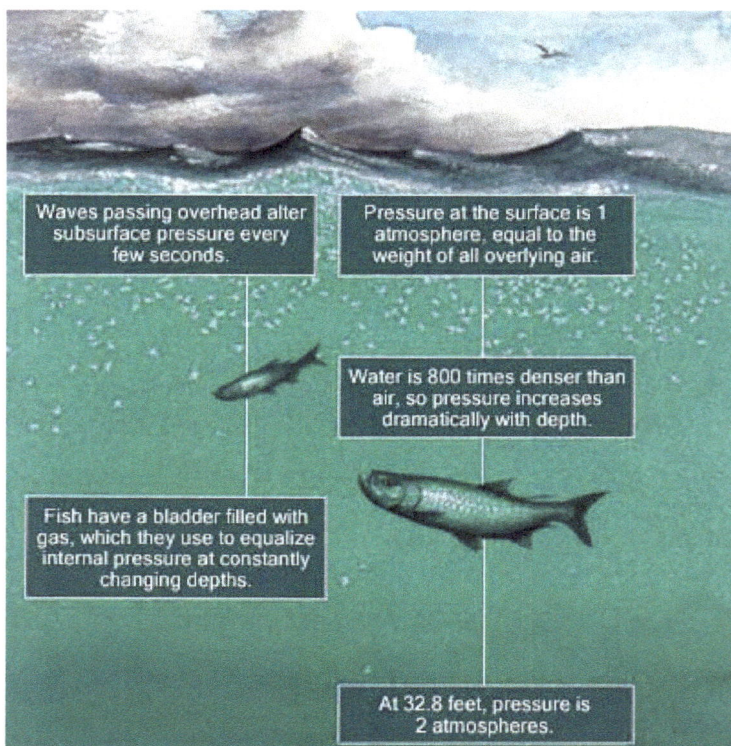

Atmospheric pressure rises quickly with greater underwater depths. Artist Jonathan Milo
media.midcurrent.com.s3.amazonaws.com/wp Creative Commons License

One informative episode occurred with the grand opening of a brand new hyperbaric facility. The grand opening was toasted with champagne that was consumed while sixty feet (twenty meters) deep. The hosts and guests were disappointed that the champagne appeared to be flat without much carbonation. They decided to celebrate by drinking it even though it was flat because it tasted good. Their discomfort on ascent was exceeded only by their embarrassment. During ascent the gas in the 'flat' champagne (which was present in the normal amounts) came out of solution and expanded in their stomachs leading to uncontrolled belching.

Another unusual way to experience the effect of a prolonged dive was part of a research effort of the National Space and Aeronautic Administration (NASA)

*Air*Veda: Ancient & New Medical Wisdom

OCEAN project to assess the effects of long term space travel, comparing the similar exposures of space travel and underwater living. The research facilities have since remained open as a tourist hotel in Key Largo, Florida, where guests enter the hotel by scuba diving over twenty feet to the entrance. The hotel maintains and atmospheric pressure of approximately one and one half atmospheres.

For those who enjoy scuba diving, you are already familiar with the effects of increased atmospheric pressure. The pressure on the ears can become intense unless you are able to equalize the pressure regularly in descent and ascent. To be a certified scuba diver you must be knowledgeable about the risk of potentially life threatening illness and conditions that can be associated with these pressure changes. When inhaled at pressures higher than four atmospheres nitrogen can act as an anesthetic agent causing nitrogen narcosis. This is a temporary semi-anesthetized state of mental impairment similar to that caused by nitrous oxide, commonly known as laughing gas.

Nitrogen also dissolves in the bloodstream and body fats. Rapid decompression in the case of divers ascending too quickly, can lead to life threatening decompression sickness formerly known as caisson sickness or the bends, when nitrogen bubbles form in the bloodstream, nerves, joints. Most scuba divers also know not to ingest carbonated beverages or legumes and other gas producing foods during a dive. It is not the descent that is a problem. Remember from Boyles law that as you go deeper underwater the atmospheric pressure is increasing and the gas bubbles are getting smaller and smaller in volume. The problem is on the ascent where after a half hour of diving time at one hundred feet underwater, you begin your ascent. Your bowel has a modest size bubble of gas at that depth, but during the ascent this bubble expands and expands and can cause significant discomfort

Even though most experienced scuba divers know better than to fly shortly after a dive, even experienced scuba divers sometimes forget the same process can occur on land. Occasionally scuba divers will travel by land in an automobile from sea level after a dive, up a mountain road to a community or destination at a much higher elevation. Various gas mixtures have been developed for divers to reduce these risks. Trimix consists of oxygen, helium, and nitrogen, and Heliox is nitrogen free with just helium and oxygen. Hydrox is hydrogen and oxygen, an explosive combination if ignited. Nitrox is nitrogen and oxygen but is usually enriched for dives to increase the oxygen content and reduce the risk of decompression sickness.

Similar conditions can occur in miners when the mine shaft is pressurized to prevent ground water from entering, flying in unpressurized or depressurized aircraft at higher altitudes, and in space travel when the pressure in a spacesuit used for extravehicular activity is lower than the ambient pressure within the spaceship. An unusual but particularly dangerous combination is a novice scuba diver returning from a diving holiday unaware than a recent dive followed by even further reduction of atmospheric pressure by flying can lead to catastrophic consequences. Even though the dive table may suggest the risk period has ended, dive tables are calculated for a return to sea level, not the common commercial aircraft pressurization at an equivalent of an eight-thousand-foot elevation. See separate entry entitled Scuba Diving for more information.

Spelunking

Spelunking, the exploration of caves, has become an increasingly popular activity and can take place above or below sea level altitudes. Some of the deepest explored caves have vertical drops in excess of one thousand feet. Although changes in atmospheric pressure are noticeable, this effect is one of the least dangerous aspects of the sport activity. The exploration of underwater caves known as cave diving, combines spelunking with scuba diving, and is a particularly demanding and challenging activity. In this activity understanding the potential effects of atmospheric pressure changes becomes critically important.

Shutterstock/DudarevMikhail

Underground Miner

Mines have been present from prehistoric times but the depth of mines continues to increase. The deepest mineshaft in commercial operation to date extends two and one-half miles below the surface. As one goes deeper into the interior of the planet the atmospheric pressure increases. Just like in the diving experience, the great depth of the mine can lead to significant reduction in the volume of gasses with the increasing atmospheric pressure. In addition, some mines are pressurized to prevent ground water from entering the mineshaft. The danger is on the return to the surface as the higher atmospheric pressure is reduced back to normal. With the reduction in atmospheric pressure the volume of the gasses increases, and may leave solution causing bubble formation in the blood stream.

One of the additional occupational hazards of miners is the exposure to toxic gasses, including methane. The technology has now advanced to sophisticated monitoring for such gasses, but the miner's canary still carries an image into present day folklore and humor. Canaries and similar birds were taken into the mines as an early warning sign of methane toxicity. The birds are extremely sensitive to methane and die promptly on exposure to the toxic gas. If the miner's canary suddenly toppled off its perch in an episode of sudden death the miners knew that they had to quickly evacuate the mine. Bathroom humor would have the canary as a warning of toxic methane fumes emanating from flatus. If the canary died someone farted.

Public Domain Creative Commons License

lunar.thegamez.net/coalmining/canary

Ayurveda Medicine

Dhanvantari (धन्वंतरी), known as an avatar of Vishnu is the Hindu god associated with Ayurveda. The above photo was taken at a recent Ayurveda expo in Bangalore titled 'Arogya'. Author HPNadig Creative Commons

Ayurveda (Sanskrit आयुर्वेद life-knowledge) also known as Ayurveda medicine is the oldest known system of traditional medicine, and is native to the Indian subcontinent. In Western cultures, Ayurveda medicine is considered a form of alternative or complementary medicine. The *Suśruta Saṃhitā* and the *Charaka Saṃhitā* are the oldest known Ayurveda texts. These classical Sanskrit encyclopedias of medicine are considered a formal compilation of the historical works of Ayurveda. A general overview of Ayurveda is offered in the introduction to this volume, on pages nine through sixteen.

Ayurveda medicine approaches health and wellness in a holistic approach, and has enjoyed renewed popularity in Western culture. It has a keen focus on digestive health. Ayurveda teaches that the human body digests not just physical nutrients, but the totality of all experiences, emotions, and sensory input. The sense of smell, touch, taste, sight, and hearing have a significant influence on digestion and health.

THREE DOSHAS

VATA	PITTA	KAPHA
Gas, Air Humor.	Fire, Bile Humor.	Water, Phlegm Humor.
Causes pain, dryness, wasting, debility, anxiety, depression, constipation, arthritis, rheumatism, over-analysation, mental diseases, cancer etc.	Causes blood and skin rashes and diseases, hepatitis, dysentery, infections, anger, desire, excess driving force	Causes obesity, diabetes, excess consumption, slowness, swelling, tumors, excess growths of bones, nails, hair etc.

In Ayurveda, a dosha is one of three bodily humors that in combination create an individual's constitution. Ayurveda medicine advocates that to be in good health one must achieve a balance between three doshas, known as Vata, Pitta and Kapha. Vata is required to activate and sustain the function of the nervous system. It affects rheumatism, gout, the windy humor, flatulence, etc. Pitta is the transforming bilious humor that is secreted through the digestive tract. It flows through the liver and in Ayurveda medicine it is believed to permeate the spleen, heart, eyes, and skin. Its primary quality is the heat and energy of bile to direct digestion and metabolism. Kapha is the body fluid associated with mucus, lubrication, nourishment and is the carrier of nutrients.

The strength and health of digestion in Ayurveda is ascribed to the Agni, a Sanskrit term for the "digestive fire". The digestive process metabolizes the food as well as environmental senses that are internalized. The body assimilates that which is useful, and produces a vital essence called Ojas, a Sanskrit word meaning strength. Ojas is the basis of physical well-being, strength, mental clarity, and immunity to illness. The digestive process also produces waste, which must be eliminated for health and wellness. When the digestive energy of Agni is weakened through physical inactivity, poor health, excess stress, or negative emotions the digestive process is impaired. The digestive process produces waste and toxins known as Ama that causes poor health and disease.

In the Ayurveda approach to digestive health the root cause of poor Agni is addressed, not just the symptoms that result. Ayurveda incorporates health practices designed to strengthen the digestive fire of Agni to improve the metabolism of food and minimize uncomfortable digestive symptoms such as gas, indigestion, bloating, and constipation. These holistic approaches include portion control to avoid overeating. The stomach should not be filled more than three quarters full as it needs internal space to allow room for the digestive process of acid, enzymes, the churning process and the gases produced. Overfilling the stomach can lead to reflux, indigestion, heartburn, and nausea.

Daily movement such as short walks, yoga, swimming, or exercise stimulate the digestive processes and enhance the peristalsis moving digestive material through the gastrointestinal tract. It also helps to maintain blood glucose levels without after meal spikes that nay cause difficulties especially for diabetics. Meditation on a regular basis for thirty minutes twice each day can be very beneficial in reducing stress and improving the Agni. Clearing away negative emotions and the deep relaxation of meditation is a practice that may provide many health benefits.

Ginger is a helpful carminative and is known in Ayurveda as the "universal remedy" due to its many benefits including relaxing the smooth muscle of the intestines. It also stimulates saliva, bile, and digestive enzyme production aiding in the digestive process. Ginger contains phenolic compounds such as gingerol, shogaol, and other volatile oils that are responsible for its potent properties. It may be taken during the day in the form of a refreshing and easy to prepare ginger tea.

The timing of meals is also important with the major meal of the day best consumed at midday. Having lunch as the major meal instead of dinner is a healthful approach allowing activity through the rest of the day to assist in the digestive process. The typical approach in the US of a large evening meal followed by inactivity and the recumbent position for sleeping leads to a propensity to reflux and a sluggish digestive process.

The Ayurveda focus on proper digestion and its central role in physical and emotional health is summarized in its philosophy. According to Ayurveda we are not what we eat, but we are what we digest. The wisdom of Ayurveda has withstood the test of many thousands years of experience well. Each individual can best judge what approaches provide benefit and chose selectively from a variety of health care disciplines.

In Sanskrit literature, Ayurveda is called "the science of eight components" (Sanskrit *aṣṭāṅga* अष्टांग). This system of classification became the basic canons of Ayurveda medicine.

Kāya-chikitsā - cure of diseases affecting the body (general medicine)
Kaumāra-bhṛtya - treatment of children (pediatrics)
Śhalya-chikitsā - removal of any substance, which has entered the body
　　　such as the extraction of darts, of splinters, etc. (surgery)
Śālākya-tantra - cure of diseases of the eye or ear etc. by sharp
　　　instruments (ophthalmology/ENT)

Bhūta (past)-vidyā - treatment of mental diseases supposed to be
 produced by past experiences (psychiatry)
Agada-tantra - doctrine of antidotes (toxicology)
Rasayana-tantra doctrine of Rasayana (elixirs)
Vājīkaraṇa tantra (aphrodisiacs)

Ayurveda medicine advocates that these ancient concepts based on the knowledge discovered by the Rishis and Munis long ago remain timeless. Ayurveda examines the homeostasis of the whole body system, and approaches good health as the ability to exist in harmony with physical reality. While people may be of a predominant dosha, it is common to have variable displays of all of their elements. The dominance of the doshas within an individual are likewise variable, and Ayurveda medicine attempts to modify the doshas to achieve the correct balance needed to achieve and maintain health.

Bacteria (see Microbiome, Pathogen)

Bacterial Overgrowth, Small Intestine

Small intestinal bacterial overgrowth (SIBO) is a condition characterized by excessive bacterial growth in the small bowel. This results in alteration of the gut flora and microbiome. Risk factors include motility or anatomical changes that lead to stasis, immune deficiencies, and the reflux of colonic bacteria into the small bowel.

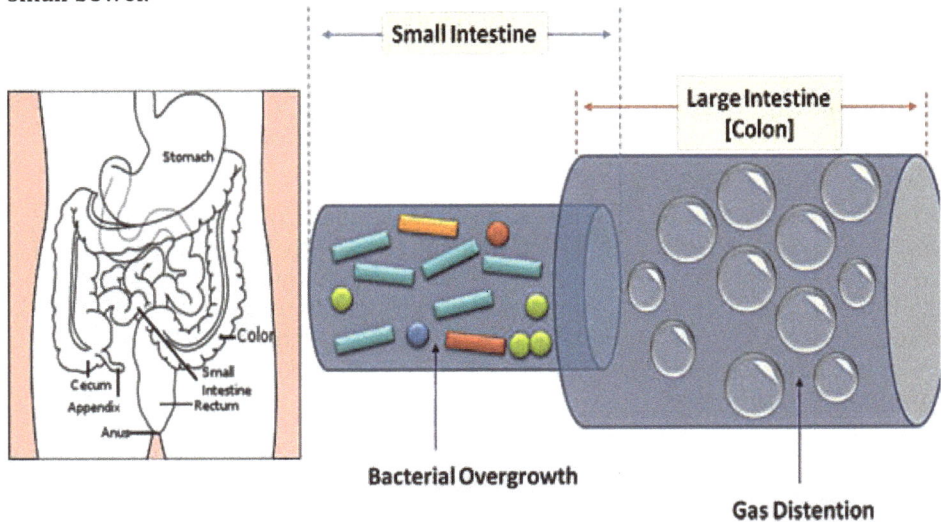

Anatomical changes, such as the surgical removal of the ileocecal valve, may predispose to small bowel bacterial overgrowth. The symptoms of bacterial overgrowth may include nausea, vomiting, bloating, flatus, chronic diarrhea, constipation, abdominal discomfort, weight loss, malnutrition, and anemia from vitamin B_{12} deficiency.

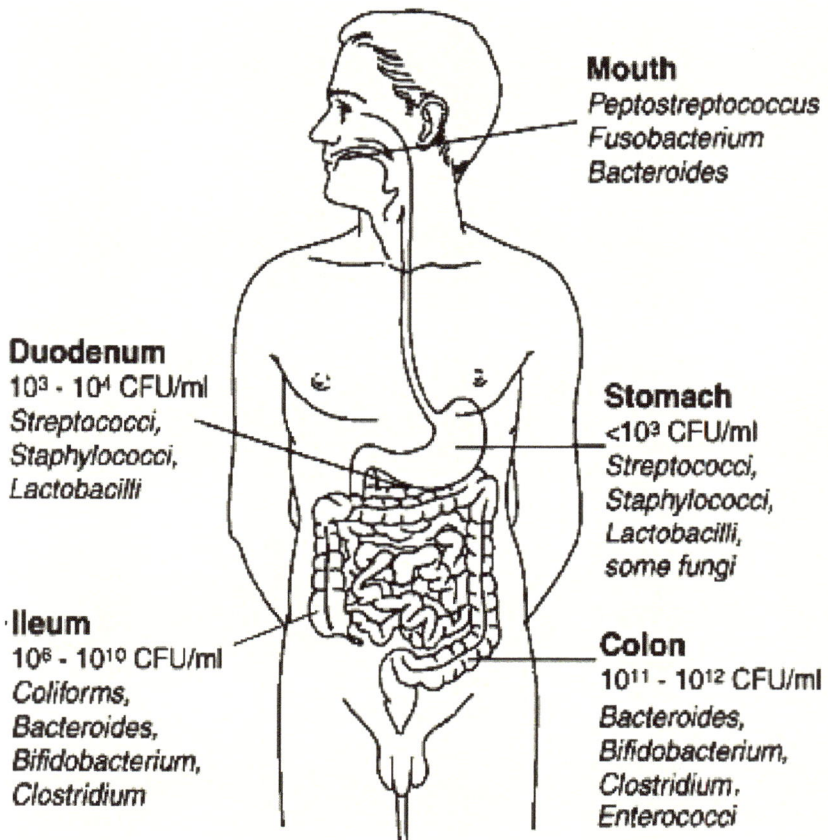

Mouth
Peptostreptococcus
Fusobacterium
Bacteroides

Duodenum
10^3 - 10^4 CFU/ml
Streptococci,
Staphylococci,
Lactobacilli

Stomach
<10^3 CFU/ml
Streptococci,
Staphylococci,
Lactobacilli,
some fungi

Ileum
10^6 - 10^{10} CFU/ml
Coliforms,
Bacteroides,
Bifidobacterium,
Clostridium

Colon
10^{11} - 10^{12} CFU/ml
Bacteroides,
Bifidobacterium,
Clostridium,
Enterococci

Irritable bowel syndrome (IBS) may have an association with SIBO with some studies showing improvement after treatment. Rosacea, a dermatological condition, also appears to have an association with improvement after treatment. Small bowel bacterial overgrowth syndrome is often treated with antibiotics. If retreatment is required, various antibiotics may be given in a cyclic fashion. Probiotics may also be of benefit in an attempt to return the microbiome to normal flora and balance.

Bariatric (Weight Loss) Surgery

Bariatric (Greek bar- weight, iatr - treatment) is the field of knowledge that deals with obesity including diet, exercise, behavioral therapy, pharmaceuticals, hormones, and surgery. Overweight and obesity are defined in relationship to the Body Mass Index, commonly referred to by its initials BMI. They are commonly associated with complicating co-morbid conditions including heart disease, diabetes, cancer, asthma, sleep apnea, and chronic musculoskeletal problems that lead to higher mortality rates.

Diet, exercise, behavior therapy, and anti-obesity drugs are first-line treatment. Bariatric surgery is the term for the surgical treatment of morbid obesity and gastric bypasses are one class of such operations. Gastric bypass surgery divides the stomach into a small upper pouch and a larger lower "remnant" pouch and then reconnects the small intestine to both. There are a variety of anatomical variations that have been developed, but all result in a marked reduction of the volume of food the stomach can receive during a meal.

Bariatric weight loss surgery is usually reserved for those who have failed more conservative approaches. It generally results in greater weight loss than conventional treatment and may lead to improvement in quality of life and obesity related disorders such as hypertension and diabetes. Unfortunately, surgical complications may occur and a poorly motivated patient may defeat the limitation of the size of their meals by continuing to ingest excess calories by increasing their daily meal frequency. The combination of approaches is best tailored to each individual patient.

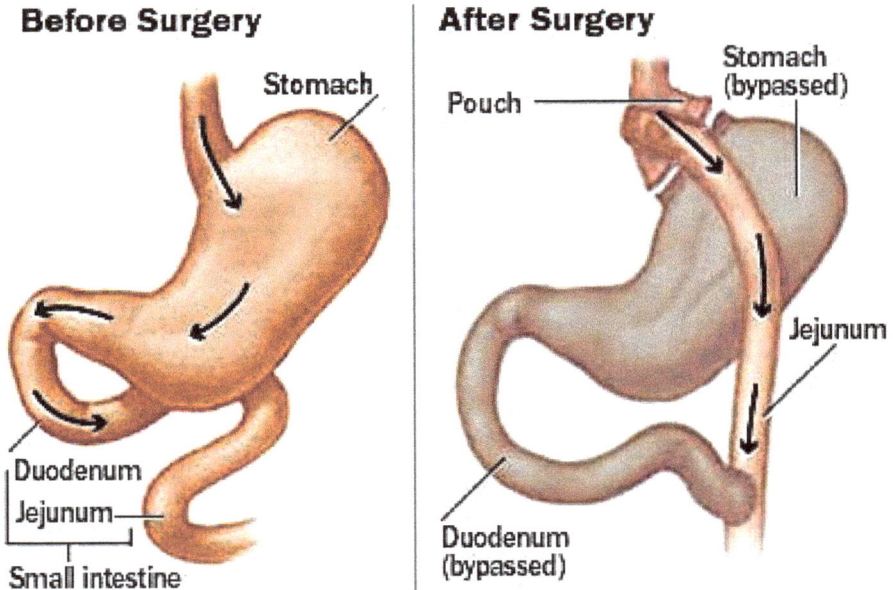

Before Surgery

Stomach

Duodenum
Jejunum
Small intestine

After Surgery

Pouch

Stomach
(bypassed)

Jejunum

Duodenum
(bypassed)

The surgery is usually undertaken to treat morbid obesity, defined as a body mass index greater than forty, when traditional dietary therapy has failed. Morbid obesity complications include type 2 diabetes, hypertension, and sleep apnea, and the rapid weight loss following surgery often results in improvement of these conditions a well. Although there are risks and complications with any surgery the benefits of weight loss can be very significant and each case must be individualized to every persons unique situation.

Graphic of a gastric bypass using a Roux-en-Y anastomosis. The transverse colon is not shown so that the Roux-en-Y can be clearly seen. The variant seen in this image is *retrocolic, retrogastric*, because the distal small bowel that joins the proximal segment of stomach is behind the transverse colon and stomach. Author: Courtesy of Ethicon Endosurgery, Inc.

Weight loss of sixty-five to eighty percent of excess body weight is common after surgery in the large series of gastric bypass operations reported. Hyperlipidemia and hypertension is corrected in over seventy percent of patients. Obstructive sleep apnea is markedly improved. Type 2 diabetes is reversed in up to ninety percent of patients. Gastroesophageal reflux disease is relieved in nearly all patients. Research publications show that overall there was an eighty-nine percent reduction in mortality over the five years following surgery in comparison to a matched group of patients treated without surgery. Surgical complications rate is approximately fifteen percent with a mortality rate of approximately zero point five percent.

With the volume the stomach can stretch reduced by approximately ninety percent when even a small amount of food is eaten it creates a feeling of fullness and satiety. For many people with morbid obesity the normal sensation of fullness and satiety does not stop compulsive overeating. After the gastric bypass surgery, they quickly learn that overeating results in nausea, vomiting and increasing discomfort. Post-operative gastric bypass patients also develop a lowered tolerance for alcoholic beverages, which are absorbed at a faster rate after surgery.

The reasons gastric bypass surgery works is multifactorial. It appears to be a combination of reduced caloric intake, behavioral changes to eating patterns and diet, and physiological changes related to the digestive process and the hormones that control appetite and satiety. More recent research suggests it leads to important changes in the gut microbiome. Human beings are creative and complex individuals and a number have managed to regain the weight loss accomplished after expensive and not without risk surgery. This often requires an excessive number of frequent small meals throughout the day. Research to elucidate the causes and approaches to obesity and eating disorders is an ongoing process.

Bean (Legume)

Beans are a legume native to the Americas that have a well-deserved reputation for contributing to intestinal gas production. The bean is rich in the sugars raffinose, verbascose, and stachyose. As humans do not produce the enzyme required for its degradation, alpha galactosidase, these sugars undergo fermentation by the gut flora.

"Beans, Beans, The Musical Fruit" is a schoolyard saying and children's song about the capacity for beans to contribute to flatulence.

Beans, beans, the musical fruit
The more you eat, the more you toot
The more you toot, the better you feel
So we have beans at every meal!

There are also several alternative versions, such as the one below:

Beans, beans, they're good for your heart
The more you eat, the more you fart
The more you fart, the happier/better you feel
So let's eat beans with every meal

The US Department of Agriculture is working on the development of a bean with lower levels of these sugars and so far the Anasazi bean has been the leading candidate, but no breakthrough yet. Thankfully there are alpha-galactosidase enzyme supplements that can provide relief. The enzyme is not heat stabile, so it will be inactivated with the heat of cooking. The enzyme should be added to the first bite of the beans consumed and if a large portion is ingested additional enzyme intake during the course of the bean meal is recommended.

An alternative approach is to soak the beans for several hours, leeching out some of the sugars into the water, which is discarded. The best approach is to soak the beans until they begin to germinate. With germination the bean itself begins to release alpha-galactosidase to break down its complex sugar content for the nutritional use of the newly germinated bean plant. With germination approximately eighty percent of the complex sugars are digested.

A legume is a plant in the family Fabaceae (or Leguminosae), grown agriculturally for their food grain seed, livestock forage and silage, and soil-enhancement. Most legumes harbor the symbiotic bacteria Rhizobia in their root nodules, which convert nitrogen in the atmosphere into ammonia and ammonium. This source of nitrogen contributes to the legumes production of amino acids and high protein content. Legumes include alfalfa, clover, peas, beans, lentils, lupins, soybeans, and peanuts and a number of trees and shrubs.

In farming crop rotation or growing legumes near non-legumes is common. Legumes are sometimes referred to as "green manure" because their symbiotic bacteria enrich the soil with nitrogenous products. A legume fruit is typically a pod that opens along a seam. They are an excellent source of protein but contain lower quantities of the essential amino acid methionine.

Beer (see Carbonation, Nitrogenation)

Belch (see Burp, Eructation)

Shutterstock/Catherine Lall

Bicarbonate Secretion

Sodium bicarbonate secretion is stimulated by the hormone secretin. Sodium bicarbonate is produced and released from the Brunner glands of the proximal duodenum as well as secreted by the pancreas. The pancreatic juices flow through the pancreatic duct, sphincter of Oddi, and ampulla of Vater into the second portion of the duodenum. The sodium bicarbonate neutralizes the acidic chyme, which has entered the duodenum from the stomach. When sodium bicarbonate interacts with and neutralizes acid, water results and carbon dioxide is released as a gas. The large quantity of carbon dioxide released when the gastric acid is neutralized in the duodenum by the addition of sodium bicarbonate may lead to temporary bloating and distension. As carbon dioxide easily diffuses across the cell lining of the small intestine, it is rapidly absorbed into the bloodstream and carried to the lungs where it is released from the bloodstream at the alveolus, and eliminated from the body by exhaling the carbon dioxide in the breath.

Baking soda and baking powder are both used to make dough rise with bubbles of carbon dioxide. Baking soda is pure alkaline sodium bicarbonate that when mixed with an acid releases CO_2 gas. That's why sodium bicarbonate is a long-standing treatment for 'acid or sour stomach' and indigestion as its alkaline nature neutralizes the stomach acid and generates carbon dioxide gas in the process.

Baking powder contains sodium bicarbonate and the acid cream of tartar, which will react when dissolved in water. A drying agent, normally a starch, is also in the mix to prevent moisture from starting the reaction prematurely. Baking powder is fine for baking but it would not be an effective antacid as it also contains acid that would consume all of the sodium bicarbonate's neutralizing capacity.

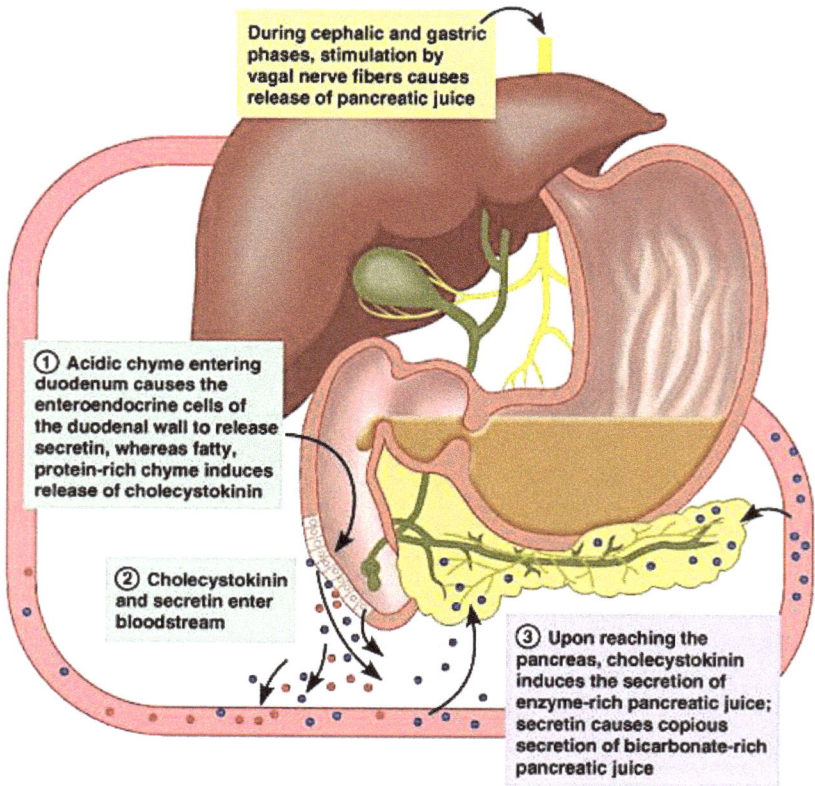

During cephalic and gastric phases, stimulation by vagal nerve fibers causes release of pancreatic juice

① Acidic chyme entering duodenum causes the enteroendocrine cells of the duodenal wall to release secretin, whereas fatty, protein-rich chyme induces release of cholecystokinin

② Cholecystokinin and secretin enter bloodstream

③ Upon reaching the pancreas, cholecystokinin induces the secretion of enzyme-rich pancreatic juice; secretin causes copious secretion of bicarbonate-rich pancreatic juice

Bifidobacteria (see Probiotic)

Bifidobacteria (previously called *Lactobacillus bifidus*) is a Gram-positive anaerobic symbiotic bacterium, which is commonly found in the gastrointestinal tract, vagina, and mouth. Some bifidobacteria have a long history of being used as probiotics. In 1899 Henry Tissier, a French pediatrician at the Pasteur Institute in Paris, identified dominant bacteria shaped like the letter Y in the bowels of healthy infants that he named Bifidobacterium. He recommended treating infants suffering from diarrhea with the bacteria. In 1907 Elie Metchnikoff at the Pasteur Institute proposed that lactic acid bacteria are beneficial to human health. He observed that the longevity of Bulgarian peasants was the result of their consumption of fermented milk products such as yogurt. He suggested that oral administration of healthful organisms would improve the intestinal microflora.

A number of Bifidobacterium strains are important probiotics and are used in the food industry. Beneficial effects may include regulation of intestinal microbiome, inhibition of pathogens, modulation of immune responses, repression of pro-carcinogenic activity, production of vitamins, and the bioconversion of dietary compounds into bioactive molecules.

Mother's milk contains high concentrations of lactose and lower quantities of phosphate a pH buffer. When bifidobacteria and other lactic acid bacteria in the infant's GI tract ferment the mother's breast milk, the pH is reduced making it more difficult for Gram-negative bacteria to grow. The genus Bifidobacterium possesses a unique fructose based pathway to ferment carbohydrates. The sensitivity of members of the genus Bifidobacterium to oxygen generally limits probiotic activity to anaerobic habitats.

Bismuth

Bismuth is a chemical element, number eighty-three on the periodic table, which has long history of being used in preparations designed to treat gastrointestinal complaints. It is a heavy metal with a low level of toxicity. Its various compounds have also been used historically to treat syphilis and the severe diarrhea from cholera. Bismuthinite is a mineral consisting of bismuth sulfide (Bi_2S_3) and is an important ore of bismuth.

Bismuth subgallate, with a chemical formula $C_7H_5BiO_6$, is the active ingredient in Devrom, an over the counter product described as an internal deodorizer. The term 'sub' refers to the high oxygen content in the molecule and the presence of bismuth oxygen compounds. It is used to reduce the fecal odor arising from flatulence and fecal incontinence. Those with gastric bypass bariatric surgery, inflammatory bowel disease, irritable bowel syndrome, and ostomy appliances commonly use it. It has also been used to treat *Helicobacter pylori* infection and is also used in wound therapy.

The mechanism by which bismuth works is uncertain. It may be related to its known antimicrobial activity, perhaps inhibiting the microbes that generate some of the more offensive gasses that contain sulfur as well as aromatic and volatile organic compounds. Bismuth also reacts directly with sulfur producing bismuth sulfide, a dark black insoluble compound. Bismuth sulfide may cause darkening or blackening of the tongue if sulfur is found in high concentrations in the saliva. It will also cause blackening of the stool as it binds with the sulfur that would otherwise give rise to hydrogen sulfide and other offensive sulfur gasses. The dark black color of the stool may be mistaken for melena, a sign of internal bleeding that results from the digestive process on blood cells and hemoglobin. The black coloration is not a health concern and is temporary, clearing with cessation of bismuth intake.

Bismuth subsalicylate has a bismuth oxide core structure with salicylate ions attached to its surface. It is used as an antidiarrheal and is the active ingredient in Pepto-Bismol, as well as the U.S. version of Kaopectate since it was reformulated in 2004. It is a popular remedy for indigestion, nausea, heartburn, and as a preventative for traveler's diarrhea. It is also used to treat some other gastrointestinal diseases and infections including the microorganism *Helicobacter pylori*, which is associated with peptic ulcer disease and stomach cancer.

Bismuth in crystalline form. Shutterstock/MiriamDoerr

The antimicrobial property may be as a result of an oligodynamic effect, where toxic small doses of heavy metal ions are toxic to microbes. Another antimicrobial effect may arise from the release of salicylic acid as the compound is hydrolyzed. It is believed that the salicylic acid acts as an antimicrobial for toxigenic *Escherichia coli,* a principal cause of traveler's diarrhea.

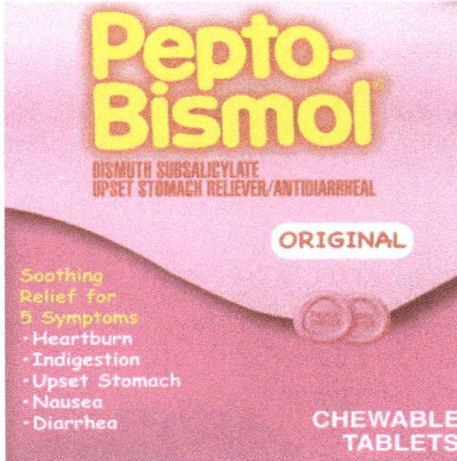

As a derivative of salicylic acid, bismuth subsalicylate also displays anti-inflammatory properties as well as some of the adverse effects of salicylates. Because salicylate levels can accumulate and lead to toxicity any use beyond a few weeks length is discouraged. Children should not take bismuth subsalicylate while suffering from a viral infection between of the associated risk of acquiring Reye's syndrome and liver failure. Nursing mothers should not use bismuth subsalicylate as it is excreted in breast milk and may pose a risk of Reye's syndrome in nursing children.

Bloat

Bloat is the common sensation that the abdomen is distended or overly full. There are many causes of bloating ranging from simple overeating and the normal production of intestinal gasses to abdominal ascites fluid buildup from an underlying tumor. Common causes of abdominal bloating include overeating, gastric distension, lactose intolerance, fructose intolerance and other food intolerances, food allergy, aerophagia (air swallowing), irritable bowel syndrome, partial or complete bowel obstruction, gastric dumping syndrome or rapid gastric emptying, gas producing foods, constipation, visceral fat and obesity.

Less common causes include splenic flexure syndrome, menstruation, dysmenorrhea, premenstrual syndrome, polycystic ovary syndrome and ovarian cysts, Alvarez' syndrome, intestinal parasites (e.g., *Ascaris lumbricoides*), diverticulosis, celiac disease, prescription medications such as phentermine, intra-abdominal tumors such as cancer of the ovary, liver, uterus, stomach, and colon.

Temporary bloating is common after gastrointestinal endoscopic procedures. Rarely a megacolon, which is an abnormal dilation of the colon, can be caused by ulcerative colitis or Chagas disease caused by the parasite *Trypanosoma cruzi*. After surgical repair of a hiatal hernia or treatment for gastro esophageal reflux with a procedure known as a Nissen fundoplication, the ability to burp and belch is restricted resulting in uncomfortable bloating and distension.

Common Foods that Cause Bloating/Gas:

- Cabbage
- Cauliflower
- Beans
- Oats
- Apples
- Milk
- Fluffy Wheat

- Broccoli
- Onions
- Corn
- Potatoes
- Pears
- Soft Cheese
- Peaches

A number of lifestyle and dietary factors can also affect the frequency and intensity of the sensation of bloating. Exercise stimulates the releases of hormones that encourage peristaltic activity in the bowels. In a similar fashion, caffeine containing beverages and food such as coffee, tea, cola, and chocolate also stimulate peristalsis and improve the transit time of food through the digestive tract. This gives the gut flora less time to ferment the material in the lumen of the bowel, with a resultant decrease in the total volume of gas produced by bacterial fermentation. Even a walk after a meal may help to move the contents along helping to ease the volume of gas produced. If nothing else, it at least allows you to release it outdoors!

Meals that are high in fat create the exact opposite effect, as fat causes the release of hormones and slows down gut motility. As the food spends more time in the digestive tract continued bacterial fermentation produces increasing quantities of gas. In addition, foods that are extremely hot or cold tend to be swallowed in smaller quantities resulting in more swallows being necessary to eat or drink the same volume at a moderate temperature. As each swallow contributes an additional quantity of air entering the esophagus and digestive tract, more swallows results in more air ingestion. Foods or snacks that require excess chewing with resultant excess swallowing of saliva, such as chewing or bubble gum, also contribute to excess air ingestion.

Certain types of vegetables and fruits contain sugars and starches, which may be poorly digested by people but happily fermented by bacteria comprising the gut flora. The most common food intolerance is lactose intolerance. The treatment is always directed at the underlying cause. Empiric trials of carminatives, probiotics, dietary restrictions, enzyme replacement therapy, simethicone etc. can be attempted. Alternative health approaches to treat bloating include acupuncture, homoeopathy and hypnosis. Sometimes the underlying bloat is not bloating from air but from the increased body fat of obesity. Now that is a real challenge, but the benefits of eliminating that bloat can be profoundly beneficial to health and longevity.

With the increasing popularity of surgery to correct hiatal hernia and reflux the gas bloat syndrome is occurring more frequently. This is a postoperative consequence of hiatal hernia repair, typically called a Nissen fundoplication. With the correction of the hiatal hernia and increasing tightness around the lower esophageal sphincter the ability to burp and belch is impaired. The inability to release swallowed air or gasses forming in the upper digestive tract can lead to bloating, distention, and discomfort. At times dilation of the lower esophageal sphincter can be performed as an outpatient to provide relief, or reoperation may be necessary if the gas bloat is intolerable.

Bariatric surgery is the term for the surgical treatment of morbid obesity, and gastric bypasses are one class of such operations. Gastric bypass surgery divides the stomach into a small upper pouch and a larger lower "remnant" pouch and then reconnects the small intestine to both. There are a variety of anatomical variations that have been developed, but all result in a marked reduction of the volume of food the stomach can receive during a meal. The surgery is usually undertaken to treat morbid obesity, defined as a body mass index greater than forty, when traditional dietary therapy has failed. Complications of morbid obesity include type 2 diabetes, hypertension, and sleep apnea, and the rapid weight loss following surgery often results in improvement of these conditions a well. Although there are risks and complications with any surgery the benefits of weight loss can be very significant and each case must be individualized to every persons unique situation.

Weight loss of sixty-five to eighty percent of excess body weight is common after bariatric surgery of the gastric bypass type operation. Hyperlipidemia and hypertension is corrected in over seventy percent of patients. Obstructive sleep apnea is markedly improved and Type 2 diabetes is reversed in up to ninety percent of patients. Gastroesophageal reflux disease is relieved in nearly all patients. Research publications show that overall there was an eighty-nine percent reduction in mortality over the five years following surgery in comparison to a matched group of patients treated without surgery. The surgical complications rate is approximately fifteen percent, with a mortality rate of approximately one-half of one percent.

Shutterstock/Zhoozha

With the volume the stomach can stretch reduced by approximately ninety percent when even a small amount of food is eaten it creates a feeling of fullness and satiety. For many people with morbid obesity the normal sensation of fullness and satiety does not stop compulsive overeating. After the gastric bypass surgery, they quickly learn that overeating results in nausea, vomiting, and increasing discomfort. Post-operative gastric bypass patients also develop a lowered tolerance for alcoholic beverages, which are absorbed at a faster rate after surgery.

The reasons gastric bypass surgery works is multifactorial. It appears to be a combination of reduced caloric intake, behavioral changes to eating patterns and diet, and physiological changes related to the digestive process and the hormones that control appetite and satiety. More recent research suggests it leads to important changes in the gut microbiome. Human beings are creative and complex individuals and a number have managed to regain the weight loss accomplished after expensive and not without risk surgery. This often requires an excessive number of frequent small meals throughout the day. Research to elucidate the causes and approaches to obesity and eating disorders is an ongoing process.

Bloat, Veterinary

Bloat, a critical veterinary medical condition also known as gastric dilatation volvulus occurs when the stomach becomes over distended by gas and cannot release it by eructation. It can also be a gastric torsion if the stomach is also twisted on its mesentery. The condition occurs in domesticated animals, especially ruminants and certain dog breeds. In dogs, gas accumulation in the stomach is usually associated with volvulus of the stomach, which prevents gas from escaping. In cattle eating in a young pasture of legumes such as alfalfa with the air bubbles becoming trapped in the rumen often causes bloating. Signs of bloat in cattle are abdominal distention, cessation of grazing, lethargy, and difficulty in urinating or defecating, and rapid breathing.

A stomach tube may be inserted to release the trapped air or a surgical incision into the flank to open the rumen and manually remove the froth and air may be required. Bloat is an emergency veterinary medical condition and has a high mortality even under professional care.

Borborygmus

borborygmus

Borborygmus (Greek βορβορυγμός borborygmós). The Greeks created this onomatopoetic word to imitate its sounds. In humans and animals peristaltic activity with the mixing, churning, and propulsion of chime, liquids, solids, and gasses can create intestinal noises audible to oneself and others nearby. The noises are described as rumbling, growling or gurgling and louder sounds may also occur with hunger. The actor Humphrey Bogart gives an Academy Award worthy demonstration of borborygmi in the 1951 movie *The African Queen*.

Bowel sounds are normally always audible with a stethoscope over a brief period of time. Partial obstruction of the intestines may also contribute to more borborygmi; the audible bowel sounds that can be heard by the unaided ear. When listening with a stethoscope the bowel sounds in early obstruction are often hyperactive, and become quiescent and diminished with longer standing obstruction. The absence of bowel sounds is frequently noted for a few hours after anesthesia, but can also be a sign of serious bowel injury or obstruction. It is common after anesthesia that eating or drinking is not allowed until the bowel sounds have returned, and the individual begins to pass gas proving that the bowels have resumed their normal motility and movement.

The word borborygmus is a type of word called an onomatopoeia. Onomatopoeia. Comes from the Greek word ὀνοματοποιία ὄνομα for "name" and ποιέω for "I make". Although its origin describes a word that literally means making up a name, in the English language it is defined as a word that imitates or phonetically reproduces the sound that it is defining. A more accurate word would be echo mimetic, from the Greek words from Ηχώ meaning "echo or sound" and μιμητικό meaning "mimetic or imitation". Common onomatopoeias are echomimetc words that reproduce animal sounds such as "oink", "meow", "roar" or "chirp". Onomatopoeias vary with languages, for example the sound of a clock may be described as tick tock in English, dī dā in Mandarin Chinese or katchin katchin in Japanese.

In the case of a frog, the variation of echo mimetic onomatopoeia is not due to the frogs speaking foreign languages but because different species of frogs make different sounds. Ancient Greece marsh frogs went brekekekex koax koax (as in Aristophanes' comic play The Frogs), English ribbit for species of the American pond frog said ribbit, ribbit, and the common English frog went "croak".

Bowel Movement (Defecation, BM)

Defecation, a bowel movement or often named for its abbreviated initials BM, is the elimination of fecal waste material from the digestive tract via the anus. The stimulus to defecate is the distention of the rectum or sigmoid colon with feces. This reflex can be triggered by manual stimulation of the rectal wall stretch receptors. Voluntary control of defecation is part of the toilet training process and is typically mastered during childhood. This control can be lost again with neurological, psychological or senescent changes. The involuntary release of feces is known as fecal incontinence, often called encopresis in children.

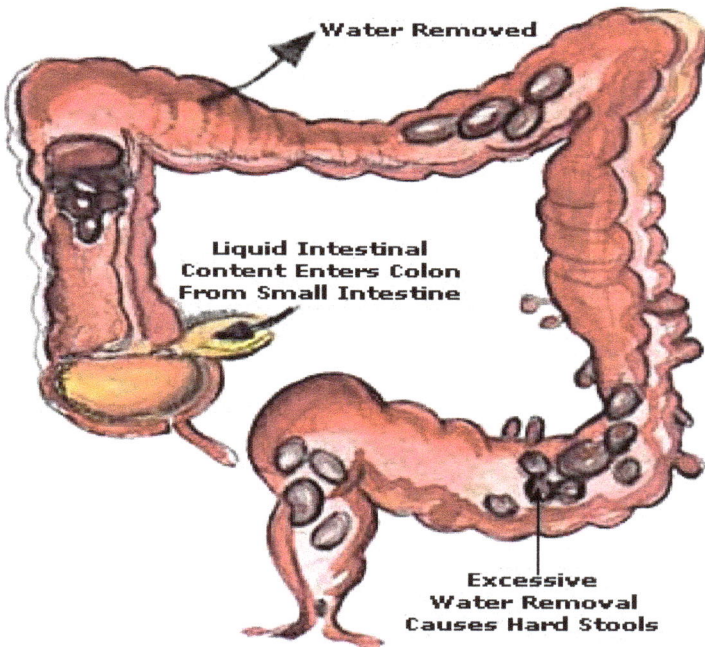

Water Removed

Liquid Intestinal Content Enters Colon From Small Intestine

Excessive Water Removal Causes Hard Stools

Creative Commons License

Defecation is a complex reflex coordination of neuromuscular activity that relaxes the puborectalis muscle straightening the normally ninety-degree anorectal angle and initiates the relaxation of the internal anal sphincters. There is a strong urge to defecate but the external anal sphincter contracts to prevent defecation until voluntarily released to initiate the process. Colonic contractions, along with increased intra-abdominal pressure by performance of the Valsalva maneuver (attempting to exhale against a closed epiglottis), then push the fecal material out of the rectum via the anus.

The frequency range of normal bowel movements is variable and can range from two bowel movements per day to once per week, often dependent on diet. The squatting position is most conducive to defecation. Using Western style sitting toilets, as opposed to squat toilets found in non-Western locales, can be problematic especially if the feet cannot reach the ground, as in young children. An elevated footrest to allow the thighs and legs to be flexed can greatly assist in the ease of elimination for both children and adults.

The puborectalis sling forming the anorectal angle is responsible for gross continence of solid stool. The internal anal sphincter is an involuntary muscle that contributes about fifty-five percent of the resting anal pressure. Together with the hemorrhoid vascular cushions, the internal anal sphincter maintains continence of flatus and liquid during rest.

SITTING POSTURE

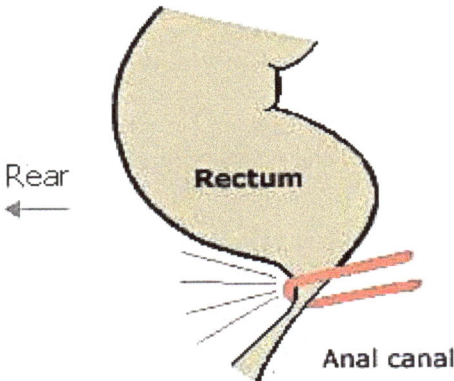

Rear

Rectum

Anal canal

Puborectalis muscle "chokes" rectum to maintain continence

SQUATTING POSTURE

Rectum

Puborectalis muscle relaxes and straightens pathway to anus

www.jcrows.com Creative Commons License

The external anal sphincter is a voluntary muscle, doubling the pressure in the anal canal during contraction. The rectoanal inhibitory reflex is an involuntary internal anal sphincter relaxation in response to rectal distention. This allows a sampling of some of the rectal contents to descend into the anal canal. Here it is brought into contact with specialized sensory mucosa to detect consistency. The rectoanal excitatory reflex is an initial semi-voluntary contraction of the external anal sphincter and puborectalis, which returns tone following the rectoanal inhibitory reflex.

Other factors include the specialized anti-peristaltic function of the last part of the sigmoid colon, the sensory ability of the lining of the rectum and the anal canal to detect the consistency and quantity of stool when present, and the normal rectoanal reflexes and defecation cycle that completes evacuation. Humans can defecate in a number of different postures. The two most common are the squatting posture and the sitting posture. The squatting posture is used for squat toilets and is also commonly used for defecation in the absence of toilets or other devices. It is commonly used in non-Western cultures. The sitting defecation posture is used in Western toilets with either a leaning forward posture or a ninety-degree sitting upright posture. The posture chosen appears to be largely a cultural decision although there is evidence that the squatting posture is more efficacious and induces the least bodily strain.

The sitting position can cause the defecating human being to repeat the Valsalva maneuver (see page 432) many times and with great force. This can lead to diverticulosis, hemorrhoids, hernias, and cardiovascular stress with defecation syncope. For those with underlying cardiac disease the additional stress induced by defecating in the sitting position as opposed to the more natural squatting position may be surprisingly life threatening. The magnitude of straining during sitting defecation is at least three times greater than with the squatting posture. Difficulty with the seated position is particularly true if the feet cannot reach the floor, as is commonly seen when small children are placed on adult height toilets. The adults may become frustrated that it is taking the child so long to defecate, not realizing that without being able to brace their feet and apply resistance that an individual is unable to generate the intra-abdominal pressure needed to promote defecation.

The affectionate term 'potty' is often used with children especially during toilet training. The term potty is also used to describe the child-size chamber pot type toilets that are at the appropriate height with a child-size seat. When a child sits on an adult-size toilet seat they may have a genuine fear of falling in, which can inhibit having a bowel movement. Regular adult toilets, which have an opening that is normally too large and frightening for a child, may be used if a child seat adapter is provided. To put in perspective that their fear is not unjustified American adults suffer forty thousand toilet related injuries per year. Falling off a toilet directly contributed to the death of King George II of Great Britain. Because the height of the adult toilet does not allow their feet to touch the ground, a foot stool can be a great help. This gives their feet a place to rest and to assume the squatting posture. This eases the initiation of a bowel movement and can accelerate toilet training.

Bowel Sound

Bowel sounds, also known as abdominal sounds, if audible at a distance by the unaided ear are known by the onomatopoeia borborygmi. Onomatopoeia is a word created to imitate the sound it is meant to describe. Bowel sounds may also have a bubbling, gurgling, rushing fluid sound and are generated by the peristaltic movement of the contents along the gastrointestinal tract.

Most bowel sounds are usually audible only by placing the listening ear on the abdominal wall or with the aid of a stethoscope. The presence of bowel sounds indicates that peristaltic activity is occurring. Changes in the bowel sounds, such as hyperactivity or absence may be indicative of a gastrointestinal disorder such as bowel obstruction or ileus. The return of bowel sounds after anesthesia are commonly required before food or drink is reintroduced.

Brain Fart

Brain fart is the popular phrase for a mental lapse, which usually results in an error while doing a repetitive activity. The actual physiological event that triggers the error has been recorded on brain scans by scientists approximately thirty seconds before the event was observed by the patient. The scientists suspect that the brain is trying to enter a more restful state to conserve energy, and have given the brain fart the more scientific name of 'maladaptive brain activity changes'. The findings were published in the *Proceedings of the National Academy of Sciences* in April 2008. Brain fart may also be used to describe a brief episode of absent-mindedness, impulsivity, or temporary inability to recall a name, word, or memory. Interestingly enough, the exact opposite of a brain fart is best described by an unusual word in the English Language, afflatus.

Oops...Brain Fart
www.flickr.com/photos/ Creative Commons License

Afflatus incorporates the root word flatus, which is a commonly used as a synonym for fart. Perhaps surprisingly the definition of the word afflatus has nothing to do with a fart. Flatus is Latin for a blowing, breathing, or a wind. Afflatus is first used by Cicero in his volume *De Natura Deorum (The Nature of the Gods)*. In his book, it is used as a phrase for a sudden rush of unexpected breath or fresh inspiration. The word inspiration is derived from the term inspire, to breath as well as to have a creative thought or new idea. Afflatus thus can mean a divine inspiration. The only way to properly associate the word afflatus with a fart is to consider it to be the exact opposite of a brain fart.

CRANIAL FLATULENCE

Bubble (see Nitrogenation, Surface Tension, Simethicone)

A bubble is a collection of gas, usually surrounded by a thin layer of fluid. The term gastric bubble is also used to describe the normal collection of gas within the stomach, and can be visualized on an abdominal radiograph (x-ray). Bubbles of gas within the digestive tract are called a burp or belch on eructation via the esophagus, or a fart or flatus on being passed out of the lower intestinal. The actual physical properties of a bubble are due to a physical property known as surface tension. This is also visually demonstrated in watching a water glider walk across water, in water forming droplets, the tears of wine in a wineglass, the water bulging without spilling above the brim of a glass, and other physical phenomena. Please see the entry on surface tension for more details.

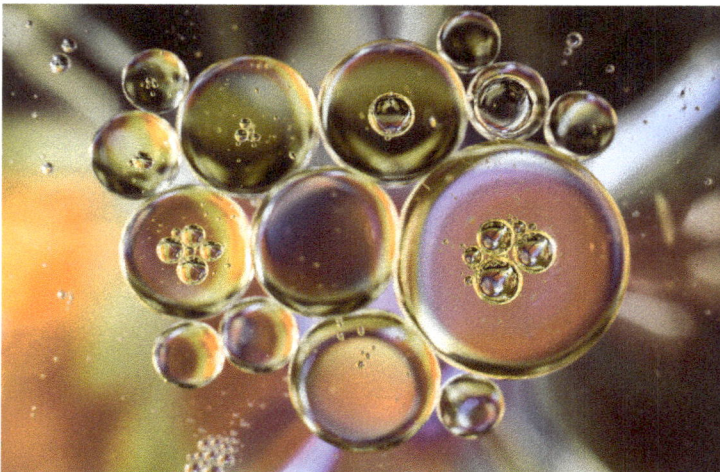

Bubbles created by surface tension. Shutterstock/GiulianoDelMoretto

Bubble. Brocken Inaglory editing user:Alvesgaspar Creative Commons License

Tears of wine, also known as Marangoni effect. Shutterstock/mountainpix

Burp / Belch (see Eructation, Gastroesophageal Reflux Disease)

The words burp and belch are the common terms used to describe the more scientific term eructation. Please see the entry on eructation as well as Gastroesophageal Reflux Disease (GERD) for more details about this common physiological event that. Other interesting word pairs of the common words with the less commonly known scientific terminology include chew for mastication, sneeze for sternutation, cough for tusis, pee for micturition, itch for pruritis, skin for integument, smell for olfaction, taste for gustation, and many others that fill a medical dictionary. When the medical rather than the common terms are used by the health care provider, proper communication may require a dictionary to translate the foreign language of medicine.

If a doctor wanted to know if you chewed your food well he might ask if you masticated a lot with every meal. Most people would respond incredulously "Masticate a lot with every meal? Are you crazy, do you think I want to go blind. I never masticate!". Medicine and English are virtually two separate and foreign languages. You need to insist that your doctor speak to you in a language you can understand. There is a famous quotation attributed to Sir Winston Churchill, a British statesmen, former Prime Minister, and Nobel Laureate for Literature. He said affectionately that the American and British people are divided only by a common language.

Loudest burp at 109.9 decibels youtu.be/Zt9rvaijpPY

The World Burping Federation located in Geneva Switzerland holds the annual World Burping Championship. The *Guinness Book of World Records* has a listing for the loudest burp on record. The record holder is Paul Hunn of the United Kingdom. His burp achieved a measurement of just under one-hundred and ten decibels, equivalent to a car horn. The world record for the longest burp is over eighteen seconds, held by Tim Janus. To achieve this record, he consumed approximately two gallons of Diet Coke and Mountain Dew. Imagine what would have happened if he swallowed a few Mentos tablets at the time of the competition (see photograph on page 33).

Butt Breathe

To butt breathe is a common term used to describe the ability to air fart. An air fart is the ability to control the anus and muscles of abdomen and respiration, to cause air to be aspirated into the colon and then released voluntarily as a fart. It is also known in more enlightened society as an air enema. The air enema has been practiced for hundreds of generations as an advanced yoga practice and as a means of achieving colonic hygiene.

Although usually considered under involuntary control, these muscles can be trained. Yogis have attained remarkable proficiency at controlling what has previously been considered involuntary muscles. At the turn of the twentieth century, the performer Joseph Pujol, under the stage name Le Pétomane, became an international sensation by demonstrating his prowess at butt breathing. This ability is not limited to trained yogi and stage performers. An internet-based survey on farting performed in 2001, had over one thousand three hundred participants. Although not a scientifically validated survey, over fifteen percent of respondents reported that they were able to fart on command.

Fart survey question for men: Can you fart on command also called "Butt Breathe"?

Only fifteen percent of the men surveyed can fart voluntarily by suctioning air into the colon. One-third of all men did not even know that this is possible!

Fart survey question for women: Can you fart on command also called "Butt Breathe"?

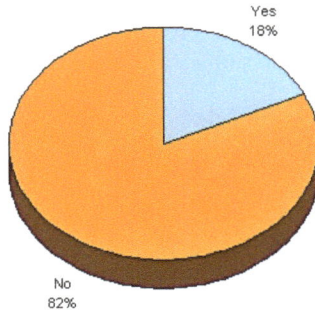

Only eighteen percent of the women surveyed can fart voluntarily by suctioning air into the colon.

Although rarely thought of as a form of butt breathe, the rare freshwater Fitzroy river turtle, *Rheodytes leukops*, found in Queensland, Australia has a unique ability. This species of turtle can breathe through its anus equivalent, the cloaca. It inspires air or, if submerged, oxygenated water into its cloaca. Through specialized highly vascular bursae it can absorb oxygen into its bloodstream. The Fitzroy turtle can obtain over two-thirds of its oxygen supply through the cloacal bursae. It pumps water in and out of the cloaca up to sixty times per minute.

Some turtles have a remarkable anaerobic capacity and can be without oxygen for up to thirty–three hours and survive. Although they are usually air breathing, they can also breathe underwater with the cloacal bursae acting like the equivalent of gills in removing oxygen from the water. This rare ability is shared with only a few other organisms, including the dragonfly nymph and the sea cucumber.

Photo by Craig Latta, freshwater turtle expert. www.tutles.net.au Used with permission.

The sea cucumber has a few other unique digestive tract features. Its anus serves as a defense mechanism and can eject sticky threads that entangle an enemy. If in danger it will expel its entire digestive and respiratory tracks that are also sticky and can ensnarl the enemy. These disgorged internal organs continue to move about independently, distracting the predator while the sea cucumber makes its escape. It then regenerates brand new respiratory and digestive tracks.

Shutterstock/C.K.Ma

Carbohydrate

A carbohydrate is an organic compound of carbon, hydrogen, and oxygen. The term is synonymous with saccharide (Greek σάκχαρον (sákkharon) "sugar". The carbohydrates are divided into monosaccharides, disaccharides, oligosaccharides, and polysaccharides. The smaller monosaccharides and disaccharides are commonly referred to as sugars ending with the suffix -ose, such as the monosaccharide glucose, the disaccharides sucrose and lactose.

Simple carbohydrates are found in foods such as fruits, milk, and vegetables

Cake, candy, and other refined sugar products are simple sugars which also provide energy but lack vitamins, minerals, and fiber

Complex carbohydrates provide vitamins, minerals, and fiber

Foods such as breads, legumes, rice, pasta, and starchy vegetables contain complex carbohydrates

Polysaccharides store linked chains of the simple sugars in the form of glycogen or starch, or as structural components such as cellulose in plants and chitin in arthropods. The monosaccharide ribose is important in coenzymes, and in the molecules of RNA and DNA dealing with protein synthesis and genetics.

Carbohydrates. www.articlesweb.org Used with permission

Monosaccharides such as glucose are the major source of fuel for metabolism. The two joined monosaccharides of a disaccharide can be released by specific enzymes such as sucrase for sucrose and lactase for lactose. Foods high in carbohydrates include fruits, breads, pastas, beans, potatoes, bran, rice, and cereals. Carbohydrates are not essential for humans as the body can obtain all its energy from protein and fats. The brain and neurons generally use glucose or ketones as an energy source.

Monosaccharides

Monosaccharides (Greek monos-single, sacchar-sugar) are simple sugar carbohydrates that are water-soluble crystalline solids, a number of which have a sweet taste. Examples include glucose (dextrose), fructose (levulose), galactose, xylose, and ribose. Monosaccharides are the building blocks of disaccharides (such as sucrose) and polysaccharides (such as cellulose and starch). Monosaccharides can be classified by the number x of carbon atoms they contain: diose (2) triose (3) tetrose (4), pentose (5), hexose (6), heptose (7), and so on. The most important monosaccharide, glucose, is a hexose.

There are a number of isomeric forms all with the same chemical formula. Most stereoisomers are chiral and therefore distinct from their mirror images. Those that rotate the direction of linearly polarized light to the right are called D dextrorotatory (rotates the polarization axis clockwise) and to the left called L is levorotatory (rotates it counterclockwise) or sys for sinister.

The Latin words dexter means right sided and laevus means on the left. Another Latin word sinister, also means on the left-hand side and in ancient times left handedness was considered a sinister (negative) characteristic. Mirror-image isomers usually have very different biochemical properties and occurrences in nature.

Disaccharides

Digestible Disaccharides in Food

Sucrose
(Glucose-fructose)

Lactose
(Galactose-glucose)

Maltose
(Glucose-glucose)

A disaccharide is the carbohydrate formed when two monosaccharides undergo a dehydration reaction and a molecule of water is removed and a glycosidic bond is formed. Like monosaccharides, disaccharides form an aqueous solution when dissolved in water. Three common examples are sucrose, lactose, and maltose. 'Disaccharide' is one of the four chemical groupings of carbohydrates (monosaccharide, disaccharide, oligosaccharide, and polysaccharide). Depending on the monosaccharide components a disaccharide may be crystalline, water-soluble, sweet and/or sticky.

Disaccharide
Sucrose: Glucose & Fructose
Lactulose: Galactose & Fructose
Lactose: Galactose & Glucose
Maltose: Glucose & Glucose, maltose is a hydrolysis product from starch
Trehalose: Glucose & Glucose
Cellobiose: Glucose & Glucose, cellobiose is a hydrolysis product of cellulose

Oligosaccharide

All carbohydrates consist of the following molecules:

Mono-saccharide
contains one saccharide molecule

Di-saccharide
contains two saccharide molecules

Poly-saccharide
contains many saccharide molecules

Oligosaccharides are carbohydrates composed of between two and ten monosaccharides joined by glycosidic linkage which can be hydrolyzed by acid to release the monosaccharide units. Some examples include maltose, sucrose, and lactose. An oligosaccharide (Greek oligos -few, and sacchar -sugar) is a saccharide containing two to ten monosaccharides. Oligosaccharides are a frequent component of glycoproteins and glycolipids and are often used as chemical markers for cell recognition. An example is ABO blood type markers where the A and B blood types have two different oligosaccharide glycolipids in the cell membranes of the red blood cells, the AB-type blood has both, while the O blood type has neither.

Fructo-oligosaccharides are also found in many vegetables and consist of short chains of fructose molecules. Naturally occurring galacto-oligosaccharides consist of short chains of galactose molecules. These compounds can only be partially digested by humans with microbial fermentation processing the residue. Mannan oligosaccharides are used in animal feed to improve digestive health, energy levels and performance. They differ from other oligosaccharides in that they are not fermentable. Other undigested oligosaccharides are fermented by the intestinal microflora and depending on the type of oligosaccharide, different microbial groups may be stimulated or suppressed. Clinical studies have shown that administering fructo-oligosaccharides, galacto-oligosaccharides, or inulin enhances the populations of symbiotic microorganisms and suppresses the populations of pathogens.

Fructo-oligosaccharides and inulin are found naturally in Jerusalem artichoke, burdock, chicory, leeks, onions, and asparagus. Fructo-oligosaccharides products derived from chicory root contain significant amounts of the polysaccharide inulin, a fiber frequently found in fruits, vegetables and other plants. Fructo-oligosaccharides can also be commercially synthesized by enzymes of the fungus *Aspergillus niger* acting on sucrose. Galacto-oligosaccharides is naturally found in soybeans and can also be synthesized from lactose. Fructo-oligosaccharides, galacto-oligosaccharides, and the polysaccharide inulin are commercially available as nutritional supplements in capsules, tablets, and as a powder.

Besides being components of glycoproteins or glycolipids some oligosaccharides, such as the raffinose family, act as storage or transport carbohydrates. Other oligosaccharides such as maltodextrins or cellodextrins, are the result of the microbial breakdown of larger polysaccharides such as starch or cellulose. Carrots can be an excellent source of oligosaccharides but this occurs only after they have been cooked for an hour as the starches need to be broken down into the shorter chains needed for bioavailability.

Polysaccharides

Monosaccharide - fruits, vegebtables, honey, nuts

Disaccharide- sugars, milk

Polysaccharides- (starchy foods) rice, potatoes, corn, wheat

Polysaccharides are polymers containing ten or more monosaccharide residues. Two common examples are cellulose the main component of the cell wall in plants, and starch, a word derived from the Anglo-Saxon stercan, meaning to stiffen. For a polysaccharide composed of a single type of monosaccharide the ending "-ose" of the monosaccharide is replaced with "-an". For example, a polymer of glucose is named glucan, a polymer of mannose is named mannan, and a polymer of galactose is named galactan. Inulin has the capacity for a much higher degree of polymerization than fructo-oligosaccharides and is categorized as a polysaccharide. It is frequently found in fruits and vegetables and is a significant source of nutrition worldwide.

Polysaccharides are sources of energy for organisms that can convert starches into glucose, however most cannot metabolize cellulose. Ruminants and termites use bacteria and protist to process cellulose. Although not digestible, dietary fiber plays a major role in digestive health by acting as a prebiotic for the gut microbiome.

Carbohydrate Digestion

The digestion of carbohydrates, which are broken down into monosaccharides like glucose, begins in the mouth with the enzyme amylase found in saliva. The pancreatic enzymes and brush border enzymes of the small intestine continue the breakdown of the various carbohydrates into monosaccharides in the lumen of the bowel. These enzymes include lactase, maltase, sucrase, dextrinase and glucoamylase. The monosaccharides are then absorbed across the mucosal surface by intestinal epithelial cell facilitated cotransport with sodium ions and facilitated diffusion. They enter the capillary bed of the villi and are then transported to the liver via the hepatic portal vein.

	Carbohydrate digestion		Protein digestion	Nucleic acid digestion	Fat digestion
	Polysaccharides	Disaccharides			
Oral cavity, pharynx, esophagus	Salivary amylase ↓ Smaller polysaccharides, maltose				
Stomach			Proteins → Pepsin → Small polypeptides		
Lumen of small intestine	Polysaccharides → Pancreatic amylases → Maltose and other disaccharides		Polypeptides → Pancreatic trypsin and chymotrypsin → Smaller polypeptides → Pancreatic carboxypeptidase → Amino acids	DNA, RNA → Pancreatic nucleases → Nucleotides	Fat globules → Bile salts → Fat droplets → Pancreatic lipase → Glycerol, fatty acids, glycerides
Epithelium of small intestine (brush border)	Disaccharidases ↓ Monosaccharides		Small peptides → Dipeptidases, carboxypeptidase, and aminopeptidase → Amino acids	Nucleotidases → Nucleosides → Nucleosidases and phosphatases → Nitrogenous bases, sugars, phosphates	

Mouth	**Dietary carbohydrates**
	↓ Salivary α-amylase
	Polysaccharides, dextrins, sucrose, lactose, maltose
Stomach	↓
Small intestine	↓ Pancreatic α-amylase
	Monosaccharides: glucose, galactose, fructose
	↓ Active transport
Intestinal lining	**Monosaccharides in blood stream**

Carbohydrates

1 Some starch is broken down to maltose in the mouth by salivary amylase.

2 Salivary amylase is inactivated by strong acid in the stomach.

3 Pancreatic amylase breaks down starch into maltose in the small intestine.

4 Enzymes in the wall of the small intestine break down the disaccharides sucrose, lactose, and maltose into monosaccharides glucose, fructose, and galactose.

5 Glucose, fructose, and galactose are absorbed into blood to be taken to the liver by a portal vein.

6 Some soluble fiber is fermented into various acids and gases by bacteria in the large intestine.

7 Insoluble fiber escapes digestion and is excreted in feces, but little other dietary carbohydrate is present.

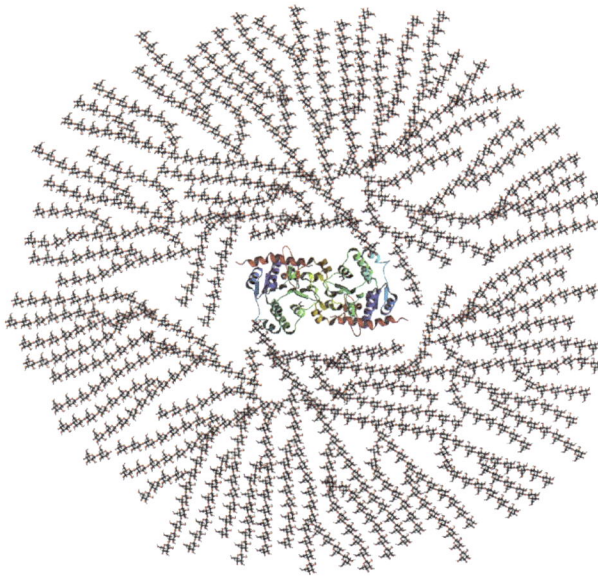

2-D cross-sectional view of glycogen: A core protein of glycogenin is surrounded by branches of glucose units. The entire globular complex may contain approximately thirty thousand glucose units. 2009 Author: Mikael Häggström Public Domain

Glucose metabolism

Intake:

Starch

Glycogen

Disaccharides

Monosaccharides
(glucose, fructose,
galactose)

Storage:
Glycogen

Distribution
and
utilization:
Free glucose

Glycogen is a polysaccharide of glucose that serves as a major form of energy storage in humans, animals, and fungi. This polysaccharide structure is the most important storage form of glucose in the body. In humans the liver and muscle are the main locations in which glycogen is made and stored. It functions as the secondary form of long-term energy storage. The primary form of energy stores are the fats held in adipose tissue. Muscle glycogen can be converted into glucose for use by the muscle cells. Liver glycogen can be converted to glucose for use throughout the body including the central nervous system.

Glycogen serves a function similar to the starch of plants. The glycogen polymer is much more extensively branched than starch allowing it to store energy in a more compact form. Glycogen is found in the form of granules in the cytoplasm of many cell types and forms an energy reserve that can be quickly mobilized to meet a sudden need for glucose. After a meal up to eight percent of the total weight of the liver cells may be composed of glycogen stores. The glycogen stored in the liver is accessible as an energy source to other organs, and for most organs is its only source of energy. An exception is muscle, which has its own limited stores of glycogen found in a lower concentration of one to two percent of the muscle mass. The muscle tissue of the uterus also stores glycogen during pregnancy to nourish the embryo.

During a meal containing carbohydrates, as the food is eaten and digested, the blood glucose levels rise. In response to the rising blood glucose levels the pancreas secretes insulin. Blood glucose from the portal vein enters the liver cells called hepatocytes. Insulin acts on the liver cells to stimulate the action of several enzymes including the key enzyme in glycogen production, glycogen synthetase. Under the influence of glycogen synthetase glucose molecules are continuously added to the chains of glycogen for storage as long as both insulin and glucose remain plentiful. In the postprandial (after meal) or fed state the liver takes in more glucose from the blood than it releases and stores the excess as glycogen.

Once a meal has been fully digested and absorbed the glucose levels begin to fall back to normal. With blood glucose returning to normal the insulin secretion is reduced and glycogen synthesis stops. When energy is required the stored glycogen is broken down and converted back to glucose. The glucose is released into the blood stream for the energy needs of other organs and cells. Glycogen phosphorylase is the primary enzyme of glycogen breakdown. For the next eight to twelve hours, glucose derived from liver glycogen is the primary source of blood glucose used by the rest of the body for fuel.

Glucagon is another hormone involved in glucose metabolism and is also produced by the pancreas. It serves as an opposite and balancing hormone to insulin. When blood levels of glucose begin to fall below the normal range the pancreas secretes glucagon in increasing amounts. Glucagon stimulates both glycogenolysis (the breakdown of glycogen), as well as gluconeogenesis (the generation of glucose from non-carbohydrates such as fatty acids). The glycogen stored in muscle cells functions as an immediate reserve source of available glucose. Muscle cells lack the enzyme glucose-6-phosphatase which is required to release glucose into the blood. As such the glycogen they store is only available for internal use by the muscle cells themselves, and cannot be shared with other cells.

Carbonation (see Nitrogenation)

Carbonated beverages are very popular worldwide. In the United States sales of carbonated beverages exceed twenty billion dollars per year, four times the sales volume of dairy products. The majority consumed today already comes carbonated with large amounts of carbon dioxide forced into solution under high pressure. As the pressure seal of the can or bottle is released the carbon dioxide forms bubbles and comes out of the solution, giving a pleasant tickling sensation on the palate, and a full at times bloated feeling in the stomach and gut.

Many soft drinks have high concentrations of simple carbohydrates such as glucose, fructose, and sucrose. Oral bacteria ferment these carbohydrates and produce acidic products, which can erode the tooth enamel beginning the dental decay process. A large number of soft drinks are already acidic and have phosphoric acid added in the manufacturing process bringing their pH level to three or lower. To put this value in perspective, neutral water has a pH of seven and gastric hydrochloric acid has a pH of two. Many dentists advocate that one should avoid the brushing of teeth shortly after an acidic beverage because the tooth enamel is more vulnerable to abrasions after being softened by acid.

Shutterstock/Radu Bercan

*Air*Veda: Ancient & New Medical Wisdom

Mineral water cures were very popular in the middle ages and beyond. Going to the source of mineral springs and the drinking of its contents was referred to as 'taking the waters'. The waters had a variety of mineral content depending on source locale and included various salts and sulfur contents. The sites of such resources became well known as spas, baths, and wells and developed into destinations for the ill and infirm, as well as those who wished to preserve their good health. The term Seltzer water was originally a trademarked name for the German town of Selter that had a famous mineral spring.

The bottling of mineral waters became a profitable enterprise by offering people the opportunity to partake of the presumed beneficial waters in their own locales. An attempt to imitate the effervescent effect of the mineral waters was made by Joseph Priestley in 1767. Some fans of carbonated beverages believe this should be his claim to fame rather than his discovery of oxygen. J. J. Schweppes of Switzerland commercialized the process in 1783, moving his factory and enterprise to England in 1783.

Before the commercial availability of already carbonated beverages, a device for home use was popular and remains commercially available. It uses canisters of carbon dioxide under pressure that are then added to and dissolved in the beverages to create the carbonation effect. The soda siphon bottles with the carbon dioxide cartridges are making a retro look comeback in today's higher technology environment. Carbon dioxide can diffuse through the plastic container over time, which is why carbonated beverages in plastic bottles go flat and lose their carbonation over a few month's time. Glass and aluminum containers hold the carbonation for longer time periods.

Have you ever wondered how much carbon dioxide gas is released from a soft drink or carbonated beverage? You have already gotten a visual demonstration if the bottle or can was dropped or shaken before being opened. This agitation accelerates the release of the carbon dioxide, and it can form a jet stream of gassy bubbles to be sprayed on everyone within a dozen feet of the demonstration. This social activity is very popular amongst preadolescent boys. The quantification of how much carbon dioxide is in a one-liter bottle of a carbonated soft drink is calculated using a formula known as Henry's Law.

William Henry was an English physician and chemist who proposed what is now called Henry's law in 1803. The law states that at a constant temperature, the amount of a given gas dissolved in a liquid is directly proportional to the pressure of that gas. As the gas pressure increases, the solubility of the gas in the liquid increases. As the temperature increases, the solubility of gas in liquid decreases. The greater the pressure, the greater the quantity of a gas that can be absorbed by a liquid. Henry's Law explains why carbon dioxide in a pressurized container, such as in a can or bottle of a carbonated beverage remains in solution until it is opened. As soon as the container is opened the pressure is reduced causing the carbon dioxide gas to lose its solubility and escape in the form of bubbles or fizz.

The gas content in a one-liter bottle is a surprising two point eight liters. In other words, there is nearly three times the volume of the original container in excess gas under pressure hidden in those tiny bubbles. Do not forget another important law of the physics of gasses, Charles' Law. This law defines the activity of gasses expanding as the temperature increases. The cooler the liquid, the greater the amount of gas that it can absorb. As the temperature of liquid increases, the solubility of the gas decreases forming bubbles that allow it to escape. If you drink a cold carbonated beverage, and after swallowing it is warmed up to body temperature, it will exhibit another substantial increase in the volume of gasses released. The burping and belching that occurs after drinking a cold carbonated beverage may seem out of proportion to the small amount consumed. Just remember that whatever the volume of liquid carbonated beverage swallowed, there is nearly three times that volume of dissolved gas waiting to be released.

CO_2 pressure released

CO_2 under pressure

CO_2 bubbles out of solution

CO_2 dissolved in solution

Creative Commons License

If you want further visual proof that Henry's Law is accurate take a look at the photographic evidence of another popular activity. The addition of a Mentos brand mint candy tablet to a liter bottle of a carbonated beverage, such as Diet Coke, sounds like such an innocent activity. This demonstration is repeated in countless elementary school science classes. The *Guinness Book of World Records* described one thousand three hundred and sixty students in the historic university town of Leuven, Belgium creating simultaneous Mentos with Diet Coke geysers.

The instantaneous foaming effect is a dramatic virtual geyser of carbonated foam shooting over twenty-eight feet into the air. This experiment is not without risk as the bottles will explode if not allowed to become a geyser. Scientific progress continues apace and Henry's Law was demonstrated with two thousand eight hundred and sixty-five simultaneous geysers demonstrated before a large crowd in a mall in Manila, Philippines, breaking the previous world record.

Mentos Geyser from carbonated beverages with the addition of Mentos. From left: carbonated water (Perrier), Classic Coke, Sprite and Diet Coke. The green marks in the background are at one half-meter increments. Photograph by K. Shimada Creative Commons License

Academic research physicist Tonya Coffey at Appalachian State University in Boone, North Carolina analyzed why the Diet Coke created the highest geyser. She determined that the aspartame in Diet Coke lowered the surface tension of the gas bubbles allowing the interaction between potassium benzoate with the gelatin and gum Arabic ingredients of the Mentos Mint. Surface tension is a physical property exhibited when certain liquids are in contact with a gas. It is particularly pronounced when liquid water is in contact with the gasses of the air.

Each water molecule contains two hydrogen atoms and one oxygen atom, giving rise to its familiar chemical shorthand of H_2O. Because of their atomic structure the negative charge of the electrons of the hydrogen atoms are attracted to the positive charge of the oxygen atom, creating was is known as a hydrogen bond. The electric charges also create an attractive force between water molecules, causing them to want to remain close together. These forces are balanced out when a water molecule is surrounded by other water molecules.

Surface tension is the physical principle, which creates islands of beaded water.
Shutterstock/Kuruneko

When the water molecules on the surface are exposed to the gasses of the air above them they are no longer exposed to balanced charges. The water molecule on the surface exposed to the air is only subject to the electric charge pulling it down, keeping it in the liquid. This resistance to leaving its fellow water molecules behind gives it the property known as surface tension, a tension that prevents it from being separated from the remaining liquid. This surface tension is visible when you see water assume the shape of a droplet, or when you fill a glass to the brim and the fluid builds up above the lip of the glass before it begins to overflow.

Pond skater using surface tension to walk on water Heteroptera suborder. Shutterstock/optimarc

It is also the principle that allows insects heavier than water, such as the water glider, to walk on water because the surface tension acts as a walkable surface.

Surface tension is the same force that allows the creation of bubbles. Surfactants are products that have the property of reducing surface tension and are used in detergents, as well as in anti-bubble and anti-gas products such as simethicone. Another principle of physics was also exhibited by the Mentos in Diet Coke geyser experiment. Because the mint has a microporous nature, the markedly increased surface area caused a rapid and vigorous foaming reaction. A single simple cube has a much smaller surface area for reactions to take place, than an identical volume cube that has been subdivided into many smaller cubes. The following illustration helps to visualize how the surface area can be dramatically increased with the same volume of material.

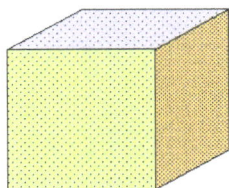

a one-meter cube has 6 square meters of suface area

pieces half the original size have twice the surface area

pieces one quarter of the original size have 4 times the surface area

pieces one-eighth of the original size have 8 times the surface area.

a cubic meter of fine sediment can have millions of square meters of surface area

Increase in surface area. Phil Stoffer, Ph.D. Geology Cafe geologycafe.com Creative Commons License

The caffeine did not accelerate the reaction. Here is the reference for those who want to read all of the scientific details. Coffey, Tonya *"Diet Coke and Mentos: What is really behind this physical reaction?" American Journal of Physics* June 2008. 76 (6): 551–557. Competitions to see which beverage will create the highest geyser are very messy affairs that again seem to attract a disproportionate number of adolescent males in their middle years. As my spouse (who happens to be a reproductive endocrinologist, an expert on the subject) likes to remind me, there are five stages of the male life cycle: infancy, childhood, adolescence, adolescence, and adolescence!

In some beverages the carbon dioxide would interfere with the taste and flavor by reacting with the ingredients, giving it an acid taste from carbonic acid. An alternative is to use nitrogen as the gas of choice as it is a neutral gas and would not interact with the beverage. The most popular example is beer, which commonly uses nitrogen, or a combination of nitrogen and carbon dioxide, under pressure in kegs.

Carbonation: The Key to the Fizz Biz

Carbon Dioxide (CO_2) consists of one carbon atom and two oxygen atoms. CO_2 is a nonpolar molecule, meaning other molecules won't stick to it easily.

Water (H_2O) consists of one oxygen atom and two hydrogen atoms. It is a polar molecule. Uneven distribution of electrons results in sticky spots — areas where molecules form weak bonds. The loose clinging results in a liquid.

Under normal conditions, it's common for CO_2 to dissolve into water. The activity of gas molecules overcomes the bonds in the H_2O chain. CO_2 escapes.

Temperature is dropped. The activity of the molecules slows. The hydrogen bonds become stronger. CO_2 can't break the H_2O chain and is retained in the water. Molecules do not, however become locked. If they did, they would become a solid — ice.

Pressure is increased. More CO_2 is crammed into the water until the mixture is supersaturated, meaning more CO_2 is dissolved in the liquid than would be possible under normal conditions. H_2O molecules squeeze in an form cages around the CO_2 molecules. CO_2 is trapped.

The water is carbonated. Syrups and flavorings are added, and the mixture then is put in a bottle. The bottle is capped, which maintains an equalized pressure inside and keeps the CO_2 in its cages until the bottle is opened.

By George Frederick for Life's Little Mysteries

i.livescience.com Creative Commons License

Carbon Dioxide (see Carbonation)

Carbon dioxide (CO_2) is a naturally occurring compound composed of two oxygen atoms bonded to a single carbon atom. It is a gas at standard temperature and pressure and exists in Earth's atmosphere as a trace gas at a concentration of 0.039 percent by volume. It is heavier than air, and when used as a fire extinguisher the dense ground-hugging layer of carbon dioxide prevents the flames from accessing oxygen.

As part of the carbon cycle, plants, algae, and cyanobacteria use light energy to photosynthesize carbohydrate from carbon dioxide and water, with oxygen produced as a waste product. However, photosynthesis cannot occur in darkness and at night some carbon dioxide is produced by plants during respiration. Carbon dioxide is exhaled in the breath of humans and land animals. It is also released from the fermentation of organic matter, volcanoes, hot springs, geysers and the combustion of hydrocarbons used as fuels. It contributes as a greenhouse gas to global warming. It is also a source of ocean acidification since it reacts with water to form carbonic acid.

Carbon dioxide in the atmosphere

Carbon is released into the atmosphere when fossil fuels are burned

Carbon is released into the atmosphere during respiration

used in photosynthesis to produce carbohydrates

plants are eaten by animals

Carbon Dioxide in decaying matter and waste

decaying plants produce

Carbon Dioxide in fossil fuels (coal & oil)

www.realtrees4kids.org Creative Commons License

A gas subsequently identified as carbon dioxide was identified by the Flemish chemist Jan Baptist van Helmont in the seventeenth century. In the 1750's Scottish physician, Joseph Black studied the gas more thoroughly. In 1772, English chemist Joseph Priestley published a paper entitled *Impregnating Water with Fixed Air*. The paper described how he forced carbon dioxide to dissolve in a bowl of agitating water, inventing what eventually became known as soda water. Soda water was the original product from which the major industry of carbonated beverages evolved.

Carbon dioxide is produced in large quantities in the digestive tract. The human stomach generates about one and one-half liters of very potent hydrochloric acid. With a pH of 1.5 it can make quick work of dissolving metal coins. The stomach lining is designed to handle the intense acidity, as well as the potent digestive enzymes released as zymogens and then activated as enzymes. The lining of the stomach is under constant attack and constant repair.

In fact, the turnover is so high that your entire stomach lining has been regenerated over the course of any three-day period. The gastric contents of food, acid, and enzymes transits through the pyloric channel and enters the duodenum. As it enters the duodenum it is in a brand new environment, and the digestive material is now known as chime. The material leaving the stomach requires prompt action from the duodenum to neutralize its high acid content. The duodenum neutralizes the acid by releasing sodium bicarbonate from its mucosal lining. It also receives a solution of pancreatic juices with a high concentration of alkaline sodium bicarbonate. The one and one-half liters of stomach acid is neutralized by one and one-half liters of sodium bicarbonate.

Do you remember from basic chemistry lessons what happens when you add an acid to an alkaline base? Did you ever perform or watch the school experiment of mixing baking soda (sodium bicarbonate) and vinegar (weak acetic acid) to create a fire extinguisher? In the demonstration a lit candle is placed on the bottom of a glass container. In a different glass pitcher, the mixture of baking soda and vinegar were reacting with an impressive display of foaming and bubbling. They were reacting as expected from the mixing of an acid and a base, generating carbon dioxide as a free gas and neutral water.

Carbon dioxide is heavier than air so although it was invisible the rising level of carbon dioxide in the glass container was pushing the lighter air out and over the top. After just minutes of bubbling, the pitcher that was now full of heavier carbon dioxide was tilted over the glass containing the lit candle. Although it appeared that the tilted pitcher was not adding anything to the glass with the candle, the heavier but invisible carbon dioxide was pouring out of the pitcher and was now displacing the air around the candle with carbon dioxide. As soon as the invisible carbon dioxide reached the level of the flame the supply of oxygen was cut off, and the candle flame went out like magic.

Main symptoms of carbon dioxide toxicity. Wikipedia. Mikael Häggström Creative Commons License

By the way there is another interesting fact about carbon dioxide and human respiration. It is the level of carbon dioxide in your blood, not the level of oxygen, that drives the respiratory center that controls breathing. The sensation of air hunger that arises when one is short of breath or suffocating is from carbon dioxide buildup, not from a lack of oxygen. That is why the trick of making your voice squeaky by breathing helium is actually very dangerous. If you breathe in and out pure helium your body continues to get rid of its carbon dioxide with each breath. It fools the body into thinking that everything is just fine, even though it is not obtaining any oxygen. The person breathing pure helium does not experience air hunger or suffocation because that sensation is only triggered by carbon dioxide which continues to be exhaled. Death occurs quickly and without warning, and because there is no sensation of air hunger it is supposedly very peaceful. As macabre as it may seem, advocates of capital punishment and euthanasia argue this would be a very humane, inexpensive, and simple way to end a life.

The one and one-half liters of potent hydrochloric acid and one and one-half liters of strongly alkaline sodium bicarbonate generate dozens of liters of carbon dioxide gas. The gas volume increases rapidly and dramatically and will lead to a bloated distended feeling within the small intestine. One may need to loosen a belt or tight clothing after a meal but fortunately the distended sensation is fairly short lived. The reason for this is that carbon dioxide gas in the intestines is rapidly absorbed and dissolved into the bloodstream. It travels to the lungs where the carbon dioxide is released via the alveoli into the airway and exhaled. The carbon dioxide present in intestinal gas is generated by colonic bacteria and other gut flora. It averages about ten percent of passed intestinal gas by volume. This figure can change significantly dependent on diet and the gastrointestinal microbiome.

Carminative

A carminative, also known as carminativum, is an herb or preparation that promotes the prevention or elimination of gas from the gastrointestinal tract. Many carminatives have been shown to work by releasing the air swallowed (aerophagia) by reducing the pressure of the lower esophageal sphincter to promote eructation (burp). This relaxation of the sphincter can also promote reflux, regurgitation and heartburn and can aggravate Gastroesophageal Reflux Disease (GERD), which may have atypical symptoms that are unrelated to heartburn.

www.flickr.com Tess Shebaylo Dewee's Carminative Creative Commons License

Many folk medicines and remedies have a long tradition of being used as carminatives. They are often mixtures of herbs, spices, and essential oils. Many foods, social, and recreational products also relax the lower esophageal sphincter and encourage eructation, although one would not ingest them specifically for this carminative effect. This category includes onion, garlic, fried foods, fatty foods, chocolate, tobacco, alcohol, and marijuana.

In Western culture, the most common product that people see and use for its carminative property is mint, which relaxes the lower esophageal sphincter to encourage eructation. Chocolate can have a similar effect, so it is common to see the two combined as a traditional after dinner chocolate mint. Indian and Asian restaurants may offer other traditional carminative herbs and seeds usually found on the counter by the exit.

Agents that may Reduce LES Pressure

Alcohol
Caffeine
Smoking

Chocolate
Fried foods
Onions
Peppermint
Fatty foods

Carminatives and other agents reduce the lower esophageal sphincter (LES) pressure, allowing the easier release of gasses and air from the stomach but at the same time make regurgitation and heartburn more likely. Restaurateurs want their customers to have enjoyed their meals, and they recognize that distension from the universal aerophagia of eating can cause discomfort. Most people have no idea that the air they swallowed, and not necessarily the meal, might be the cause of their distress. The carminative mint is offered to give prompt relief, but notice how it is offered on leaving the restaurant. The restaurant management does not want eructation to occur where others are dining in their refined accommodations. They prefer that the eructation occurs later to impress your 'significant other' or in the presence of your family and friends.

The following have all been described as having value as carminatives: Alcohol, Angelica, Anise, Asafetida, Basil, Black Pepper, Caffeine, Calamus, Capsaicin, Caraway, Cardamom, Chili (Cayenne) Pepper, Chocolate, Cinnamon (potency decreases with cooking), Cloves, Coriander, Cumin, Curcumin, Dill, Epazote,

Eucalyptus, fatty foods, Fennel, Garlic (potency increases with cooking), Ginger, Goldenrod, Hops, Lemon balm, liquorice (also spelled as licorice), Lovage, Marjoram, Mint, Motherwort, Muña, Mustard, Nigella, Nutmeg, Onion, Oregano, Parsley, Pepper, Pennyroyal, Peppermint, Rosemary, Saffron, Sage, Savory, Spearmint, Theobromine, Thyme, Tobacco, Turmeric, Valerian, Wintergreen, Winter Savory, Wormwood, and others.

Herbs & Spices Shutterstock/KrzysztofSlusarczyk

As this exhaustive list confirms, a large number of herbs and spices have been described as having carminative benefits. The problem with anecdotes and folk traditions is that it is hard to separate true beneficial properties from those that do so as a result of a placebo effect. The business of selling spices and supplements is very lucrative, so there is a strong financial interest to keep the status quo and not investigate these herbs scientifically. Although many prescription drugs can affect the tone of the lower esophageal sphincter and promote eructation the carminative property is a side effect, and not an indication that the product should be used for that purpose. To encourage eructation avoid lying down after a meal. Sitting upright lets the air swallowed rise above the food in the stomach and when the lower esophageal sphincter relaxes air, rather than food, can then escape the stomach.

Carminatives relax the lower esophageal sphincter and can be used to allow burping or belching of swallowed air to give relief of gastric distension and bloat. Others drink a carbonated beverage or an effervescent product such as Alka-Seltzer to induce eructation by increasing the gas pressure within the stomach to overcome the resistance of the lower esophageal sphincter pressure. Fried foods, greasy, fatty foods, alcohol, onion, and tobacco can also act as carminatives as can a number of herbal preparations. A number of pharmacologic agents used in the treatment of a wide variety of medical disorders can also act as carminatives by relaxing the lower esophageal sphincter. Female hormones such as progesterone and estrogen are in this category. During natural periods of higher hormone levels, such as during a pregnancy, reflux is more common. One reason is that the hormones have an effect on the lowered esophageal sphincter, causing relaxation that may lead to reflux. A second reason is the increasing intra-abdominal pressure from a growing child and uterus.

Celiac Disease (see Gluten Sensitive Enteropathy, Sprue)

Chewing (Mastication)

Chewing or mastication (Greek mastikhan-gnash the teeth) is the process of crushing and grinding food by the teeth. Mastication can be unconscious, or subconscious but can be modified by conscious control. This process increases the surface area of foods increasing the efficiency of enzymes and the absorption of nutrients. The bite pressure generated in the average human is one hundred and sixty-two pounds per square inch.

As impressive as the bite strength is, it is equally impressive how sensitive the chewing process is to recognizing when pressure should be released or withheld. It senses when a particle as small as a grain of sand is found in clam chowder, or a fragment of eggshell in an omelet. There is a very substantial amount of crushing and grinding power that macerates the food and disrupts the cellular structure of ingested plant and animal material. The disruption of cell structure often releases enzymes within the cells themselves that assist in the degradation of cellular tissue and the process of digestion.

Chewing is obviously helpful in the digestive process. but it can inadvertently lead to excessive gas swallowing. With chewing the salivary glands are actively secreting more saliva. With the increased volume of saliva more swallows will take place. Each swallow allows the ingestion of excess air, on average three to five milliliters (about one teaspoon) per swallow. Chewing gum, ill-fitting dentures, drinking from a straw or bottle, tilting the head back while drinking, chewing tobacco, mouth candies and lozenges, etc. can contribute to excess aerophagia which may result in excess burping, bloating, and farting.

After chewing the food bolus is swallowed exiting the pharynx, transiting the esophagus via peristalsis, and entering the stomach. Chewing developed to handle the herbivorous diet, as carnivores generally engage in very little chewing activity and swallow their food whole or in large chunks. Cattle and other ruminants chew food more than once to allow further enzymatic digestion and bacterial fermentation to extract more nutrients. The regurgitated food bolus is called cud.

As a physician, I often ask if a patient has any difficulty chewing their food, such as from ill-fitting dentures. Chewing food well really helps the digestive process and can lead to less aerophagia, the swallowing of air, which can contribute to intestinal gaseousness. Medical words can be like a foreign language and easy to misinterpret. I always wondered what the response from some people would be if used the medical term for chewing and I encouraged them to masticate a lot with each meal. I imagine the response would be one of shock and indignation. What's the matter with you doctor, do you think I want to go blind!

Greg Erickson, left, a paleobiologist on faculty at of Florida State University and Kent Vliet of the University of Florida measure the bite force of a saltwater crocodile in Australia. Contributed photo to St. Augustine Record, Florida

"The noise of the jaws coming together was like a gunshot. The power of the animal was astounding," said paleobiologist Greg M. Erickson of Florida State University. The crocodilians had a bite force of twenty-three thousand pounds per square inch, about double that of *Tyrannosaurus rex*, the scientist's estimate.

Dr. Brady Barr sponsored by the National Geographic Society measured comparative bite pressures of a sampling across the animal kingdom. Although humans have a very substantial bite pressure of one hundred and sixty-two pounds per square inch (psi), other species far exceed this amount of pressure generated.

Human: 162 psi
Dog: 310 psi
Lion: 600 psi
Shark: 600 psi
Hyena: 1000 psi
Turtle: 1000 psi
Crocodile: 2500 psi
Lion: 600 psi
Tiger: 1050 psi
Bear: 1200 psi
Gorilla: 1300 psi
Hippopotamus: 1821 psi
Jaguar: 2000 psi
Alligator: 2125 psi
Crocodile: 5000 psi

Chili Con Carne

Chili con carne is the Spanish name for a meal made as a stew that usually contains beans, chili peppers, tomato, and meat. Often other seasonings are added such as onions, garlic, and cumin. A wide variation of the ingredients and recipes often leads to competitions typically known as chili cook-off. It is often referred to by its abbreviated name chili in American English. It is the official culinary dish of the US State of Texas.

The high legume content has led to its recognition as a potent source of intestinal gas. The variety of spices, seasonings, and animal fat leads to an equally intense variety of subsequent farts and aromas, often of startling pungency. The use of chili as a staple of the diet of cowboys on the range has led to several comedic scenes. A famous example includes the infamous campfire scene in Mel Brook's movie *Blazing Saddles*.

Crepitation Contest

Attributed to the staff of the Canadian Broadcast Corporation in the 1940's, a recording called *The Crepitation Contest* was produced. Canadian Broadcast Corporation sportscaster Sidney S. Brown narrated it, with sound effects credited to his producer, Jules Lipton. The recording is a parody of a radio broadcast of a live sporting event with pre-game interviews of the contestants.

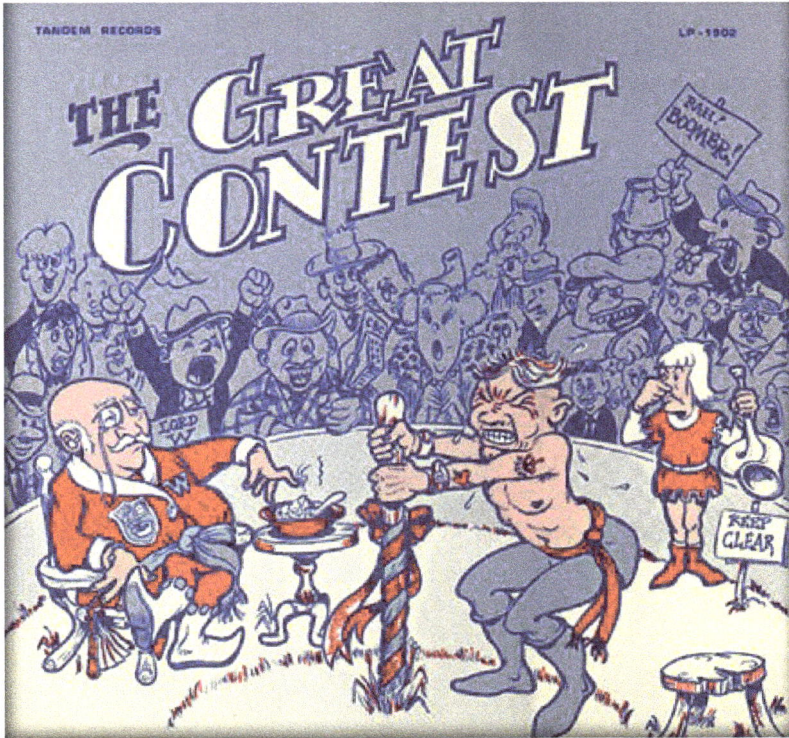

www.wfmu.org

The reigning champion is Lord Windesmear, and the challenger is Paul Boomer. The broadcast parody includes detailed descriptions of the competition including the rules, traditions, play-by-play reporting of the event and audience sounds and reactions. Reportedly the original recording was played at a New Year's Eve party in 1943 that was attended by an admiral of the United States Navy. He believed it would be a great morale booster for American serviceman. The original master recording at RCA Victor Studio in Toronto was obtained, and lacquer, and vinyl 78-rpm discs were pressed.

Diet

Diet obviously plays a major role in intestinal gas production. Certain types of vegetables and fruits contain carbohydrates with sugars and starches that may be poorly digested by people but happily fermented by bacteria comprising the gut flora. The starches, including potatoes, corn, noodles, and wheat are the source of the majority of gas generated by the gut microbial flora.

Rice is the one starch exception and rarely contributes to gas production. Wheat has the other 'distinction' of having the protein glutamate, which contains the nitrogen base product from which you generate ammonia-like aromatic compounds.

Common Foods that Cause Bloating and Gas

- Cabbage
- Cauliflower
- Beans
- Oats
- Apples
- Milk
- Fluffy wheat
- Broccoli
- Onions
- Corn
- Potatoes
- Pears
- Soft cheese
- Peaches

www.34-menopause-symptoms.com Creative Commons License

There are many specific enzymes required in the process of digestion, and deficiency in the quantity or activity of an enzyme can lead to food intolerance. The most common food intolerance is for the milk sugar lactose when an individual has decreased amounts and activity of the necessary enzyme for its digestion, lactase. The age of discovery is still in its infancy. Dozens of hormones, over one thousand and six hundred enzymes, over ten thousand species of gut microbes, and over one million genomes identified to date are just the beginning. Of the thousands of variables, we still have a clear understanding of only a few dozen. By the way, with so much remaining unknown and awaiting discovery, opportunity abounds if you have an interest in pursuing or supporting research activities.

If you are looking for a novel, practical, legitimate, and socially responsible way to avoid jury duty this may be your answer. A sincere desire to avoid inflicting your fart issues on fellow jurors may provide you with an excellent reason to be excused from jury duty. If you honestly believe you have excessive gas from an inherited enzyme deficiency you can bring the matter up with the clerk of the court and the presiding judge. If the court wants further clarification describe the scene of your intestinal gas leading the other jurors to flee the jury box complaining that it was a cruel and unusual exposure to a gas chamber. The judge just might have to declare a mistrial, stating that although justice is blind, she has not lost her sense of smell or hearing. A letter explaining the nature of your condition can go a long way to securing a permanent excuse from jury duty, and probably an invitation to use an absentee ballot to stay out of the voting booth on Election Day!

Chili con carne

Chili con carne is the Spanish name for a meal made as a stew that usually contains beans, chili peppers, tomato, and meat. Often other seasonings are added such as onions, garlic, and cumin. A wide variation of the ingredients and recipes often leads to competitions typically known as chili cook-off. It is often referred to by its abbreviated name chili in American English. It is the official culinary dish of the US State of Texas.

The high legume content has led to its recognition as a potent source of intestinal gas. The variety of spices, seasonings, and animal fat leads to an equally intense variety of subsequent farts and aromas, often of startling pungency. The use of chili as a staple of the diet of cowboys on the range has led to several comedic scenes. A famous example includes the infamous campfire scene in Mel Brook's movie Blazing Saddles.

Refueling station and restaurant. Cindy Cornett Seigle www.flickr.com Creative Commons License

Legumes

"Beans, Beans, The Musical Fruit" is a schoolyard saying and children's song about the capacity for beans to contribute to flatulence.

Beans, beans, the musical fruit
The more you eat, the more you toot
The more you toot, the better you feel
So we have beans at every meal!
There are also several alternative versions, such as the one below:

Beans, beans, they're good for your heart
The more you eat, the more you fart
The more you fart, the happier/better you feel
So let's eat beans with every meal

143

Beans have a well-deserved reputation for contributing to intestinal gas production. Recent medical literature suggests that the degree of subjective complaints that legumes cause gas may be somewhat exaggerated. The bean is rich in the sugars raffinose, verbascose and stachyose. As humans do not produce the enzyme required for its degradation, alpha-galactosidase, these sugars undergo fermentation by the gut flora. The US Department of Agriculture is working on the development of a bean with lower levels of these sugars, and so far the Anasazi bean has been the leading candidate but no breakthrough yet. With genetically modified organisms (GMO) and foods being introduced in the marketplace, it is only a matter of time before products labeled as low-gas are promoted.

www.flickr.com Creative Commons License

Thankfully there are alpha-galactosidase enzyme supplements that can provide relief. The enzyme is not heat stable, so it will be inactivated by the heat of cooking. The enzyme should be added to the first bite of the beans consumed and if a large portion is ingested additional enzyme intake during the course of the bean meal is recommended. An alternative approach is to soak the beans for several hours, leeching out some of the sugars into the water, which is discarded. The best approach is to soak the beans until they begin to germinate. With germination the seed itself begins to release alpha-galactosidase to break down its complex sugar content for the nutritional use of the newly germinated bean plant. With germination approximately eighty percent of the complex sugars are digested.

A legume is a plant in the family Fabaceae (or Leguminosae) native to the Americas, grown agriculturally for their food grain seed, livestock forage and silage, and soil enhancement. Most legumes harbor the symbiotic bacteria Rhizobia in their root nodules, which convert nitrogen in the atmosphere into ammonia and ammonium. This source of nitrogen contributes to the plant's production of amino acids and high protein content. Legumes include alfalfa, clover, peas, beans, lentils, lupins, soybeans, and peanuts and a number of trees and shrubs. In farming crop rotation, the growing of legumes near non-legumes is common. Legumes are sometimes referred to as 'green manure' because their symbiotic bacteria enrich the soil with nitrogenous products. A legume fruit is typically a pod that opens along a seam. They are an excellent source of protein but contain lower quantities of the essential amino acid methionine.

Like many legumes, the seemingly innocent lima bean should not be eaten raw, doing so can be lethal. Also known as butter beans, the legumes can contain a high level of cyanide, which is part of the plant's defense mechanism. In the United States there are restrictions about cyanide levels in commercially grown lima bean varieties, but not so in less developed countries, and many people can get sick from eating them. Even so, lima beans should be cooked thoroughly and uncovered to allow the poison to escape as gas. Also, drain and discard the cooking water to be on the safe side.

Many a granny came armed with a spoonful of castor oil to heal all ills, and studies show that it does indeed have health benefits to offer. Just be sure not to eat the beans from which the oil came. If castor beans are chewed and swallowed, they can release ricin, one of the most toxic poisons known to man. Eating just one or two castor beans can easily cause the demise of the eater. Ricin has been investigated as a warfare agent and has even been employed by secret agents and assassins.

Pumpernickel (Devil's Farts)

Pumpernickel (German Devil's Fart) is a heavy dark brown bread traditionally made with coarsely ground rye flour and whole rye berries and has been associated with the Westphalia region of Germany for over five hundred years. Like most rye breads, it is traditionally made with an acidic sourdough starter, which inhibits the rye amylase enzymes. The name is associated with the coarse bread-giving rise to flatulence. With its sourdough origins it can serve as a probiotic.

Shutterstock/eclipticblue

Pets de Nonne (Nun's Farts)

Pets de Nonne, also called Pets de Sœur, is translated as a nun's farts. They are a dessert puff pastry dating from medieval times and made from butter, milk, flour, sugar, eggs and sometimes honey is added. They are traditionally pan-fried in lard and then baked. Their lightness inspired their name in French, pets de nonne and Pets de Sœurs, suggesting that the farts of a nun were somewhat angelic.

Pets de Nonne, also called Pets de Sœurs (Nun's Farts) French and Canadian Dessert Food photo by Ziga Creative Commons License

Digestion

The purpose of the digestive tract is to support life by providing the nutrition and energy we need for all of our body functions. Intestinal gas is simply a natural waste product and is rarely of consequence. Perhaps the analogy is not the best one, but think of the digestive tract as the reverse of the assembly line, a disassembly line. A factory has a goal to be efficient and profitable, and may not win too many awards for architectural beauty. So too with the digestive tract, the process has been refined over eons of evolution, yet still have its primitive origins and end products.

We begin our factory tour with a view much like you would get sitting in your car going through an automated car wash. Before you even go to the car wash, your brain has to make the conscious decision that this activity is what it wants to do. In the same manner, the mind begins the digestive process with the decision to satisfy its hunger call, or because an appetizing opportunity presents itself. When thinking about food and eating, the brain may activate the secretion of saliva and prime the digestive processes of the stomach and internal organs.

Much like the water hoses and spray that greet your vehicle as you enter the beginning of the car wash tunnel, the entrance of food to the mouth receives a similar welcome. Jets of saliva are secreted from the ducts of the salivary glands located strategically around the oral cavity of the mouth. Saliva that is in the resting mouth is viscous and coats and protects the teeth and the inner surface of the mouth. The secreted saliva with eating or drinking is of a thinner waterier consistency. It has digestive enzymes including amylase to digest carbohydrates and lipase to digest fats.

If your carwash is as sophisticated as your digestive tract, it will have a crew to make sure your side mirrors are tucked in. It will also provide a prewash scrub of your tires to remove residue that would otherwise be difficult for the machinery to reach. The teeth, jaws, and tongue work together in a remarkable and powerful dance with very few of the missteps which would be the dance equivalent of stepping on toes, the biting of the tongue.

The food has to be processed into smaller more manageable portions than that what is found on your plate. Your dining utensils of fork, knife, and spoon are just the preliminary, as the teeth do the real work in preparing food for the process of digestion. The teeth are subdivided into distinct categories that have unique functions. The incisors cut the food as you bite into an apple and the canines tear the food apart as you dig into your pastrami sandwich. The molars crush and grind the salad and crunchy vegetables that you have as a side dish. The grinding and crushing break the plant cell walls apart that would otherwise protect its internal nutritious content from our digestive enzymes. They also increase the surface area of the food increasing their exposure to digestive acid and enzymes.

The chewing process assures that the saliva and its active enzymes are well mixed with the increased surface area of the food. They begin the process of breaking down the carbohydrates and lipids into their essential components to ready them for further digestion and absorption. The saliva also moistens the food and lubricates it for the coordinated swallowing motion of the tongue, teeth, palate, and pharynx. These muscles and organs work together to roll it into an easy to swallow food bolus. The muscles of the swallowing process include those that protect the larynx and airway. The epiglottis closes off the passageway to the trachea, bronchi, and lungs, to prevent aspiration into the airways as the food and saliva swallow takes place.

The coordinated action is developed with age, which is why small children should avoid foods, such as nuts, grapes, larger oval or rounded candies. These foods, if inappropriately swallowed into the airway, can lead to fatal choking episodes. Tragically a number of children die because the oval or rounded shape can completely block the airway. An irregular shaped object, which can be life threatening, rarely completely obstructs the airway and usually allows some air to pass. The complicated swallowing neuromuscular coordination can also be affected by neurological disorders, stroke, surgery or other conditions, which may lead to the risk of aspiration. Once swallowed, the food bolus is propelled down the esophagus by coordinated snakelike muscular action, known as peristalsis. It is not recommended, but the swallowing mechanism is so efficient that you can swallow against gravity while standing on your head.

The muscular valve at the junction of the esophagus and stomach is called the lower esophageal sphincter. The lower esophageal sphincter is designed to allow food and fluid to enter the stomach, with the door closed behind them once they leave the esophagus. If the valve opens at the wrong time, gastric acid, digestive enzymes, and food can flow back into the esophagus. The reflux of stomach contents into the esophagus can lead to symptoms of heartburn or mucosal damage. If the refluxed material goes all the way into the airway hoarseness, sore throat, aspiration, choking, or pneumonia can develop. If it occurs frequently gastroesophageal reflux disease (GERD) can predispose to a change in the normal flat squamous epithelium cell tissue lining the esophagus. The growth of columnar epithelium, more of an intestinal type tissue, in place of the squamous epithelium gives rise to a condition called a Barrett esophagus. This type of cell lining is at a higher risk for abnormal atypical cell changes and a higher risk of cancer development. Individuals with Barrett esophagus are frequently treated for GERD and monitored carefully with surveillance endoscopy and biopsy for pre-malignant changes.

The stomach is a churning caldron of muscular mixing contractions, concentrated acid secretion, and potent digestive enzymes. The vagus nerve and gut hormones play a crucial role in the intricate balance of enzymes, acid, nutrients, and motility. When the conditions are right, the pyloric sphincter of the stomach opens to allow the acid, enzyme, and food mixture to exit. This digestive material is now called chyme as it enters the first portion of the small intestine, known as the duodenum. In Greek, this means the width equivalent to twelve fingers, which is what its small size would measure using your digits. For its small size, the duodenum plays an amazing and complex part.

The highly acid chyme would quickly damage the lining of the duodenum if it did not respond quickly with the pouring on, much like a fire extinguisher, of sodium bicarbonate. The sodium bicarbonate is produced in the duodenum as well as by the pancreas. The sodium bicarbonate produced in the pancreas is released through the pancreatic duct, which empties into the duodenum through the Ampulla of Vater. The fire extinguisher analogy shares another aspect of the story. Perhaps you made a fire extinguisher in a science class, or home experiment, by adding baking soda that contains sodium bicarbonate and vinegar that contains acetic acid. This neutralization of acid is the same type of reaction that takes place in the duodenum, when the hydrochloric acid of the stomach meets the sodium bicarbonate released to neutralize it. When the two react they produce water, sodium chloride (salt), and large quantities of carbon dioxide. The carbon dioxide is released as large volumes of gas that appears as bubbles arising from the reaction. The carbon dioxide is used as a fire extinguisher in the science experiment since it is heavier than air and cuts off the oxygen supply that the flame requires.

In the human duodenum, the carbon dioxide generated as a side product of acid neutralization only serves to bloat and distend the gut with gas. The body is pretty remarkable in getting rid of the bloat relatively quickly, in that it absorbs the carbon dioxide into the bloodstream where it travels to the lungs and is exhaled. The bile ducts from the liver join the duct from the pancreas bringing digestive enzymes and bicarbonate that enter the duodenum through the Ampulla of Vater. Within the ampulla lies the muscular sphincter of Oddi. The name sounds like a character from the story of *The Wizard of Oz*, and that would be an appropriate analogy. The coordinated release of hormones, enzymes, motility and vagal input is nothing short of wizardry.

Subconsciously, your body can sense what nutrients you have ingested. The body responds by releasing the correct recipe of enzymes, potent acid in the stomach, and bicarbonate in the duodenum, adjusting the pH as necessary. It adds just the right amount of bile to the mix, controls the timing and volume of stomach emptying, and controls the speed of transit and intensity of mixing contractions through the length of the intestinal tract. The majority of the sensing and control feedback takes place in a small confined space the width of twelve fingers, the duodenum.

The breakdown products of the digestive process are absorbed by a sea of finger-like projections called the villi. It looks like a field of waving wheat stalks; each upstanding villus is ready to use its enzymes and absorptive capacity to absorb nutrients. If you looked under the microscope, you would find that each villus has thousands of even smaller villi on its surface, given the appropriate name of microvilli.

Villi Shutterstock/modella

All of these folds of absorptive tissue, if flattened out, would provide the equivalent absorptive capacity of a championship tennis court. A quote from Mark Twain also illustrates the concept of surface area: "If Switzerland were ironed flat it would be a very large country". The long intestinal tunnel of eagerly awaiting absorptive villi is about twenty feet long, and it is an amazingly efficient system of digestion and absorption. If injured, the ability of the small bowel to digest and absorb nutrients is compromised. A condition that temporarily damages the small intestine, such as a viral or bacterial gastroenteritis often called stomach flu, can cause a blunting or shortening of the villi. The villous blunting will also lead to the loss of digestive enzymes that reside on the villi.

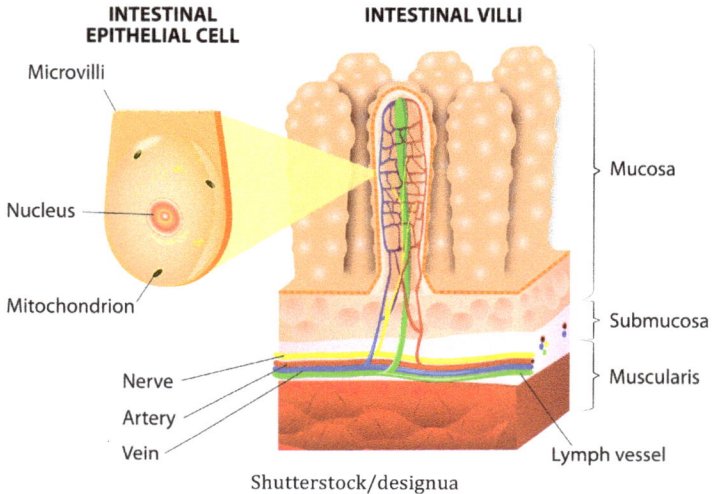

Shutterstock/designua

Without the ability to digest and absorb nutrients, the unabsorbed material can cause what is known as an osmotic diarrhea. People are often advised to avoid dairy products for a week or so after stomach flu to allow the villi and enzymes to recover. If you eat or drink lactose without waiting until the recovery is complete, you may end up with symptoms of temporary lactose intolerance such as gas and diarrhea. When the liquid chyme leaves the jejunum and ileum of the small intestine, it goes through the ileocecal valve to enter the colon. In the cecum of the colon lies the infamous appendix, which for thousands of years mystified science as to its purpose. It looks like its function has finally, and only very recently, been identified. It stores a reservoir of intestinal bacteria, representing the healthy gut microbiome, from which the gut flora can be replenished after a bout of intestinal dysentery.

The gut microbiome is much more important than most people realize. The microbes of the body far outnumber the number of human cells. In fact, if you just go by the number of cells and not their mass, they outnumber human cells by ten to one. In other words, you as a living system are only ten percent human and ninety percent microbes! The vast majority of the microbes living within and on us are commensals. The term commensal is used to describe a symbiotic relationship from which both parties benefit. They are able to process foods that would otherwise be indigestible, and convert them to absorbable nutrients and metabolites. It is not an understatement to say that they are a requirement for our health and well-being. The gut microbiome also plays a critical role in the gut-brain-microbiome-axis, which provides for the communication of information between the three. Many experts now include food as the fourth component of this important communication axis.

The colon, unlike the small intestine, is less involved in the digestion of foods and nutrients. It is primarily involved in the absorption of water and sodium, as well as some fat-soluble vitamins such as vitamin K. The colon removes the excess moisture from the watery chime solidifying the stool as it transits the gut. The ability to conserve water is necessary, and without this ability the risk of dehydration would be substantially increased. The fecal material of the stool is stored in the rectum, and sigmoid colon, awaiting the right opportunity to be eliminated through defecation. A process or illness that impairs the colon's absorption of water will lead to more fluid in the stool and diarrhea. The loss of water and electrolytes as a consequence of diarrhea, unfortunately, remains a life-threatening condition in many parts of the world, especially for infants and children.

If the elimination of the feces is delayed, the moisture continues to be absorbed, and the stools can become harder resulting in constipation. Constipation itself can be self-perpetuating as it aggravates the situation because the stools become harder and more difficult to pass the longer they remain in the colon. The more common treatments for constipation attempt to increase the moisture content of the stool. The feces excreted can provide information about bowel health. For most people going about their daily activities, the passage of the feces itself is the end of the story of digestion. The human digestive system, like that of other animals, does not remove all of the contained nutrients from food. For other organisms, including the common housefly, the feces are thus an available source of nutrition. For them, the elimination of feces is just the beginning of their story of digestion and can play an important role in the transmission of disease back to humans.

Farts are ubiquitous, all living creatures generate gas from the cellular respiration of metabolism, and humans are no exception. The bacteria in your colonic flora produce microscopic nanofarts and microfarts, which collect into larger bubbles of gas in the bowel. They are intermixed with the atmospheric air swallowed throughout the day and particularly at meals. The nature of the intestinal gas may provide clues to digestive health and disease.

Distension (see Bloat)

Distension and its synonymous term bloat are the familiar sensation that the abdomen is distended or overly full. There are many causes of bloating ranging from simple overeating and the regular production of intestinal gasses to abdominal ascites fluid buildup from an underlying tumor. Common causes of abdominal bloating include overeating, gastric distension, lactose intolerance, fructose intolerance and other food intolerances. Other causes include food allergy, aerophagia (air swallowing), irritable bowel syndrome, partial or complete bowel obstruction, and gastric dumping syndrome or rapid gastric emptying. The list continues with gas-producing foods, constipation, visceral fat, and obesity.

Less common causes include splenic flexure syndrome, menstruation, dysmenorrhea, premenstrual syndrome, polycystic ovary syndrome and ovarian cysts, and Alvarez' syndrome. The possibilities are an extensive list of ailments, infections, and disorders including intestinal parasites (e.g., *Ascaris lumbricoides*), diverticulosis, celiac disease, prescription medications such as phentermine, intra-abdominal tumors such as cancer of the ovary, liver, uterus, stomach, and colon. Temporary bloating is common after gastrointestinal endoscopic procedures. Rarely a megacolon, which is an abnormal dilation of the colon, can be caused by ulcerative colitis or Chagas disease caused by the parasite *Trypanosoma cruzi*. After surgical repair of a hiatal hernia or treatment for gastroesophageal reflux with a procedure known as a Nissen fundoplication, the ability to burp and belch is restricted resulting in uncomfortable bloating and distension.

A number of lifestyle and dietary factors can also affect the frequency and intensity of the sensation of bloating. Exercise stimulates the releases of hormones that encourage peristaltic activity in the bowels. In a similar fashion, caffeine containing beverages and food such as coffee, tea, cola, and chocolate also stimulate peristalsis and improve the transit time of food through the digestive tract. A rapid gastrointestinal transit gives the gut flora less time to ferment the material in the lumen of the bowel, with a resultant decrease in the total volume of gas produced by bacterial fermentation. Even a walk after a meal may help to move the contents along helping to ease the volume of gas produced. If nothing else, it at least allows you to release it outdoors!

Meals that are high in fat create the exact opposite effect as fat causes the release of hormones and slows down gut motility. As the food spends more time in the digestive tract continued bacterial fermentation produces increasing quantities of gas.' In addition, foods that are extremely hot or cold tend to be swallowed in smaller quantities resulting in more swallows being necessary to eat or drink the same volume at a moderate temperature. As each swallow contributes an additional quantity of air entering the esophagus and digestive tract, more swallows results in more air ingestion. Foods or snacks that require excess chewing with resultant excess swallowing of saliva, such as chewing or bubble gum, also contribute to excess air intake. Certain types of vegetables and fruits contain sugars and starches, which may be poorly digested by people but happily fermented by bacteria comprising the gut flora. The most common food intolerance is lactose intolerance.

The treatment is always directed at the underlying cause. Empiric trials of carminatives, probiotics, dietary restrictions, enzyme replacement therapy, simethicone, etcetera can be attempted. Alternative health approaches to treating bloating include acupuncture, homeopathy, and hypnosis. Sometimes the underlying bloat is not bloating from the air but from the increased body fat of obesity. Now that is a real challenge, but the benefits of eliminating that bloat can be profoundly beneficial to health and longevity. Another contributor to gastrointestinal bloat is reduced gut motility. With the reduction in peristaltic activity, the intestinal gasses accumulate and distend the bowel. Diabetes mellitus, neuropathy, various drugs including opiates, and other causes may lead to a reduction in peristaltic activity. Bowel obstruction leads to distension of proximal portions of the gastrointestinal tract because of accumulating gas, fluids, and undigested food residue.

Shutterstock/sisacorn

Bloating and distension continue even after death. As there is no longer any gastrointestinal peristalsis or motility, the gasses rapidly accumulate. In the cases of victims of drowning the body, which initially descended deeper into the water, begins rise as the gasses accumulate. After a day or so enough gas has collected so that the body floats to the surface and remains there for a week or so. In cold water or colder climates, the microbial metabolism is slowed so it takes longer for sufficient gas to be produced to float a body from submerged depths. In the San Francisco Bay area, the Golden Gate Bridge is a frequent location for tragic suicide leaps into the frigid waters below. The water is so cold it often takes a week for gasses to accumulate to allow retrieval of the body. The cold temperature also involves Charles Law, which dictates that the lower the temperature the smaller the volume the gas will occupy.

At some point the pressure of the gasses that are accumulating through the microbial metabolism and the decomposition process result in rupture of the body. This event can be explosive in nature and injury and death have occurred from proximity to decomposing bodies and animal remains. In most societies, early burial prevents exposure to the decomposition process. In Western and other cultures, a body may be displayed prior to burial. As the intestinal gas production does not cease with death, and indeed accelerates, gas may continue to escape as an audible fart. Part of the mortician practice is to perform a procedure that seals and secures the anus of the deceased so that the audible release of gas does not occur. Most people are not aware that the dead can fart, and when an uninformed person is exposed to a deceased person farting they are frightened, often believing that they are at least partly alive. Perhaps this has given rise to a belief in a zombie like state between life and death.

Diverticulosis

Diverticulosis is the presence of out pockets, called diverticula, of the colonic mucosa and submucosa through weaknesses of muscle layers in the colon wall. These are more common with advancing age and typically are most pronounced in the sigmoid colon. The incidence of ten percent of Americans having diverticulosis at age forty, to over fifty percent at age sixty is thought to be due to progressive weakening of the colon wall connective tissue. Diverticula are typically asymptomatic and the first sign of the condition may be painless lower intestinal bleeding. The bleeding can be brisk and life threatening or subtle presenting as an anemia of undetermined cause. The diverticula can also present as an infection called diverticulitis and if untreated abscesses, perforation, and life threatening peritonitis may develop. Diverticula can be visualized on colonoscopy and barium enema, but if an infection is suspect CAT scan or MRI is the preferred study to reduce the risk of perforation.

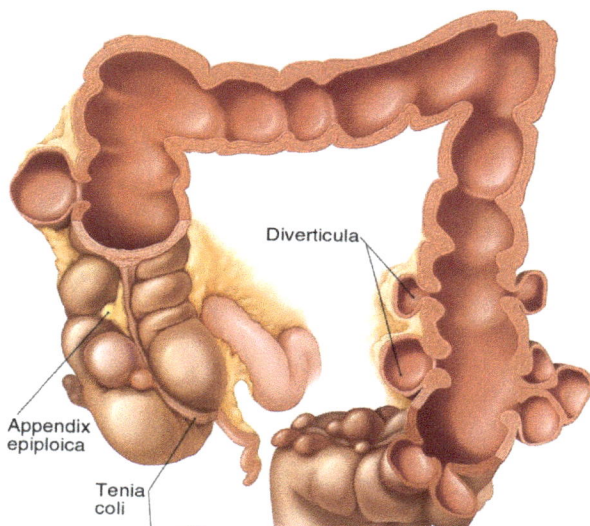

The passage of intestinal gas in African culture is basically a nonevent. It is considered part of the normal digestive process and not the cause of any embarrassment or suppression. It even came to be mentioned in a prestigious medical journal during a discussion of the cause of diverticular disease of the colon, discussed below. The development of diverticula has been ascribed to the high pressure generated within the bowel with the mass motion of feces. This is thought to cause herniation at the vulnerable location where blood vessels enter the colonic wall. Dr. Denis Burkitt, already famous for his identification of Burkitt Lymphoma a pediatric tumor seen in Africa, suggested an explanation for why diverticulosis is so common in Western society but rare in Africa. He theorized that because Africans eat a higher fiber diet than Westerners and use the natural squatting position for defecation, they pass soft bulky stools without straining. He wrote a book advocating his position and it became an international best seller

Another scientist challenged his theory with a letter to the editor published in the prestigious British medical journal, The Lancet. He theorized the reason Africans do not get diverticulosis was because they look upon farting as a perfectly normal activity and do so whenever the urge arises. In Western society, he argued, we sit in our office cubicles all day long holding on to internal gasses under very high pressure and only when we get into our cars at the end of the day do we allow ourselves to release the pent up high pressure gas and toot our way home. The fact that the incidence is identical in black and white Americans excluded a racial factor as a possible explanation.

An old theory ascribed diverticulitis to seeds ingested and lodged in the diverticula, because this was often seen in surgical specimens with the condition. More recent analysis concludes that these were just coincidental findings and those previous dietary restrictions of nuts, popcorn hulls, sunflower seeds, pumpkin seeds, caraway seeds, and sesame seeds were unnecessary. Although there is no scientific evidence showing statistical improvement, most scientists believe that a higher fiber diet may well be helpful in diverticulosis and has the added advantage that it may reduce cholesterol levels and the risk of colon cancer as well. Fiber is also an important prebiotic, and thus may be beneficial to improving the health of the gut microbiome.

Elevator (see Atmospheric Pressure, Fart Aroma, Fart, Diffusion)

Elevators are a source of frustration and humor when it comes to intestinal gas in confined small places. There is an underlying science as to why farts are more likely to occur when going up as opposed to coming down. Additional insights can be gathered by reading the entries on atmospheric pressure, altitude, ideal gas laws, fart aroma, and diffusion.

Shutterstock/g-stockstudio

Enzyme

Enzyme deficiencies can lead to inadequate digestion of foods, which can result in excess material for the gut microbes to ferment with excess gas production. Enzymes are large molecules that are highly selective catalysts that greatly accelerate metabolic reactions. These range from the digestion of food to the synthesis of proteins and DNA. They are often described as being analogous to a lock and key. Most enzymes are proteins that have specific three-dimensional structure that acts like a key, with the substrate acting as a lock.

| Substrate entering active site of enzyme | Enzyme/substrate complex | Enzyme/products complex | Products leaving active site of enzyme |

The molecules at the beginning of the process are called substrates, and are converted into different molecules called products. Most enzyme reaction rates are millions of times faster than reactions without the presence of the enzyme catalyst, and the enzymes are not consumed by the reactions and can be reused. Enzyme activity can be affected by other molecules such as inhibitors that decrease enzyme activity and activators that increase activity. Many pharmaceutical products, active ingredients from plants, and poisons are enzyme inhibitors or activators.

Five food Enzyme Families

Digesting sugar sources requires
the enzyme Maltase

Digesting fat from all sou
requires the enzyme lipa

Lipase

Digesting sources of carbohydrates
requires the enzyme
Amylase

Digesting sources of da
requires the enzyme Lac

Cellulase

Amylase

Amylase

Lactase

Protease

Digesting Fiber from grains
requires the enzyme
Cellulase

Digesting protein
nuts, beans, and
requires an enz
like protease

Grains | Vegetables | Fruits | Milk | Meat & Beans

Many believe that raw food contains it's own specific enzymes to
assist the body in breaking it down into nutrients for proper digestion.

PROTEIN DIGESTION

Substrate	Extracellular enzymes		Intestinal mucosal enzymes	End Products
Protein	Pepsin Trypsin	Carboxypeptidase A	Aminopeptidase Tripeptidase	Amino Acids
	Chymotrypsin Elastases	Carboxypeptidase B	Dipeptidase	
Nucleoprotein	Protein	Ribonuclease	Oligonucleotidase 5' Nucleotidase	Purine Bases Pyrimidine Bases Pentose-1-PO_4
	Hydrolysis	Deoxyribonuclease	Alkaline Phosphatase Adenosine Deaminase	

CARBOHYDRATE DIGESTION

Substrate	Extracellular enzymes	Intestinal mucosal enzymes	End Products
Amylose Amylopectin Glycogen	α Amylase	Maltase Isomaltase	Glucose
Chitin	Chitinase	Chitobiase	Glucosamine
Sucrose		Sucrase	Glucose Fructose
Lactose		Lactase	Glucose Galactose
Trehalose		Trehalase	Glucose

LIPID DIGESTION

Substrate	Extracellular enzymes	Intestinal mucosal enzymes	End Products
Triglycerides	Lipase Colipase		β-mono-glyceride Fatty Acids
Phospholipids	Phospholipase	Phosphatase	Alcohols Fatty Acids Phosphate
Cholesterol Esters	Cholesterol Esterase		Cholestrol Fatty Acid
Waxes	Lipase		Monohydric Alcohol Fatty Acid

Enzyme Type	Enzyme	Function
Carbohydrate-Specific Enzymes	Amylase, Alpha-Amylase	Converts complex starch in root vegetables and grains into maltose (a disaccharide), maltotriose (a trisaccharide), dextrins, and oligosaccharides
	Glucoamylase	Converts maltose, maltotriose, and oligosaccharides into glucose
Sugar-Specific (Disaccharide) Enzymes	Lactase	Converts lactose (milk sugar) into glucose and galactose
	Maltase	Digests maltose in malt, cereal grains, and processed foods into glucose
	Sucrase (Invertase)	Converts sucrose (table sugar) into glucose and fructose; forms sucrase-isomaltase complex in the intestinal lining that breaks down dextrins
	Pullulanase	Breaks down amylopectin starch molecules resistant to degradation that may otherwise remain trapped in the microvilli and contribute to inflammation
Vegetable/Fiber-Specific Enzymes	Cellulase, Hemicellulase	Liberates nutrients from fruits and vegetables, making them more bioavailable
	Alpha-Galactosidase	Breaks down hard-to-digest carbohydrates found in legumes and cruciferous vegetables
	Pectinase	Hydrolyzes pectin; reduces the bulking effect of some fibrous foods
	Phytase	Breaks down phytates in grains (wheat, oats, barley) and legumes
	Beta-Glucanase	Breaks down glucans in cereal grains and in yeast cell walls
	Galactomannase	Degrades hemicellulose, cellulose, and cell walls with mannose
Protein and Peptide-Specific Enzymes	Acid and Alkaline Protease	Breaks down plant, vegetable, and meat derived proteins
	Peptidase and Dipeptidyl Peptidase IV (DPP-IV)	Breaks down casein (dairy products) and gluten (wheat, barley, rye) and their exorphin peptides
Fat-Specific Enzymes	Lipase	Hydrolyzes fats in meat and dairy products, oils in nuts and seeds, and triglycerides
Specialty Enzymes	Lysozyme (highly purified from egg white)	Degrades polysaccharides found in the cell walls of many bacteria, yeast, and other pathogens
	Serratia Peptidase	Breaks down casein protein peptides; breaks down fibrin and protects sensitive GI tissues from irritation and inflammation

There are a wide variety of enzyme deficiencies and food intolerances that can be major contributors to gaseous distension and flatulence. Taking a Sherlock Holmes approach and trying an elimination diet is certainly reasonable. Enzyme supplements are commercially available and are another approach for an empiric trial if the suspect foods are not well defined. Medications can also interfere with enzyme activity and give rise to flatulence. Enzymes include proteases that digest proteins such as pepsin, pepsinogen, trypsin, trypsinogen, chymotrypsin, and chymotrypsinogen. Other enzymes include amylase, lipase, invertase, sucrose, maltase, lactase, and about one thousand six-hundred others!

It is important to take the appropriate enzyme with the appropriate food. The right enzyme for the wrong food, or the wrong enzyme for the right food, will not make a bit of difference in helping your digestion. The most common enzyme deficiency is lactase resulting in lactose intolerance. With over one thousand six-hundred known enzymes it is best to do your own Sherlock Holmes detective work with elimination diets or challenges to identify the foods you are best to avoid, or others will be avoiding you because of the intestinal gas that results.

*Air*Veda: Ancient & New Medical Wisdom

All plants harbor the ability to generate digestive enzymes to break down the starch content of their own seeds and fruit. That is how the fertilized seed gets its nutrition for growth. In fact, we can take advantage of this property to ease our digestion of plants by letting them germinate before ingesting them. For some plants like sprouts and beans that is a very doable suggestion. For other fruits and plants by the time they germinate the starches have lost all culinary appeal to us. What may be surprising is the variety and diversity of enzymes the plants generate across various species. They number in the thousands and the vast majority have yet to be identified and analyzed. The development of plant genomics has accelerated our understanding of the vast diversity of enzymes we are exposed to. A number of plants also generate proteases to digest the plant storage proteins that a number of varieties have a rich storehouse of. For example, wheat has many endopeptidases. The plant world also uses proteolytic enzymes in defense against insect pests, to avoid being consumed by animals that do not assist them in their propagation.

Eructation (Burp, Belch) (see Aerophagia, Gastroesophageal Reflux Disease)

Commonly called a burp or belch the words are now synonymous with the medical term eructation. The English language, as all living languages, continues to evolve. Today the words are interchangeable but they were not always synonymous. In older times, a burp was considered an involuntary release of gas from the stomach. Encouraged and admired in infants and young children, tolerated in most cultures and societies if not in mixed company, and frowned upon by the female spouse, it was recognized as an involuntary act of nature. The belch however took on a more sinister demeanor being considered a voluntary and thus controllable outburst of gastric gasses. Although considered a talent worthy of development by adolescent males and those who remain in that mindset through their adult years, most of society frowns upon the activity.

Burping or belching may be a symptom of a hiatal hernia, GERD, or of lower esophageal sphincter dysfunction. The other dysfunction that is often associated with GERD and can lead to burping and belching is a motility disorder of the esophagus known as transient relaxation of the lower esophageal sphincter. As you can imagine, the lower esophageal sphincter (LES) isn't supposed to be tightly closed all of the time. The lower esophageal sphincter needs to relax every time you swallow to allow the material ingested to enter the stomach. It also needs to relax whenever you need to burp, belch, or vomit to allow for material to exit as well. The condition of transient relaxation of the LES is where the relaxation occurs for unknown reasons at an abnormal time, often without warning. It is much as if a security gate that is only supposed to open for authorized traffic opens on its own at random times. Many food products, herbs, pharmaceuticals, and social habits can contribute to relaxation of the lower esophageal sphincter by their carminative properties. The ability to identify and avoid these products may be the key to controlling gastroesophageal reflux disease without requiring expensive prescription therapy with potential side effects.

Baby bottles are a common source of aerophagia, air swallowing. Burping the baby after the feeding helps to release the swallowed air. Shutterstock/JohannaGoodyear

Burping the baby after the feeding helps to release the swallowed air.
Shutterstock/GoldenPixels

Air swallowing is a universal event in humans and is also known as aerophagia. We do it with every one of the on average two thousand swallows we take every day, ingesting approximately five milliliters (one teaspoonful) of air with every swallow. Air is seventy-eight percent nitrogen, which is a poorly absorbed gas. If it is not released in a burp, it will contribute to bloating and distension. The volume of air swallowed is impressive, but is only a small percentage of what the digestive process can generate in terms of gas production.

Aerophagia is the swallowing of air, allowing it to enter the digestive tract, and it occurs naturally and without thinking in every individual. There is a variation of aerophagia in which the behavior becomes a purposeful, and at times obsessive-compulsive, behavior. More often, when excessive spontaneous aerophagia is occurring it is a subconscious or unconscious behavior, much like a nervous tic. The volume of air swallowed in these conditions can be impressive, and a plain x-ray of the abdomen may demonstrate that the entire digestive tract is filled with air from esophagus to rectum.

The important fact is that seventy-eight percent of air is nitrogen and the gastrointestinal tract poorly absorbs the nitrogen, unlike the oxygen and carbon dioxide. Once the nitrogen is swallowed it has only two ways to get out of the digestive tract. Coming up as a burp or belch is its closest exit, but it has to overcome the lower esophageal sphincter, the upper esophageal sphincter and the oncoming rush with peristalsis and gravity of more food, fluid, drink, saliva, and yes even more air being swallowed.

4.bp.blogspot.com Creative Commons License

Eructation is common after the ingestion of carbonated or nitrogenated (also called nitrogenized) beverages. The gas is kept in solution in the beverage while under the high pressure generated at the time of bottling or canning. Once the vessel pressure is released the release of gas is visible as bubbles arising in the beverage. When the beverage is ingested the bubbles of gas escape within the stomach. The common increase in temperature from a cold or room temperature beverage to higher internal temperature of the body also contributes to increasing the gas volume. The stomach will expand along with the gas accumulation until the intra-gastric pressure exceeds the pressure maintained by the lower esophageal sphincter. Once the sphincter pressure is exceeded the gas escapes as an eructation. The aroma of the gastric contents may escape with the eructation, so alcohol and the most recent meal ingested may discerned by those in near proximity.

A hidden source of swallowed air is the air content present within many foods. Many fruits contain a great deal more air than you would have imagined. If you take an apple and press all of the juice out, you would have all of the air removed. When you add the volume of the juice and the pressed fruit together you will find that it was only sixty percent of the volume of the original fruit. In other words, of the entire fruit that you ate forty percent was air.

We have been in love with ice cream for thousands of years. All ice creams are not prepared in an identical manner. There is another important factor that leads to differences besides the ingredients such as cream or milk fat content, flavorings, sweeteners, stabilizers, emulsifiers, lactose, whey, casein, etcetera. It may be surprising to learn that the two largest ingredients in ice cream by volume are water (between fifty-five percent and sixty-four percent) and air (between three percent and fifty percent).

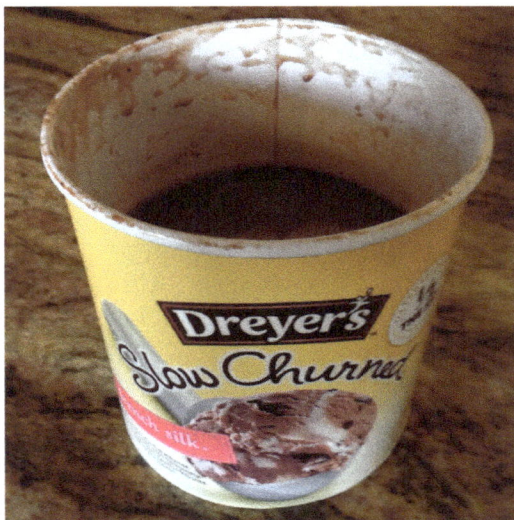

Overrun is the term used to describe air that is added into the finished food product to expand its volume as well as for texture. Air content of ice cream ranges from three percent to fifty percent and has a significant influence on texture, taste, and the value of the product purchased since ice cream is typically sold by volume, not weight. Photo by Lizabeth Weiss.

The same proposition is true for bread and most baked goods. The baking process often uses baking powder or yeast. When the dough rises you are seeing the additional volume of gasses such as carbon dioxide being produced by the yeast fermentation process. While we are on the subject of yeast, microbes of this type including *Candida albicans* are a normal constituent of the gut microbiome. Just like one sees with the rising of dough, the yeast organisms ferment carbohydrates and starches resulting in the release of gas. Excess yeast may lead to increase gaseousness. One of the thoughts as to why beer is known for producing intestinal gas are the residual yeast and carbohydrates, in addition to the nitrogen and carbon dioxide gasses already added to the beverage.

Many foods are whipped with air to increase their volume, which adds to the smoothness and creaminess of the product. It also adds to the bottom line of profitability to the manufacturer, as you are paying the commercial price for a product typically sold by volume, for extra air that virtually did not cost them anything. As long as they don't push it to the detriment of flavor and texture the more air added to a product increases its volume and profitability.

*Air*Veda: Ancient & New Medical Wisdom

Carbonated beverages are very popular worldwide. In the United States sales of carbonated beverages exceed twenty billion dollars per year, four times the sales volume of dairy products. The majority consumed today already comes carbonated with large amounts of carbon dioxide forced into solution under high pressure. As the pressure seal of the can or bottle is released the carbon dioxide forms bubbles and comes out of the solution, giving a pleasant tickling sensation on the palate, and a full at times bloated feeling in the stomach and gut.

Nitrogen is poorly soluble in liquids, and the high density of bubbles contributes to a smooth creamy mouth feel. Most beers are saturated with a combination of thirty percent carbon dioxide and seventy percent nitrogen. The head serves both an aesthetic purpose, as well as accomplishing the dispersal of the beer aroma. You can get an idea of how high the nitrogen content is by looking at the size of the head created. A significant percentage of the volume of your drink is the head, and a friendly bartender will discard some of the head to give you more drink for your money, as well as to encourage a larger gratuity. Beer drinkers are famous for the burping and belching generated. The added nitrogen gives them an edge up in competitive burping and belching contests since it is not as rapidly absorbed and eliminated via the lungs as is carbon dioxide.

Yeast microbes including *Candida albicans* are a normal constituent of the gut microbiome. Just like one sees with the rising of dough, the yeast organisms ferment carbohydrates and starches resulting in the release of gas. Excess yeast may lead to increase gaseousness. One of the thoughts as to why beer is known for producing intestinal gas are the residual yeast and carbohydrates, in addition to the nitrogen and carbon dioxide gasses already added to the beverage. Nitrogen is also used in iced coffee beverages, providing a head of bubbles very similar to that of beer. Aerophagia is common with the use of chewing tobacco and even smoking tobacco whether as cigar, pipe, cigarette, or electronic smokeless cigarette. If you hold a conversation while you are eating it will cause even more air swallowing, as will drinking from a straw or tilting your head back to drink from a bottle or can. Rush through your meals and you swallow more air. See entry on aerophagia for more details

Longest burp at 18.1 seconds. youtu.be/gU3jBonhsrQ.

The World Burping Federation located in Geneva Switzerland holds the annual World Burping Championships. The *Guinness Book of World Records* has a listing for the loudest burp on record. The record holder is Paul Hunn of the United Kingdom. His burp was recorded with a car horn equivalent rating of nearly one hundred and ten decibels. The longest burp, by Tim Janus, has been recorded at over eighteen seconds. To achieve this record, he consumed approximately two gallons of Diet Coke and Mountain Dew. Imagine what would have happened if he swallowed a few Mentos tablets at the time of the competition.

Esophagus (Gullet, Foodpipe)

Esophagus (Greek oisophagos "entrance for eating.") (gullet) is a muscular passageway from the pharynx to the stomach. During swallowing, food passes from the mouth through the pharynx into the esophagus and travels via peristalsis to the stomach. There is an upper esophageal sphincter where it adjoins the pharynx and a lower esophageal sphincter where it joins the stomach, typically just below the diaphragm.

The lower esophageal sphincter is also referred to as the cardiac sphincter and gastroesophageal sphincter. It is a ring shaped area of high muscle tone at the distal esophagus typically just below the diaphragm that acts as a one valve to prevent gastroesophageal reflux except when vomiting is necessary. The lower esophageal sphincter is under involuntary control and is usually in a closed position. It relaxes during a swallow to allow the passage of the food bolus. In cases of gastroesophageal reflux disease, it may also relax inappropriately allowing acidic gastric contents back into the esophagus causing heartburn and mucosal damage. Lower esophageal sphincter pressure and relaxation are regulated by excitatory (e.g., acetylcholine, substance P) and inhibitory (e.g., nitric oxide, vasoactive intestinal peptide) neurotransmitters. Disorders of the lower esophageal sphincter can lead to the common disorder of gastroesophageal reflux disease (GERD) and its frequent symptom of heartburn. It also plays a major role in other conditions such as achalasia, nutcracker esophagus, and diffuse esophageal spasm.

The esophagus is normally lined by squamous epithelium similar to the mucous membrane lining the inside of the mouth. This epithelium is sensitive to acid and digestive enzymes and a competent lower esophageal sphincter is critical to protect it from reflux if gastric contents.

The symptom of heartburn is typically ascribed to the reflux or regurgitation of acidic stomach contents and may be a sign of gastro esophageal reflux disease (GERD). A number of esophageal disorders are associated with reflux and abnormalities of its motility. Unfortunately, cancer of the esophagus is not uncommon and its hallmark symptom of difficulty swallowing due to partial obstruction may make its first appearance when the disease is already incurable.

Pressure differential between intra-thoracic negative pressure of 5 mm of mercury vs. intra-abdominal positive pressure of 5 mmm of mercury, and lower esophageal sphincter (LES) pressure of positive 25 mm of mercury. Author presentation image.

Fart (Flatus)

The word fart is the correct word to use in the English language, and indeed is one of its oldest words. The alternative terms used, such as flatus and flatulence are not original English words as they have been borrowed from the Latin. There is controversy as to the derivation of the word fart. It is thought to have Indo-European roots in the Germanic language word farzen. One thought is that it originated as an onomatopoeia, a word that phonetically imitates the sound of the event it describes. Another thought is that it was related to the term for partridge, as the bird makes a similar sound when it is disturbed in its natural habitat and takes flight.

Farts are ubiquitous, all living creatures generate gas from the cellular respiration, and humans are no exception. The microorganisms in your intestinal flora produce microscopic nanofarts and microfarts, which collect into larger bubbles of gas in the bowel. They are intermixed with the atmospheric air swallowed throughout the day and particularly at meals, when chewing gum, when chewing tobacco, or when smoking tobacco or other recreational products.

onpasture.com Creative Commons License

Aerophagia is universal, and we swallow on average three to five milliliters (one teaspoonful) of air with every swallow. Even when we are not eating or drinking, we regularly swallow the saliva we produce. The average human swallows over two thousand times a day. Chewing gum, hard candies, and use of chewing or smoking tobacco or other recreational products increase the volume of air swallowed. Drinking through a straw, directly from a can or bottle, or talking while eating, will also increase the amount of air swallowed.

Another common source of swallowed air is within the foods we eat. An apple is forty percent air by volume, and bread is over sixty percent air by volume. If you compress an apple or a loaf of bread, you will see that a sizeable portion of their total volume is air. Whipped foods, soufflés, and baked goods, all have high air content. Have you ever forgotten to put an ice cream container back in the freezer? Ice cream is typically forty percent air by volume and when it melts the air escapes, and the full container is no longer full. By the way, the ice cream industry knows that adding air, known in the industry as overage, enhances the mouth feel texture of the ice cream. They also know that it adds up to forty percent to the profit margin, because ice cream is sold by volume, not by weight.

Besides the swallowed air, additional gasses are produced during the enzymatic digestive processes, as well as the neutralization of gastric hydrochloric acid and pancreatic and duodenal bicarbonate. The result is that a large volume of gasses transits the bowel and a portion may be eliminated as a fart. Fortunately, the vast majority of the gasses produced are absorbed by the gut and then through diffusion into the bloodstream where it enters into solution. The gasses leave the blood when they arrive at the alveoli of the lungs where they are exhaled. The chemical component gasses have very different properties of diffusion through the bowel wall and into solution in the bloodstream.

Carbon dioxide readily diffuses and enters solution and is readily exhaled. It is the largest component of the volume of gas generated in the proximal intestinal tract. It is a major contributor to the temporary distension and discomfort that commonly occurs after a meal. Carbonation is also utilized as a common beverage enhancer and adds to the volume of carbon dioxide gas in the stomach. Carbon dioxide is the most rapidly absorbed component of intestinal gas and is the easiest to eliminate by simply exhaling it in the breath. As very little remains in the bowel, it is only a relatively minor component of a fart.

Average Fart Composition

Nitrogen 59%, Hydrogen 21%, Carbon Dioxide 9%, Methane 7%, Oxygen 4%

Creative Commons License

The volume of gasses in the gastrointestinal tract is dependent on many factors. The volume of gas produced is determined by the amount and nature of foods ingested, and the body's ability to synthesize and utilize specific enzymes for the various food types. The nature and quantity of the bacteria in the gut flora influences the nature of intestinal gas both by their active metabolism and by their ability to aid or hinder the digestive enzymes and processes.

*Air*Veda: Ancient & New Medical Wisdom

One of the most common causes of excess gaseousness is the deficiency of the enzyme lactase. Lactase hydrolyses the complex disaccharide dairy sugar lactose into the readily absorbable monosaccharide sugars glucose and galactose. With insufficient lactase, the sugar molecule is not metabolized by the digestive system but is instead metabolized by the gut flora, also known as the microbiome. Lactase deficiency results in gas production and may also give rise to cramps and diarrhea. Another food sugar that can cause excess gaseousness is commonly seen in fruit and is thus known as fructose. The human digestive system can handle only a limited quantity of fructose at a time. If the fructose intake exceeds this capacity the gut flora ferments this sugar, with the release of gas, and often cramps and diarrhea.

That the microbes within our digestive tracts ferment foods that we have not fully digested is to our advantage, which is why the microbiome is considered essential to our good health. We can absorb some of the nutrients the microbes release in the fermentation process, including vitamins and bioactive molecules. We even use microbe fermentation in the preparation of many foods. When you add yeast to flour and watch the dough rise you are seeing the result of the release of gasses from the fermentation process. The spongy character of bread and cakes, and why they are sixty percent air by volume, is the result of the gas production of the yeast fungus. The characteristic holes in Swiss cheese are the result of microbial gas production. The entire production of wines, beer, and other alcohol beverages are based on microbial fermentation. In a very literal sense, we are ingesting the waste product of microbial fermentation.

Before you develop an opinion that a delicious baked good dependent on yeast farts loses some of its culinary appeals, recognize that this paradox was addressed hundreds of years ago. A French pastry delicacy is known as Pets de Nonne, also called Pets de Sœurs and translated as nun's farts. They are a dessert puff pastry dating from medieval times and made from butter, milk, flour, sugar, eggs and sometimes honey is added. They are traditionally pan-fried in lard and then baked. Their lightness inspired their name in French, pets de nonne and Pets de Sœurs. Another baked good named for its association with the fart is Pumpernickel (German: Devil's Fart) bread. It is a heavy dark brown bread traditionally made with coarsely ground rye flour and whole rye berries. It has been long associated with the Westphalia region of Germany for over five hundred years. Like most rye breads, it is traditionally made with an acidic sourdough starter, which inhibits the rye amylase enzymes. The name is associated with the coarse bread-giving rise to flatulence.

Beans are known as the musical fruit because of the gas they produce in all humans. The reason for this is that legumes contain complex sugars known as raffinose, verbascose, and stachyose. Humans and other animals lack the enzyme, called alpha-galactosidase, needed to metabolize these complex sugars into absorbable simple sugars. Without the enzyme, the complex sugars are fermented by the gut microbiome producing gas. Alpha-galactosidase is now commercially available as a dietary enzyme supplement to reduce the gas production associated with particular foods such as legumes. Another enzyme that humans do not possess is cellulase, without which we cannot digest the cellulose found in most plants and grasses. Herbivorous animals do have those enzymes, which is why they can subsist on grazing of grasses and forage.

Another factor in gas production is the speed of gastrointestinal transit. Drugs, hormones, food products, and illness may influence this. The absorptive capacity and health of the mucosal lining, and the physical length of the individual's gastrointestinal tract also play a role. The often-quoted figure of twelve farts per day is a reasonable approximation of the average number of farts passed, but there is a very wide range of what is considered normal. Besides the numerical quantity of farts passed per day is the question of what is considered an average volume of gas passed. If you are familiar with physics, a series of natural laws were defined that express the relationship between temperature, pressure, and volume. The relationship between temperature and pressure is direct, i.e. the higher the temperature, the larger the volume of space a gas would occupy.

The expansion to a larger volume of occupied space may result in intestinal bloating, discomfort, and increased burping and farting. The relationship with pressure is inverse, i.e. the greater the pressure, the smaller the volume. We experience a change in intestinal gas volume based on temperature when we drink a cold carbonated or nitrogenated beverage. As the temperature of the gas increases from refrigerated to body temperature the gas volume increases dramatically. We will also often experience significant changes in volume due to pressure changes, as beverages from highly pressurized containers are exposed to the much lower pressures found within the intestinal tract they expand dramatically. Increases in pressure reduce the volume of gas, which is not a problem when it comes to the gut and our symptoms of gas if atmospheric pressure is increasing, such as with scuba diving or going down a mine shaft. It can become a major problem when the pressure decreases and the gas volume increases such as upon ascent from a dive or a mine, or going higher in altitude such as air travel or mountain climbing.

The atmospheric pressure changes as we go higher or lower from sea level. The effects on intestinal gas are seen in scuba divers, pilots, airplane passengers, mountain climbers, living at higher elevations, and even taking an elevator to the top of a skyscraper. When the pressure change is rapid, for example, a scuba diver returning to the surface, or an astronaut on the ascent to orbit, the consequences can be dramatic and life threatening and are known as barotrauma. Most gasses that are commercially available (oxygen, helium, air, etc.) are compressed and contained in hardened metal canisters that can withstand very high pressure. Compression of the gas allows for significant savings of space, for example allowing scuba divers to have the equivalent of a roomful of air within a single tank. The intestinal tract is flexible and expandable to a degree, more like a balloon than a metal container. As such changes in the surrounding atmospheric pressure can result in significant volume changes, which in the extreme of barotrauma may lead to perforation and rupture.

The fart would not be as notorious as it is if it were not for its aroma. Over ninety-nine percent of the gasses in a fart are odorless. While a number of individuals may have methane present in their farts, methane is odorless. If you smell a natural gas (methane) leak, it is not the methane you smell, but an odorant gas added by the gas company as a safety precaution to give notice of danger. The majority of the aroma from a fart comes from hydrogen sulfide, skatole, indole, and aromatic fatty acids, the majority coming from the digestion of animal fats. While vegetarians may fart more than carnivores, the aroma is not nearly as pungent or offensive.

Aerophagia is universal, and we swallow on average three to five milliliters (one teaspoonful) of air with every swallow. Added into the mixture are the gasses produced during the enzymatic digestive processes as well as the neutralization of gastric hydrochloric acid and pancreatic and duodenal bicarbonate. The result is a large volume of gasses transiting the bowel that may be eliminated as a fart. Fortunately, the vast majority of the gasses produced are absorbed by the gut, then into the bloodstream through diffusion dissolving into solution. They are finally released when they reach the alveoli of the lungs and are exhaled. The component gasses have very different properties of diffusion through the bowel wall and into the bloodstream.

Carbon dioxide readily diffuses, enters solution, and is readily exhaled. It is the largest volume of gas generated and is the major contributor to distension and postprandial (after meal) discomfort. The good news is it is the easiest to eliminate from the bowel because of its rapid diffusion into the bloodstream. Carbon dioxide is only a minor contributor to flatulence. The volume of gasses in the gastrointestinal tract is dependent on the quantity and nature of foods ingested, and the body's ability to synthesize and utilize specific enzymes for the various food types.

The nature and number of microorganisms in the gut flora also play a major role. It may also be affected by the speed of gastrointestinal transit, which likewise may be influenced by drugs, hormones, food product, illness, absorptive capacity, and the physical length of the individual's gastrointestinal tract. The often-quoted figure of eleven and one-half farts per day is a reasonable approximation of the average number of farts passed, but there is a very wide range of what is considered normal. There are so many variables that what is reasonable for an individual can only be determined over a longer period than a single day.

Fart, Art

The fart has been the subject of numerous works of art over the ages. It has been represented in virtually all of the artistic media including literature, music, paintings, sculpture, cinema, photography, etcetera. It has been the material for live and stage performances for thousands of years, and of course is notorious for personal and up-close entertainment. The following images are just a few of the visual representations over the years. A thorough review of the fart through the arts is found in the unique companion volume to this book, entitled *Artsy Fartsy, Cultural History of the Fart.*

James Gillray, *Scientific Researches! New Discoveries in PNEUMATICKS! or an Experimental Lecture on the Powers of Air*. Public Domain

Louis-Léopold Boilly *Thirty-Six Faces of Expression*. Public Domain

Richard Newton, Public Domain

Fart, Diffusion

The word Fart in northern European languages including German and the Scandinavian languages means speed. In you go by a school or hospital you may go by a no farting zone. Or you might receive a police citation for exceeding the fart limit! The sense of smell requires that molecules from the source material travel to the nasopharynx and touch the olfactory nerve receptors. The detection of a fart by odor requires the direct contact of the odorant molecule and the cilia of the nerve cell. Most people do not realize that a fart actually contains odorants as well as transmissible microbes, so although not as well recognized as a source of communicable disease like a sneeze or a cough, a fart could reasonably be considered a public health hazard, as well as a nuisance.

It is possible to become ill and acquire a pathogenic infection from a fart, similar to what can occur with a cough or sneeze. Coughing and sneezing release a large plume of aerosolized droplets impregnated with microbial pathogens. A single sneeze can disperse up to forty thousand aerosol droplets, which can transmit pathogens and disease. The sneeze is a much more effective dispersant of infectious material than a cough, speaking, or squeaking a fart. On the other hand, the farts plume of microbes is of fecal origin, giving rise to an entirely different microbial exposure, consistent with the fecal oral contamination route of many communicable diseases.

Shutterstock/JamesKlotz

Sneezes reach a velocity of up to five hundred miles per hour (eight hundred kilometers per hour) Some sneezes are so loud the volume may give the impression that they have broken the sound barrier! Shutterstock/RioPatuca

A sneeze, or sternutation, is a powerful rapid expulsion of air from the lungs through the nose and mouth. The average velocity of a sneeze is forty-two meters per second), equivalent to approximately ninety-five miles per hour. The average speed of a cough is fifteen meters per second and the average velocity of the breath of ordinary speech is four meters per second. The sneeze and cough can quickly reach a velocity of over one hundred miles per hour (one hundred and fifty kilometers per hour) and has been recorded at speeds up to five hundred miles per hour (nine hundred and fifty kilometers per hour). These discharges will spread contaminants throughout a large size room. The flushing of a toilet will aerosolize fecal microbes that would cover a room with dimensions of twenty feet by twenty feet in a matter of seconds.

The mechanism of increasing intra-abdominal pressure for a fart is similar to generating intra-thoracic pressure for a sneeze. The size of the exit orifice is a major determinant of velocity. No one has voluntarily gotten close enough to a fart blast to measure its ejection velocity or count the vapor droplets. The brave soul who does so may not get a Nobel Prize, but would certainly be worthy of nomination for an IgNobel Prize.

Farts have been recorded with the speed of aroma travel at a conservative ten miles per hour. It was not clear if this was from an individual wearing clothing at the time. Science or a dedicated researcher somewhere will one day answer the question about fart speed. Perhaps a luxury watch company will sponsor a competition for the *Guinness Book of World Records* which has a number of fart categories already entered into the competitive arena, but somehow missed out on the exciting competition of fart speed!

Back in the 1946 a spoof recording of the International Crepitation Contest was created, and it is still commercially available today. It was produced by recording engineers for the Canadian Broadcasting Corporation and was supposedly held on February 31, 1946 as the World Championship Crepitation Contest. The fictitious location of the Maple Leaf Auditorium at Thunderblow, Canada between competitors Paul Boomer and Lord Windesmear completed the scene for the blow-by-blow description of the announcer.

Fart, Etymology

English is the richest language on the planet, with more words by far in its vocabulary than any other. This richness is due to the significant influence of its history of occupation by foreigners, especially during the days of the Roman Empire. Unlike other conquerors, the Romans did not impose their own language, in this case Latin, on the inhabitants of the British Isles. The population adapted their native tongue to include words borrowed from the occupiers and foreign influences. This led to the rapid expansion of the English vocabulary, including many different words that are synonyms.

The word fart is the correct word to use in the English language, and indeed is one of its oldest words. The alternative terms used, such as flatus and flatulence are not originally English words as they have been borrowed from the Latin. In Latin these words have the general meaning of a wind or a blowing.

There is controversy as to the derivation of the word fart. It is thought to have Indo-European roots in the Germanic language word farzen. The word fart may have originated as an onomatopoeia, a word that phonetically imitates the sound of the event it describes. Another thought is that it was related to the term for partridge, as the bird makes a similar sound when it is disturbed in its natural habitat and takes flight. How it made that transition may be an enlightening example of the evolution of words and language.

The Indo-European word *perd* means fart, and this led to the Latin word *pedere* the verb form of fart, and *peditum* the noun form of fart. The Indo-European *perd* led to the Greek word for fart πέρδομαι *perdomai*. It is also cognate with Sanskrit *pardate*, Avestan *pərəδaiti*, Italian *fare un peto*, French "péter", Russian пердеть (perdet') and Polish "pierd". The related Greek word *perdix* referred to a type of bird that made an explosive fart-like sound when it was flushed from the brush when startled. While being incorporated from Greek to Old French it became *perdriz*, then Middle English *partrich*, and finally Modern English *partridge*. The final step that has yet to be taken would be to complete the circuitous history and modify the name of the partridge to *fartridge*!

The word fart is also found in other languages, but there it often has a different and unrelated meaning. In the Scandinavian languages, it usually denotes speed or motion. In Danish and Norwegian, it is often used in combination with other words that obscures the meaning even more. For example, in Danish a *fartcertifikate* means a trade certificate. In Norwegian, a *fart plan* means a schedule. The Norwegian phrase *stå på fartin* pronounced as stop-a–fartin means ready to leave. Likewise, the phrase *farts måler* pronounced as fart smeller refers to a speedometer. In Swedish, a speed bump is called a *farthinder*. *Fartlek* is speed training for athletes by running at alternate intervals of fast and slow paces.

Likewise, if you travel on a Scandinavian marine vessel, you may see the control of engine speed labeled as *half fart* and *full fart* for half speed and full speed respectively. Fart kontrol zones are speed zones. In Germany, a similar word *fahrt* means a journey, trip, tour, or passage. It is often seen in signs that say *einfahrt* (sounds like in-fart) and *ausfahrt* (sounds like out-fart) denoting entrance and exit respectively.

In Spanish and Portuguese *fart* means an excess of anything, especially food. One of the richest desserts they offer is called a *farte*, which means a fruit tarte in Spain, and usually a sugar almond or cream cake in Portugal. In Italy, the word *farto* means mattress. In Hungary, *fartaj* means buttocks. In Poland, if you want to buy a local favorite candy bar with a name that that means lucky, you will be looking for a *Fart* bar.

Several languages have a number of different words for variations on a theme for which there is only one word in English. The word snow is one example where we have a singular word, but the Inuit, Eskimo, Aleut, Sami and other languages of the native people of the Arctic and northern latitudes may have hundreds of words. When it comes to the word fart, the English language is very limited with just the singular word. I will not leap to the conclusion that the language that has the most words for fart needed to do so for necessity. Their population may or may not have the world's highest rate of fart production, but they certainly have the most descriptive fart words.

The Russian words for fart include *perdyozh* (first act of breaking wind), *perdun* (perpetrator and outcome), *perdil'nik* (place from where it comes), *Perun* (ancient God of wind), *bzdun* (silent fart), *bzdyukha* (silent fart as well as a stupid jerk). Some of the Russian verbs for the action of farting are particularly colorful. *Perdet'* (to fart with or without sound), *bzdet'* (to fart silently), *pereperdet* (to fart repeatedly), and my favorite word *nabzdet'sya* (to fart silently to one's complete and utter satisfaction!).

The word fart is one of the oldest words in the English language. One of the most influential dictionaries in the long history of the language is Samuel Johnson's *A Dictionary of the English Language* published in 1755. An important innovation in his dictionary was the use of quotations from literature to illustrate the usage of the word defined.

SAMUEL JOHNSON, L.L.D.
Public Domain

The word fart is proper English and was in use for hundreds of years before relatively recent polite and civil society considered it taboo. Without an alternative term, euphemisms were created and used. The number of terms that were synonymous with fart numbers in the many hundreds.

FART. *n. f.* [ꝼeꞃꞇ, Saxon.] Wind from behind.

Love is the *fart*
Of every heart;
It pains a man when 'tis kept clofe;
And others doth offend, when 'tis let loofe. *Suckling.*

To FART. *v. a.* [from the noun.] To break wind behind.

As when we a a gun difcharge,
Although the bore be ne'er fo large,
Before the flame from muzzle burft,
Juft at the breech it flafhes firft;
So from my lord his paffion broke,
He *farted* firft and then he fpoke. *Swift.*

Public Domain

The origins of these phrases and their acceptance into the cultural lexicon, are often obscured. Sometimes new words are added directly by an author creatively using a newly invented word in a literary work. I am fond of a new word coined by David Gilmour, an entrepreneur, and philanthropist. He described a word that combines the sense of anticipation and subsequent disappointment, when the experience is not as satisfying as expected. The word he created 'anticipointment' is a portmanteau that should stand the test of time.

I am tempted to add to new words in the lexicon as well. I am using the author's prerogative to place the word in print below, and although I have not heard them elsewhere before, someone may well have created them before me. The word is fartigenic, or its alternative, fartogenic. Fartigenic is a portmanteau combining the word fart, with the Latin root suffix -genic of Genesis and creation fame. The term describes a substance, which induces the creation of a fart. Refried beans and chili con carne would be good examples of fartigenic foods.

The colloquialisms, idioms, and synonyms that for better or for worse, are part of the lexicon can be found in a number of resources including the unique companion volume to this book *Artsy Fartsy, Cultural History of the Fart.* This volume provides an informative and entertaining overview of the fart through human history and culture, including works of literature, music, and the arts.

Fart, Flammable (see Methane, Hydrogen, Oxygen)

The individual gasses that make intestinal gas flammable (inflammable and flammable are synonyms and interchangeable words, their antonym nonflammable means the exact opposite) and explosive are hydrogen, methane, and oxygen. Hydrogen is a chemical element which has the symbol H and atomic number one. It is the lightest element and in its single atom form it is by far the most abundant element in the universe, comprising approximately seventy-five percent of its total identifiable mass. In the earth's atmosphere as the diatomic H_2 molecule, it is a colorless, odorless, tasteless, non-toxic, highly explosive gas. Most of the hydrogen on Earth is in molecules such as water and organic compounds because hydrogen readily forms covalent bonds.

Public Domain

Hydrogen is lighter than air and lighter than helium. Unfortunately, it is also explosively flammable. Hydrogen fires are less destructive to immediate surroundings because of the buoyancy of H_2, which causes the heat of combustion to be released upwards as it ascends in the atmosphere. On May 6, 1937, the hydrogen-filled German airship Hindenburg burst into flames while attempting to land at Lakehurst, New Jersey. In little more than thirty seconds, the largest object ever to soar through the air was incinerated with a tragic great loss of life.

In 1766, Henry Cavendish was the first to identify hydrogen gas. In 1783 Antoine Lavoisier gave the element the name hydrogen (Greek ὕδρω hydro water and γενῆς genes creator) when he and Laplace confirmed Cavendish's finding that water is produced when hydrogen is burned. Methane is produced in the human intestinal tract by microbial organisms. Methanogens are microorganisms of the Kingdom Archaea, not bacteria as previously thought. They produce methane as a metabolic byproduct in anaerobic conditions when oxygen is not present.

Methanogens have been found in a variety of extreme environments, and can thrive and reproduce in boiling water as well as in ice cores taken miles down in arctic glaciers. They are common in wetlands, where they produce marsh gas, and in the digestive tracts of animals and humans where they generate the methane content of flatulence as well as the ruminant belch. It was discovered by Carl Scheele Sweden in 1773, but his publisher delayed publication for two years. The delay in publication inadvertently allowed British clergyman Joseph Priestley, who independently discovered it a year later, to be given priority as its discoverer because his work was published first.

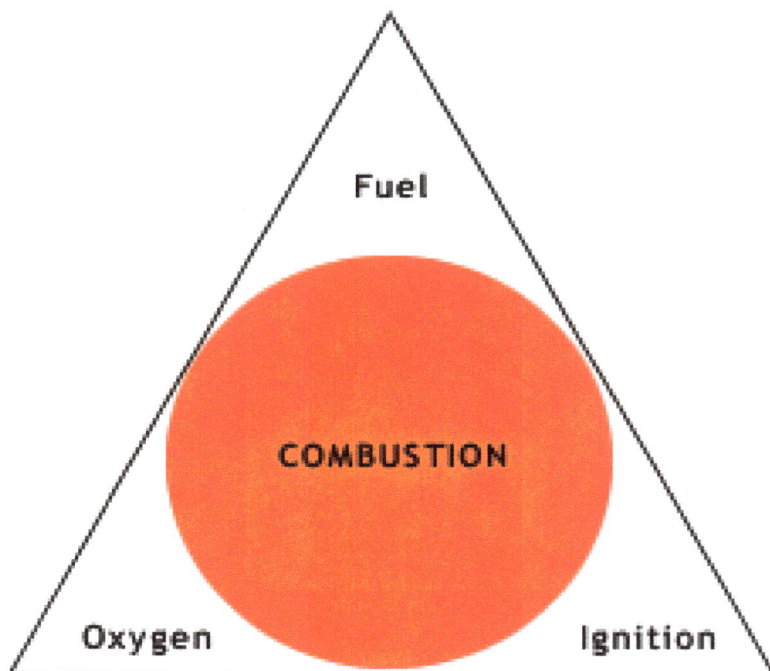

www.omega.com Creative Commons License

Oxygen is a chemical element with symbol O and atomic number eight that forms dioxygen a colorless odorless and tasteless gas. It was mistakenly named Oxygen (the Greek ὀξύς (oxys) "acid", and γόνος (gonos) "producer"), by Antoine Lavoisier because he incorrectly thought that all acids required oxygen. Acids actually require the element hydrogen, not oxygen.

Oxygen is a highly reactive element that forms compounds with most elements except the noble gases. Oxygen is a strong oxidizing agent, and only fluorine has greater electronegativity. Oxygen is the third most abundant element in the universe, after hydrogen and helium. On the surface of the Earth, it is the most abundant element making up half of the earth's crust and nearly twenty-one percent of the air.

AirVeda: Ancient & New Medical Wisdom

Intestinal gas that contains hydrogen or methane, in addition to oxygen, is potentially combustible. Electrical cautery devices used during routine colon and intestinal surgery can potentially ignite these gasses. With the advent of colonoscopy electro-cautery loop snares to remove colon polyps was developed. A few cases of fatal colonic explosions occurred before the danger of explosive intestinal gas was recognized as a risk of the procedure. The bowel preparation solution was found to increase hydrogen and methane gasses and raised the risk of explosion. The bowel preparation has been changed, and carbon dioxide is often used to inflate the colon to reduce the risk of explosion even further.

hydrogen and methane are combustible gasses and in the presence of oxygen and an ignition source, you have a potent flammable commodity. When methane burns, it has a characteristic blue flame that you may see in a pilot light if you have a gas stove or furnace. Adolescent males and those who remain as adolescents intellectually have a fondness for demonstrating their dragon like ability to be human flamethrowers by igniting their farts. The lighting of farts is not a recommended activity, and severe injury has resulted from the successful ignition of flammable gasses near exposed sensitive anatomy.

Shutterstock/Nomad_Soul

One of the more unusual injuries from a lit fart was second and third degree burns on the buttocks and a broken arm. The stout gentlemen was sitting on the toilet defecating and farting extensively for some time. Being overweight his buttocks formed a firm seal around the toilet seat, retaining all of the gasses in the enclosed space of the toilet bowl. He was smoking at the time and made a little space under his cheeks to innocently toss the lit cigarette into the toilet bowl. It promptly ignited blowing him off the seat, shattering the porcelain toilet bowl, and causing extensive burn injuries to his buttocks. His wife called the paramedics, and as he was being carried down the stairwell to the waiting ambulance he told them what caused the explosion. They laughed so hard they dropped the gurney thus breaking his arm.

Moment of ignition of a fart, video is at youtu.be/Zt9rvaijpPY

Hydrogen and methane are the two flammable gasses that may be found in a fart making them flammable. Lighting a fart to see if one produces these gasses is a dangerous activity. Significant burns to the anogenital area have occurred, especially when ignited without a clothing barrier. The popular television show *Mythbusters* filmed an episode confirming that many farts are indeed flammable. It appears that the network found the episode too provocative and, perhaps for liability concerns that children watching might attempt their own demonstrations, decided to not 'air' the episode.

Lighting a match to a pile of cow dung is not a sign of higher intelligence. The methane and hydrogen generated by the microbes active in the manure pile may accumulate to explosive levels.
youtu.be/bZI1eeV88lQ

On occasion dung and excrement can be more than just flammable, it can be explosive. The microorganisms that produce hydrogen and methane that lead to ignitable farts continue their activity while sitting in a pile of manure. For those foolish enough to light a match in a pile of cow dung to see what happens up close and personal the link to the video above should be convincing.

Now that you know intestinal gasses are flammable see if the numbers from the following Internet survey surprise you with how many people already knew this from personal experiments.

Women: Have you ever considered lighting one of your pass intestinal gas?

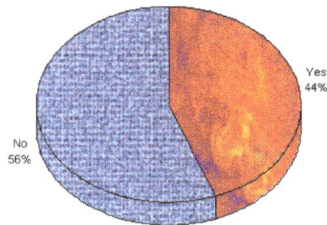

No
56%

Yes
44%

Almost half of the women surveyed indicate that they have considered an attempt to ignite their release of intestinal gas. They may not have done it or tried it, but they have thought about it.

Women: Have you ever attempted lighting one of your passages of intestinal gas?

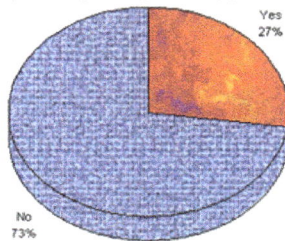

Yes
27%

No
73%

About a quarter of the women surveyed have attempted to ignited their passed intestinal gas.

Women: When you attempted to light your passed intestinal gas, did it ignite?

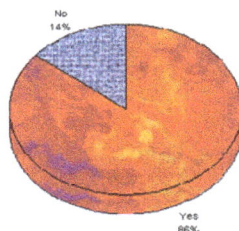

No
14%

Yes
86%

The large majority of women that have made the attempt were successful in confirming that the gas was flammable. The other fourteen percent may not have tried to ignite enough gas, or their diet and gut flora did not generate a flammable mixture of gasses. It appears that most women in the survey passed intestinal gas that burned with a blue flame due to the methane. Those who produced hydrogen had intestinal gas that burned with a yellow flame. Yellow flame was the second most common flame color.

Women: If you have lit your pass intestinal gas have you ever gotten burned?

Women: If you lit your own pass intestinal gas and been burned was the of burn of your body, hair, or pants:

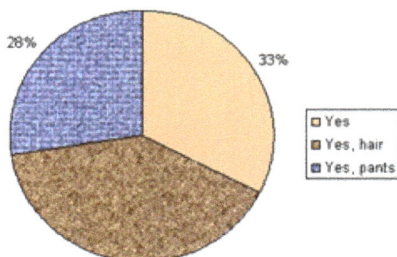

Lighting passed intestinal gas can be very dangerous. About a third of the women that admit lighting their intestinal gas ended up getting some type of burn. About half of these burns consisted of just the singeing of hair. Twenty-eight percent of these burns consist of burning a hole in one's underwear, and thirty-three percent are unfortunate enough to burn their skin.

Women: Have you ever lit another person's intestinal gas?

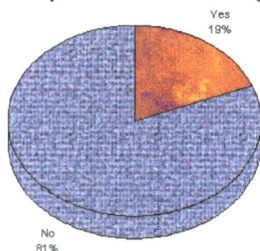

About one-fifth of the women surveyed were brave or foolish enough to light another person's intestinal gas. Most of these experiences were with friends or spouses. About half of the women surveyed admit seeing someone light a fart.

Spontaneous Human Combustion

As explosive and flammable farts are a well-recognized phenomenon, a theory has developed that they may also be responsible for spontaneous human combustion. A rare and bizarre event, spontaneous human combustion has been a proposed explanation of cases where a human body is consumed by flame without an external source of ignition. Typically, the body is incinerated but the surrounding area has not been damaged by fire. Once a body begins to burn the tissue can continue to fuel the flames with a wick effect drawing on melted fat and other tissues.

img.gawkerassets.com

Although the external source could not be identified, there are several potential explanations. Combustible fuel is undoubtedly present, perhaps as the gases methane and hydrogen, flammable clothing and alcohol, as well as body fat. Human fat is similar to the animal fats that were used in tallow candles. The external ignition source may have been a cigarette or spark of static electricity. Curious rural phenomena with similar spontaneous combustion effects include swamp gas, St. Elmo's fire, ball lightning, gamma ray discharges, and others.

Static electricity is an imbalance of electric charges between objects. As the imbalance is discharged with the transfer of electrons between the objects, most people can feel, see, and hear the spark of the static shock. Lightning is a static discharge, different only in its intensity. A spark, which is responsible for the majority of industrial fires and explosions, occurs between objects at different electric potentials.

The energy released in a static electricity discharge may vary over a wide range and the charge buildup increases as the humidity decreases. As little as 0.2 millijoules is the ignition energy required for methane, and a miniscule 0.017 mJ is the ignition energy for hydrogen. The low spark energy is often below the threshold of auditory, visual, or sensory perception of humans and may the source of the ignition that appears to be spontaneous.

The ignition of the flammable gasses of hydrogen and methane often present in a fart may thus appear to be a spontaneous occurrence. Of course, there may have been a more obvious source such as a lit cigarette that was consumed in the event, never to be found. There is a saying in medicine that is used as analogy for the search for a disease that will explain the symptoms. When you hear hoof beats, look for a horse, but be prepared for a zebra.

In spontaneous human combustion, the most likely explanation is an accidental fire from a cigarette. The cigarette may ignite the clothing and then the wicking effect continues to burn fueled by human tissue and fat until the body fire has exhausted itself. To be a bit more creative one can imagine a large fart with hydrogen and methane attracted the pet dog to come over and investigate the noise and smell. Close contact of the pet may have released a static spark and the rest is history. When in doubt, the standard excuse is to simply blame the poor dog.

Fart, Frequency

The fact is that all living creatures create gas from the cellular respiration, which is ubiquitous through a variety of life forms. The bacteria in your intestinal flora generate microscopic nanofarts and microfarts, which collect into larger bubbles of gas in the bowel. They are intermixed with the atmospheric air swallowed throughout the day and particularly at meals, when chewing gum, chewing tobacco, or smoking tobacco or other recreational products.

Aerophagia is universal, and we swallow on average three to five milliliters (one teaspoonful) of air with every swallow. Now add into the mixture the gasses produced during the enzymatic digestive processes as well as the neutralization of gastric hydrochloric acid and pancreatic and duodenal bicarbonate. You now have a virtual windstorm of voluminous gasses transiting the bowel.

Fortunately, the vast majority of the gasses produced are absorbed by the gut. They then enter into the bloodstream through diffusion, finally being exhaled when they reach the alveoli of the lungs. The component gasses have very different properties of diffusion through the bowel wall and into the bloodstream. Carbon dioxide readily diffuses and enters solution and is exhaled. Carbon dioxide is the largest volume of gas generated, and is a major contributor to distension and postprandial (after meal) discomfort. It is also the gas most readily absorbed and eliminated from the bowel. Carbon dioxide is thus only a relatively minor contributor to flatulence.

*Air*Veda: Ancient & New Medical Wisdom

Nitrogen is the largest volume component of atmospheric air, and as would be expected, represents an identically high proportion of the gasses swallowed through aerophagia. Once in the body the carbon dioxide of the air is absorbed and eliminated as discussed above. The nitrogen however, is a very poorly absorbed gas, and will either come back up as a burp or come out the other end as a fart.

The oxygen in the air, representing nearly twenty-one percent of the air gasses swallowed during aerophagia, is absorbed slowly, as the gut is not nearly as efficient at oxygen absorption as the lungs are for respiration. As the carbon dioxide and oxygen are absorbed the percent of the gastrointestinal tract air that is nitrogen increases. As soon as the digestive process begins, the hydrochloric acid of the stomach is neutralized by bicarbonate of the duodenum and pancreas. Large volumes of carbon dioxide gas are generated, as are smaller quantities of hydrogen, methane, and other aromatic gasses.

The amount of gas in the gastrointestinal tract is dependent on the quantity and nature of foods ingested, and the body's ability to synthesize and utilize specific enzymes for the various food types. It is also dependent on the nature and number of the microorganisms in the gut flora, and the speed of gastrointestinal transit. Gastrointestinal transit may be influenced by drugs, hormones, food product, illness, the absorptive capacity of the mucosal lining, and the physical length of the individual's gastrointestinal tract.

The question of what is the average number of farts per day is similar to the question if what is an average price for a typical used car. To answer that question, you would need more information, such as which year, make, model, condition, diesel or gas or electric or hybrid, mileage, etcetera. The quoted figure for fart production of eleven and one-half farts per day is a reasonable approximation. It came from a very small sample size of male medical students, but how one defines normal is subject to a very wide range depending on the variables. The female medical students were too smart to participate in the study, so as far as science knows, women do not fart.

Later suggestions that they fart, but less than the guys, is just as suspect. The differences in the physical attributes of the male and female of a species represent their sexual dimorphism. The theory of sexual selection advanced by Charles Darwin in 1871 is closely associated with sexual dimorphism. On average, adult humans males are four percent taller and eight percent heavier than females. In a number of other species, it is the female that is larger, occasionally dramatically so. The triple wart sea devil, an anglerfish, exhibits extreme sexual dimorphism. The male becomes little more than a stunted sperm-producing body permanently attached to the female. It lives a parasitic existence off of the females hard work and effort in providing livelihood and producing the next generation of offspring. Some human males appear to have evolved their behavioral patterns from the anglerfish modus operandi.

In most mammals, humans included, the males are larger in size, mass, and caloric intake. In most species is the female that is diminutive in size, sometimes dramatically so. It would only make sense that males would generate more gas, but how do the two compare if the caloric intake and composition were identical. Since there are no identically comparable cases studies, one would have to study averages from large populations of each gender and minimize the variables as much as possible.

As curious as we may be to know the answer to this question vital to gender politics and security, no studies are planned or anticipated. There have been reports of extreme flatulence in the medical literature of what may be considered the upper limits of the normal range, up to one hundred and fifty farts in a twenty-four-hour period. There are probably more accurate reports of what is the upper limit of spousal tolerance in divorce court proceedings and depositions.

For general health we talk about achieving our target heart rate during exercise. Is there an equivalent for a target fart rate? For harmonious relationships, ideal would be below the quoted figure of eleven and one-half farts per day, that way you could reasonably suggest that you fart less than average. You could also argue that the twenty-three farts you passed were each only a half-fart so you still are within the normal range.

As we age, we produce less digestive enzymes, and there is an argument to be made that there should be an adjustment and tolerance allowed for 'old farts'. The sheer number of variables allow many explanations for why you fart much less than expected for your given circumstances. But perhaps the best excuse is that you did not do anything, it is the billions of nanofarting and microfarting microorganisms that are to blame. If you are told to pick on someone closer to your own size, you could blame the dog and claim it is a talented ventrilo-farter.

Trying to arrive at a definition of what constitutes a discrete individual fart is a challenge worthy of drafting and getting unanimous approval of a United Nations resolution. Is a staccato stutter, often very small farts completed in rapid succession, to count as one single fart or as ten? Is one large long loud fart the equivalent of four small farts over thirty seconds. Should a loud eardrum shattering tuba blast count the same as a faint and dainty toot? Perhaps the nebulous definition should allow the creator of the uniquely individual fart poetic license.

Fart, Global Warming

Global warming due to greenhouse gas production from human activity is mainly due to deforestation, the combustion of fossil fuels, livestock enteric fermentation and manure management, and landfill emissions. In terms of biomass, bacteria would be the main contributors to global warming by their methane production. A ruminant (Latin *ruminare* - to chew over again) is a mammal that digests plants in a multi compartment stomach through bacterial fermentation. It regurgitates the semi-digested mass, called cud, and chews it again and repeats the swallow.

The process of re-chewing the cud is called "ruminating". There are about one hundred and fifty species of ruminants, which include both domestic and wild species. Ruminating mammals include cattle, goats, sheep, giraffes, yaks, deer, camels, llamas, and antelope.

Other contenders nominated have been termites, which have over two thousand species and are prolific methane producers (initial reports suggested that they produce forty percent of global methane), livestock such as cows, sheep, and pigs, and lastly dinosaurs, which are no longer around to defend their reputations.

Creative Commons License

Ruminant bacterial fermentation is a significant contributor to global methane production, which is over twenty times as potent a greenhouse gas compared to carbon dioxide. To incentivize efforts to reduce livestock methane production a number of countries have proposed taxes on the release of greenhouse gasses. University of Alberta, Canada, Professor Stephen Moore is examining the genes from ruminant stomachs with the goal of developing a cow breed which burps less to reduce methane in the greenhouse gases responsible for global warming. A different approach is being undertaken by Professor of Animal Nutrition Winfried Drochner at the University of Hohenheim, Stuttgart, Germany. A fist-sized plant-based pill bolus combined with a special diet and strict feeding times reduces the methane produced by cows. "Our aim is to increase the wellbeing of the cow, to reduce the greenhouse gases produced and to increase agricultural production all at once. It is an effective way of fighting global warming. We could use the energy to boost the cow's metabolism, the fist-sized tablets mean that microbiotic substances can slowly dissolve in the cow's stomach over several months," said Professor Drochner.

Another method being used to reduce methane emissions is reducing the grass and low efficiency foods the livestock are receiving that require excessive fermentation. Replacing the feed with a diet higher in energy and rich in edible oils can reduce methane production by up to twenty-five percent. New Hampshire-based Stonyfield Farm reduced emissions from their cows an average of twelve percent by adding alfalfa, flax, or hemp to livestock feed. "If every U.S. dairy farmer reduced emissions by twelve per cent it would be equal to about half a million cars being taken off the road," said Nancy Hirshberg, Vice-President of Stonyfield's Natural Resources department. It took extensive scientific experimentation to collect the intestinal gasses of herds of cattle before it was discovered that the methane production was coming from the other end of the cows and other ruminants. It is the burps and belches from the multi compartment ruminant stomach that is the primary source of methane.

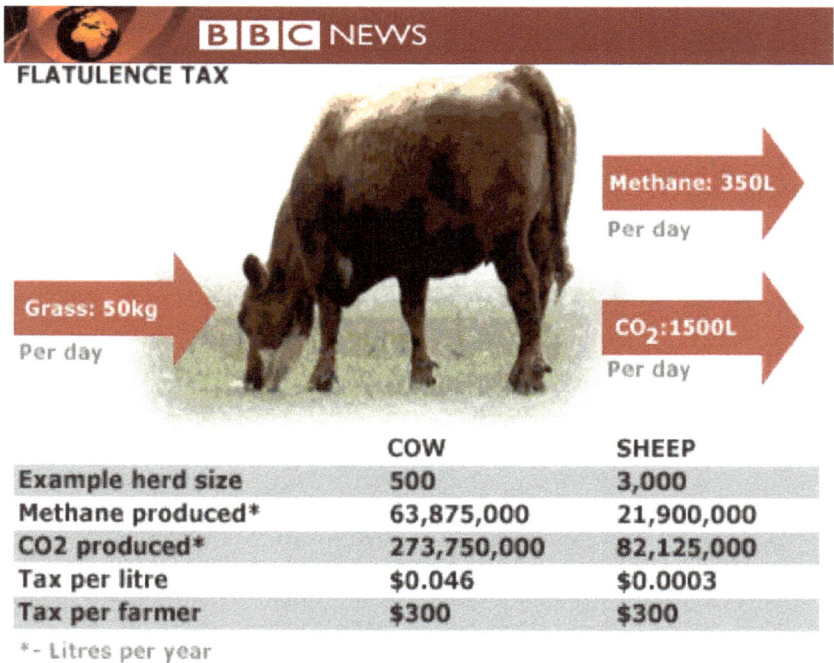

BBC NEWS

FLATULENCE TAX

Methane: 350L Per day

Grass: 50kg Per day

CO_2:1500L Per day

	COW	SHEEP
Example herd size	500	3,000
Methane produced*	63,875,000	21,900,000
CO2 produced*	273,750,000	82,125,000
Tax per litre	$0.046	$0.0003
Tax per farmer	$300	$300

*- Litres per year

In spite of it being labeled as a flatulence tax, the predominant source of global warming from ruminants comes from fermentation in their multi compartment stomachs. It should really be called a burping and belching tax, but that is not as newsworthy.

Kangaroos are herbivores and as marsupial their burps and farts contain little or no methane, a potent greenhouse gas. It appears that the reduced methane emissions are due to the microbes in the kangaroos' gut flora. Australian researchers hope that introducing a similar gut flora to other methane producing herbivores such as cattle and sheep will contribute to a reduction in greenhouse gasses and the resultant global warming. Methane can cause about twenty times as much atmospheric warming as an equivalent volume of carbon dioxide.

Kangaroos, like cattle and sheep, are ruminants that re-chew their cud with the assistance of the gut flora to digest and metabolize their cellulose based grazing diet. In the foregut the meal is broken down by fermentation with carbon dioxide and hydrogen released. In cows and other ruminants, microbes called methanogens transform these gases into methane. But in the kangaroos' guts the same hydrogen and carbon dioxide may be utilized by bacteria called acetogens to produce acetate, a volatile fatty acid.

These microbes compete with methanogens to use the carbon dioxide and hydrogen, so the more acetogens the less methane production. The odds are in generally in favor of methanogens, since the process of methane production is generally more energy efficient than producing acetate. One of the acetogen microbes, *Blautia coccoides,* is in the gut flora of cows as well as in kangaroos. Further research is being undertaken to understand why the organism is more successful in competing with the methanogens in kangaroos than in other herbivores.

It is the burps and belches from the multi compartment ruminant stomach that is the primary source of methane. Shutterstock/AlisaBurkova

Carbon dioxide, methane, nitrous oxide (N_2O), and three groups of fluorinated gases (sulfur hexafluoride (SF_6), hydro fluorocarbons (HFCs), and per fluorocarbons (PFCs)) are the major greenhouse gases impacted by human activity. These are regulated under the Kyoto Protocol, an international treaty that was adopted in 2005. Nitrogen dioxide (NO_2) warms the atmosphere three hundred and ten times more than carbon dioxide and methane twenty-one times more than carbon dioxide. Although CFCs are greenhouse gases, regulations were initiated because CFCs' cause ozone depletion, not because of their contribution to global warming. Ozone depletion itself has a relatively minor effect on greenhouse warming.

Dinosaurs are no longer around to defend themselves and have been accused of contributing to global warming. We do not know if they were ruminants and contributed by belching up gasses as well, but there should be no doubt that they were big time farters. Their nickname "thunder lizards" may have more to do with their farts than their footsteps. For more information about fart contributions to global warming see entries on methane and carbon dioxide.

Fart, History & Culture (Art, Music, Literature)

Artsy Fartsy: Cultural History of the Fart is a fascinating and factually correct review of the common fart through human culture and history. The cough, sneeze, hiccup, stomach rumble, burp, belch, and other bodily sounds simply cannot compete with the notoriety of the fart. Whether encountered live and in person or through the medium of literature, television, film, art, or music it may leave a powerful and lingering memory.

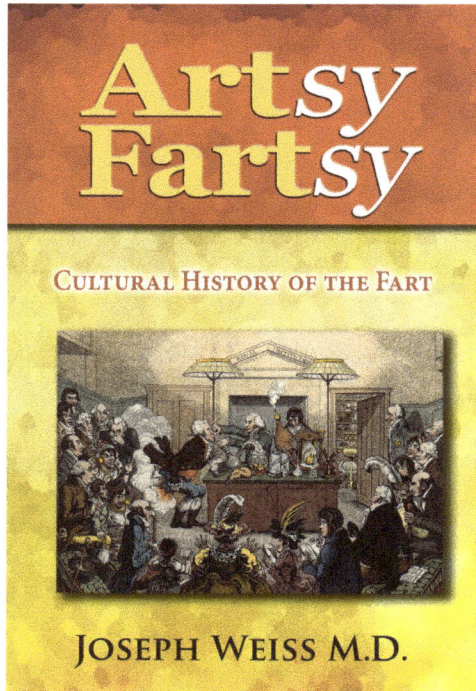

The history of the fart in culture and society is a seldom told but fascinating tale. The very same fart that has triggered wars and the deaths of thousands of innocents (see entry on Flavius Josephus) has also led to the laughter and entertainment of millions worldwide (see entry on Joseph Pujol and Cinematic

Arts). Even today the response to a fart can reach from the extremes of triggering violence to inducing spasms of uncontrollable laughter.

The intent of **Artsy Fartsy: Cultural History of the Fart** is to demonstrate that the ubiquitous fart has a more illustrious story to share than just lowbrow humor. The societal standards and cultural acceptance of this normal physiologic event have evolved over the years, and it is currently popular as a point of humor even in sophisticated circles. *Artsy Fartsy*, is a chronological survey of some of the high and low points in the cultural history of this ubiquitous but inherently controversial activity. Rather than an exhaustive and long-winded discourse, this volume is meant to introduce the reader to the colorful and extremely varied response to the fart over the course of human history.

The book provides an entertaining overview of the fart in human culture and history, not an extensively referenced academic treatise. The number of references to farts in the arts, especially over the recent years, is so numerous that a complete list is not practical or possible. The good news for those wanting more in depth information about any author, artist, or topic of interest is the powerful reference resource of the Internet. I expect that many will be surprised that the fart was a subject near to the hearts and minds of many illustrious and enlightened notables over the course of thousands of years of human history. The cultural mores of Western society have evolved and the fart has become a normal physiological event that has become more tolerated, although not yet universally accepted.

Fart Non-Human

Blue Whale

The Blue Whale is the largest animal on Earth, up to one hundred feet (thirty meters) long and three hundred and forty thousand pounds (154,545 Kilograms or one hundred and seventy tons). The blue whale is a mammal that ingests and digests up to sixteen thousand pounds (7,272 kilograms or eight tons) of plankton per day. The whale digestive tract generates large quantities of gas and when the blue whale releases a fart the bubble expands as it rises to the surface. The decreasing atmospheric pressure as it continues to rise contributes to its expansion as described in physics by Boyle's Law. When it just reaches the surface of the ocean the fart bubble is so huge it could easily enclose and asphyxiate a large horse. The smell is just as powerful as its size would predict.

Cat

Cats fart just like dogs, but they are wiser and more discreet. Because they are generally more diminutive in size than dogs they are not as easily identified or innocently blamed as the source of the fart. The alpha-galactosidase enzyme has also been marketed as a veterinary product with the brand name Curtail. It has been offered as a solution for dogs and cats that have farted one time too many. Although that particular product is no longer actively being marketed, the active ingredient is alpha-galactosidase. That is the same enzyme found in other products marketed for human consumption to reduce intestinal gas production.

<u>Cow, Sheep, & Ruminant</u>

A ruminant (Latin *ruminare* - to chew over again) is a mammal that digests plants in a multi compartment stomach through bacterial fermentation. It regurgitates the semi-digested mass, called cud, and chews it again and repeats the swallow. The process of re-chewing the cud is called "ruminating". There are about one hundred and fifty species of ruminants, which include both domestic and wild species. Ruminating mammals include cattle, goats, sheep, giraffes, yaks, deer, camels, llamas, and antelope. Ruminant bacterial fermentation is a significant contributor to global methane production, which is over twenty times as potent greenhouse gas. Please see the entries on Global Warming and Methane for more details about ruminant gas production.

<u>Dinosaur</u>

Dinosaurs are no longer around to defend themselves and have been accused of contributing to global warming. We do not know if they were ruminants and contributed by belching up gasses as well, but there should be no doubt that they were big time farters. Their nickname "thunder lizards" may have more to do with their farts than their footsteps.

The hulking sauropods were widespread about one hundred and fifty million years ago, and methane-producing microbes aided the sauropods' digestion by fermenting their plant food. Dave Wilkinson of Liverpool John Moores University, Graeme Ruxton from the University of St Andrews, and methane expert Euan Nisbet at the University of London studied the implications. Wilkinson, Ruxton, and Nisbet calculated global methane emissions from sauropods to have been approximately five hundred and twenty million tons per year. By comparison modern livestock ruminant animals produce methane emission of up to one hundred million tons per year.

There is a common public misperception that petroleum is predominantly derived from the organic remains of the great dinosaurs. Rather than the enormous dinosaurs, it was microscopic bacteria that produced the petroleum reserves of our time period. Single-celled bacteria evolved in the earth's oceans about three billion years ago, and were the dominant life form on the planet until about six hundred million years ago. In fact, if dominant is qualified as largest by biomass, bacteria retain that distinction today.

As microscopic as the individual bacteria may be, the bacterial colonies known as "mats" were of enormous proportions. They had masses of millions of tons compared to the hundred tons for the largest dinosaur, the sauropods. As these massive colonies died off and decayed they subsided to the bottom of the sea and were covered by layers of accumulating sediments. Over millions of years these layers of sediment thousands of feet underground were compressed under tremendous pressure and temperature, and developed into the liquid hydrocarbons we recognize as petroleum.

The vast majority of the world's coal deposits date back to the Carboniferous period, about three hundred million years ago. The first dinosaurs would not make their grand entrance in the evolutionary timetable until seventy-five million years later. During the Carboniferous period the earth was heavily forested. With the death and decomposition of these trees and plant life buried under great pressure and temperature under heavy layers of sediment, they were transformed into solid coal rather than liquid petroleum. As the search for petroleum and coal preserves often entails drilling and excavation of deep layers of sediment, it is not uncommon for fossils of dinosaurs and other prehistoric forms of life to be uncovered. The discovery of a theropod dinosaur during fossil fuel exploration in China has been given the appropriate name Gasosaurus. It looks as though Dino's story may have come full circle.

Dog

Dogs are just like any other organism, they do fart. Some breeds fart more than others especially the short snouted English bulldog and similar breeds that are serious air swallowers and farters. Several hundred years ago lap dogs were specifically bred to be small enough for a lady to keep with her at all times and if intestinal gas ruffled her undergarments it would not ruffle her composure as she would simply excuse her dog for the emission

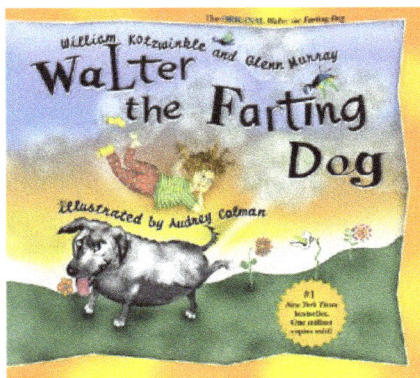

Walter the Farting Dog by William Kotzwinkle & Glenn Murray.

Hippopotamus

The hippopotamus (Greek hippos-horse and potamus-river) is considered by many experts to be the most dangerous animal in Africa (excluding the malaria carrying mosquito) having killed many more people than lions have. The hippo is extremely aggressive with its huge canine teeth and sharp incisors, unpredictable and fearless of humans. Most deaths occur when the victim gets between the hippo and deep water or between a mother and her calf.

Hippopotamus Shutterstock/IvanMateev

Hippos weigh up to eight thousand pounds, gallop at eighteen miles per hour (twenty-nine miles per hour), sleep or lounge around on riverbanks and in the water most of the day, and graze on the grasslands at night. Their skin secretes a sticky pinkish oil that helps protect them from the sun. They defecate generous amounts of excrement into the rivers and ponds in which they wallow all day, punctuated by voluminous farts. They also participate in marking territory by what the hippo experts refer to as "dung showering." They blow feces mixed with urine over a large area around their watering hole, twirling their relatively short tails like fans to distribute the aromatic spray.

Horse

The well-known phenomenon of horse farts has been exploited on television with an episode of the comedy series *Seinfeld* entitled *The Rye*. Cramer feeds the horse a beef and pasta meal pulling a hansom carriage in Central Park in New York City. It makes the horse so extremely flatulent that Cramer and the passengers in the carriage cannot bear the gas exposure.

mapsaboutnothing.wordpress.com

A similar equine theme took place in a prime and extremely expensive American football Super Bowl advertisement for Budweiser beer. A man and a young woman are in a romantic horse drawn carriage. He presents her with a lit candle and reaches down to pull up some bottles of Budweiser beer. As he is out of the way getting the beer the horses tail lifts, releases a fart, and the candle explodes in a ball of flame singeing her features. When he resurfaces he smells smoke and asks if she smells a barbeque.

critbritlit.blogspot.com Creative Commons License

Ronald Wilson Reagan (1911–2004) was the fortieth President of the United Sates. I heard an apocryphal story from a normally reliable source that served in a high position in the administration of former president Ronald Reagan. Then again the source was a politician, which should automatically double the suspicion that this story was just the continued passage of excessive hot air. Her Majesty, Queen Elizabeth II was visiting the presidential ranch, Rancho Cielo, in the Santa Ynez Mountains of California. The ranch is at a high elevation (Rancho Cielo is Spanish for Sky Ranch) and as both the president and queen are horse aficionados they went for a ride on the ranch trails. At higher altitude, as you may recall from Boyle's Law of the physics of gasses, the atmospheric pressure is less than at sea level and the volume of gasses expands. The horse's intestinal tract likewise experienced expanding gasses and being natural animals they release it at will, even if they are in the presence of a Royal Queen and President.

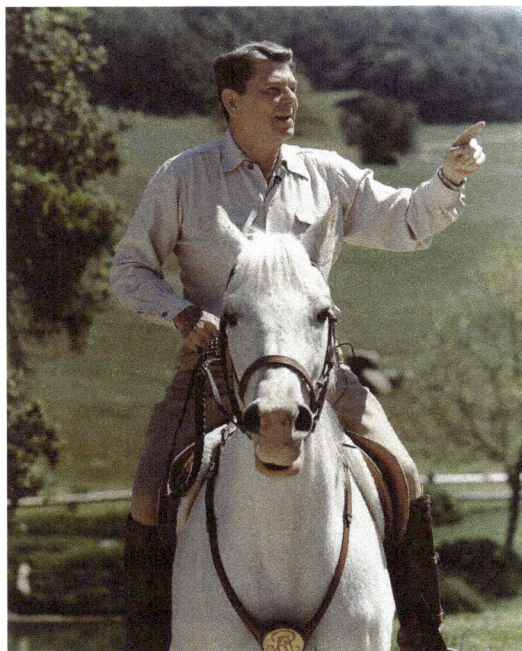

US President Ronald Reagan riding a white horse. 2004 Pete Souza official White House photographer Public Domain

Along the trail the Queen's horse in particular became increasingly flatulent with noisy and pungent emissions. At one point the aroma became particularly strong and the Queen said to Mr. Reagan. "Mr. President I really must apologize for the terrible aroma." Some observers thought that perhaps President Reagans Alzheimer Disease was beginning to take hold, but much more likely it was his quick wit that rose to the occasion. Mr. Regan responded, "Your Majesty, you needn't have apologized at all. In fact, if you hadn't said anything, I would have thought it was the horses!"

Kangaroo

img1-azcdn.newser.com Creative Commons License

Kangaroos are herbivores and as marsupials their burps and farts contain little or no methane, a potent greenhouse gas. It appears that the reduced methane emissions are due to the microbes in the kangaroos' gut flora. Australian researchers hope that introducing a similar gut flora to other methane producing herbivores such as cattle and sheep will contribute to a reduction in greenhouse gasses and the resultant global warming. Methane can cause about twenty times as much atmospheric warming as an equivalent volume of carbon dioxide.

Kangaroos, like cattle and sheep, are ruminants that re-chew their cud with the assistance of the gut flora to digest the and metabolize their cellulose based grazing diet. In the foregut the meal is broken down by fermentation with carbon dioxide and hydrogen released. In cows and other ruminants, microbes called methanogens transform these gases into methane. But in the kangaroos' guts the same hydrogen and carbon dioxide may be utilized by bacteria called acetogens to produce acetate, a volatile fatty acid.

These microbes compete with methanogens to use the carbon dioxide and hydrogen, so the more acetogens the less methane production. The odds are in generally in favor of methanogens, since the process of methane production is generally more energy efficient than producing acetate. One of the acetogen microbes, *Blautia coccoides,* is in the gut flora of cows as well as in kangaroos. Further research is being undertaken to understand why the organism is more successful in competing with the methanogens in kangaroos than in other herbivores.

Microbe

Microbes including bacteria, Archaea, fungi, viruses, protist, and parasites are a major component of the gastrointestinal tract flora, also known as the gut microbiome. These organisms play a major role in the metabolism of the diet, and thus play a direct role in intestinal gas production. Although the organism's microfarts may seem to be inconsequential, the trillions of their numbers make them major contributors to the intestinal gasses of all larger organisms. The methane production that used to be blamed on bacteria is actually generated by the non-bacterial microbes from the Kingdom Archaea.

domesticlabrat.files.wordpress.com Creative Commons License

The gastrointestinal tract flora, is influenced by many environmental factors. These include diet, water purity, antibiotic exposure, chemicals, pesticides, and exposure to the microbiome of others. The gastrointestinal tract of the newborn is sterile at birth, but rapidly becomes colonized by microbes that are swallowed. Infants born via a normal vaginal delivery have a markedly different microbiome than those delivered by Cesarean section. Those born by Cesarean section have a higher incidence of allergies, asthma, and immune disorders. Many experts now suggest swathing the infect in its mother's vaginal secretions to expose it to the microbiome it would have been naturally exposed to.

Plant

Plant placed underwater to demonstrate the production and release of oxygen gas bubbles
www.pinterest.com Creative Commons License

Plant life also contributes to gas production, but one of the most important gasses they produce as far as humans are concerned is oxygen. Although not described as a fart, the plant release of gas is analogous to a fart, as it is a gas waste product of their metabolism. It just so happens that their waste product of oxygen is one humans and other animals require for life. Plants are also critically important in taking carbon dioxide out of the atmosphere as well as fixing nitrogen into products that the other life forms can access and utilize. With plant death the decay of decomposing organic matter adds gasses that can contribute to global warming.

Stinkbug

The stinkbug is an agricultural pest which has caused significant losses of fruit and vegetable crops in numerous countries including the United States. They invade human domestic dwellings during cold winter months. When they find a comfortable habitat they release an aggregation pheromone to attract other stinkbugs, which huddle closely together. The pheromone does have an aroma which most find unpleasant. They lay about four hundred eggs which hatch in less than a week, which can lead to large populations of stinkbugs in a home. One home was found to be harboring over twenty-six thousand stinkbugs. They do not damage the house structure and they do not bite humans. The stink glands are located on the underside of the thorax, between the first and second pair of legs, and on the dorsal surface of the abdomen. Although the stink glands are associated with the insect's abdomen they are not an intestinal gas, although some incorrectly believe this is the source of odor.

The odor from the stink gland is due to its release of chemicals including the aldehydes trans-2-decenal and trans-2-Octenal, both of which have a pungent odor similar to cilantro and coriander. Most people find the aroma offensive but others do not, perhaps due to a genetic basis. Some species also release a cyanide compounds with a rancid almond scent. The odor is a defense mechanism and the insect can control the quantity ejected as well as whether just one or both glands are activated. Stinkbugs are commonly eaten in Laos, where the extremely strong odors are believed to enhance the flavor. The insects are crushed and mixed with seasoning including chilies and herbs creating a paste known as cheo.

Termite

Termites are major producers of methane, and because of the enormous size of the termite population and biomass they are thought to be significant contributors to global warming, producing over twenty-five percent of the world total methane production. Of interest, termites trapped in the sap of a tree have often been found frozen in time as the sap turns to amber over the ages. The tiny bubble of gas at the tail end of the termite entrapped in amber has been analyzed and is indeed methane produced thousands of years ago from the bacterial fermentation of the wood termites ingest. The termite gut microbiome flora generates tiny bacterial nanofarts, which coalesce into the termite microfarts that have been captured in amber eons ago.

Termite farts trapped in amber have been analyzed for gas composition and indeed it is methane.
1.bp.blogspot.com Creative Commons License

*Air*Veda: Ancient & New Medical Wisdom

Fart, Smell (Aroma, Olfaction)

Olfaction, also known as olfactics, is the scientific term for the sense of smell. Olfaction occurs when odorant molecules bind to specific sites known as the olfactory receptors. The olfactory receptors are specialized sensory cells in the nasal cavity of vertebrates. Invertebrates, such as insects, typically house their olfactory sense organ on their antennae. In the snake the olfactants are acquired by the tongue, which taking advantage of its forked anatomy deposits them on the olfactory cells on the respective sides of the nasal cavity. The difference in concentration of the olfactants on each side of the nasal cavity allows the receptors to discriminate and localize the source of the scent, much like binocular vision allows depth perception. Because humans and other animals have two nostrils, each with separate inputs to the brain, it is possible for them to have perceptual rivalry in the olfactory sense akin to binocular vision.

Many vertebrates, including most mammals and reptiles, have two distinct olfactory systems. The main olfactory system identifies general odorants while the accessory olfactory system is used mainly to detect pheromones. For air-breathing animals the main olfactory system detects volatile aerosolized chemicals, and the accessory olfactory system detects chemicals usually in the fluid phase. Olfaction, along with taste, is a form of chemoreception. Although taste and smell are separate sensory systems in land animals, water-dwelling organisms often have one combined chemical sense.

Odors are also commonly called scents, and these terms can refer to both pleasant and unpleasant stimuli. The terms fragrance and aroma are used primarily by the food and cosmetic industry to describe a pleasant odor, often referred to as a perfume or bouquet. In contrast malodor, stench, reek, and stink are used specifically to describe an unpleasant odor. The sense of smell gives rise to the perception of odors, mediated by the olfactory nerve. The olfactory receptor cells are neurons present in the olfactory epithelium, a small patch of tissue in back of the nasal cavity. There are millions of olfactory receptor neurons, each neuron has hair-like projections known as cilia. The cilia have receptor proteins that are in direct contact with air and bind directly with the odorant chemicals and molecules initiating a neuron mediated electric signal. Volatile small molecule odorants, non-volatile proteins, and non-volatile hydrocarbons may all produce olfactory responses and sensations. Much like some animal species are able to visualize ultraviolet or infrared beyond the spectrum visible to humans, a number of species can smell carbon dioxide and other odorants that are not detectable and thus considered odorless based on human sensitivity.

Olfaction, taste, and trigeminal receptors with a property known as chemesthesis together contribute to flavor. The human tongue is able to distinguish five distinct qualities of taste, salt, sweet, acidic, bitter, and umami. The nose and olfactory sense of smell has a much greater sense of discrimination and can distinguish among hundreds of substances, even in extremely minute quantities. The olfactory sense of smell takes place during inhalation, while the olfactory contribution to flavor occurs during exhalation. The olfactory system is unique among the human senses in that the neural pathway bypasses the thalamus and provides neural input directly to the forebrain. In human females the sense of olfaction is strongest around the time of ovulation, significantly stronger than during other phases of the menstrual cycle and stronger than the sense in males. The association of heightened olfactory sensitivity in association with ovulation has raised speculation about pheromone activity in humans but it has yet to be scientifically confirmed.

Scent hounds as a group can smell one to ten-million times more acutely than a human. Bloodhounds, which have the keenest sense of smell of any dogs, have noses ten to one-hundred-million times more sensitive than a human's. They were bred for the specific purpose of tracking humans, and can detect a scent trail a few days old. The second most- sensitive nose is possessed by the Basset Hound, which was bred to track and hunt rabbits and other small animals. The silvertip grizzly bear found in parts of North America, has a sense of smell seven times stronger than that of the bloodhound. This keen sense of smell is essential for its skill in locating food underground. Bears can detect the scent of food from up to eighteen miles away.

Olfaction, the sense of smell, is a form of chemoreception that in humans occurs when odorant molecules bind to olfactory receptors. The stimulation of olfactory and taste receptors is through a process known as chemesthesis. Cloning of olfactory receptor proteins and identifying that odor molecules bind to specific receptors led to the 2004 Nobel Prize award to Linda B. Buck and Richard Axel.

Shutterstock/bimka

Females have greater olfactory sensitivity than males, particularly at the time of ovulation. More than pheromones are involved and females can detect by olfaction potential mates that have a genetic diversity that would be beneficial for their offspring. Odor information is retained in long-term memory and the olfactory system is anatomically associated with the regions of the brain associated with emotion. It has been long recognized that odors can trigger memories and emotions from remote times.

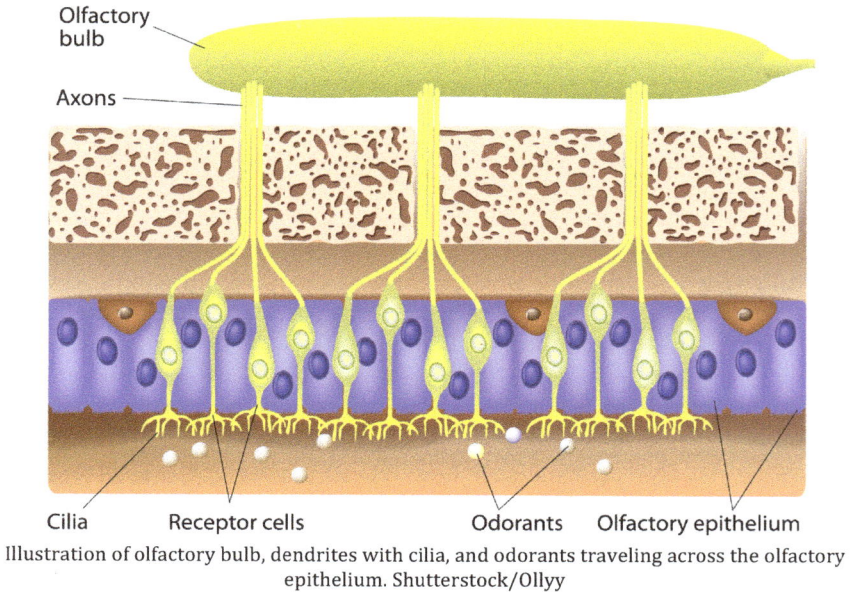

Illustration of olfactory bulb, dendrites with cilia, and odorants traveling across the olfactory epithelium. Shutterstock/Ollyy

The sense of olfaction is the most sensitive of all human senses. The nose can identify the single scented molecule hiding amongst two billion unscented ones. To use a visual analogy, paint one single square sheet of a toilet paper roll the

color red. Now wrap that unlimited length roll of toilet paper around the twenty-five-thousand-mile long equator of the planet earth, and go around a second time, a third, a fourth, and a full fifth time.

Your nose can instantaneously identify the single red square of a one hundred and twenty-five thousand mile roll of toilet paper. Are you impressed with our sense of smell? Just like wealth and beauty there is always someone who has more to keep us from being number one. Human's olfactory epithelium is less than ten percent of the surface area of a dog's olfactory epithelium, which also has one hundred times more receptors per square centimeter. Bloodhounds have olfactory receptors up to one hundred million times the sensitivities of humans, and are trained to track a human trail several days old. North American grizzly bears have the keenest sense of smell seven times greater than the bloodhound. Salmon utilize their keen sense of smell in ocean waters to locate the stream from which they hatchlings years earlier to return to spawn. A mosquito smelling the "odorless" carbon dioxide that mammals exhale to locate their next blood meal illustrates the specialized olfactory sensitivity located on their antennae.

Composition of Intestinal Gas

Major gases (non-odorous)

65% nitrogen (N_2)

20% hydrogen (H_2)

10% CO_2

3% methane (CH_4)

2% oxygen (O_2)

Trace gases (odorous)
Hydrogen sulfide (H_2S)
Indole
Skatole (3-methylindole)

The vast majority of the gasses in intestinal farts including nitrogen, hydrogen, carbon dioxide, methane, and oxygen contributing 99.9% by volume are odorless. So what on earth is in that other tiny but overwhelming fraction of less than one percent? Indole skatole, thiol, sulfhydryl, mercaptan, and aromatic fatty acids are the major culprits. The aromas generated by farts are normally considered unattractive or offensive. There is a surprising percentage of the presumably normal population (predominantly males) who profess enjoyment and pleasure with the olfactory stimulation generated by their own farts, but not those of others. The utility of specific odors to diagnose a limited number of diseases has been a part of the diagnostic medical armamentarium for thousands of years. When it comes to farts, particularly offensive aroma has been associated with fat malabsorption and inflammatory bowel conditions.

AirVeda: Ancient & New Medical Wisdom

Indole

Indole is an organic compound known as an aromatic heterocyclic because it consists of a six-membered benzene ring fused to a five-membered nitrogen-containing pyrrole ring. Indole is often used as a component of fragrances and is used in the production of a number of pharmaceutical products. The amino acid tryptophan is the precursor of the neurotransmitter serotonin and is an example of an indole derivative. Tryptophan is one of the twenty-two amino acids, and is also considered an essential amino acid. Essential amino acids are those amino acids that cannot be synthesized by humans, and therefore must be obtained through the diet. Because of its importance as an essential amino acid, tryptophan is a common constituent of most protein foods and supplements. A diet rich in tryptophan can contribute to the fecal aroma of intestinal gas.

Indole occurs naturally in human feces and contributes to the characteristic fecal odor. Surprisingly, at very low concentrations it has a flowery smell and is a constituent of many perfumes. The name indole was created from the words indigo and oleum. Indole was first isolated by the dye industry in treatment of the deep blue indigo dye with oleum. Jasmine is a climbing shrub native to northern India and China that has a delicate night blossoming white star like flower that is highly prized for its fragrance. It is harvested only at night and an experienced picker can collect ten thousand blossoms a night. It takes three and one-half million jasmine blossoms to make one pound (half a kilogram) of natural jasmine oil, which is less than three percent indole. It is priced at over one thousand times as much as synthetic jasmine, which takes advantage of the commercial production of indole.

Skatole

Skatole (from the Greek το σχατος = feces), or methylindole, is a mildly toxic organic compound belonging to the indole family. It is the primary source of the odor of feces and is produced from the breakdown of the important amino acid tryptophan, the precursor of the neurotransmitter serotonin. Surprisingly, in low concentrations skatole has a very pleasant flowery smell and is found in orange blossoms, jasmine, and other flowers and essential oils. It is used as a fragrance in many perfumes. Skatole is attractive to males of various species of bees, who gather the chemical to synthesize pheromones. It is also an attractant to gravid (pregnant) mosquitos. The U. S. military has used skatole as a non-lethal malodorant weapon. The German physician Ludwig Brieger, who also identified cadaverine and putrescence, discovered skatole in 1877. His neighbors were probably not pleased with the smell coming from his laboratory as the names he gave his discoveries were derived from their source material.

Skatole also plays a major role in the aroma of pork obtained from mature male pigs (boars). After puberty, under the influence of the male hormone androstenone, the gut microbiome of the male pig generates skatole. This odorant is deposited in the fat and muscle giving it an offensive smell and taste known as taint. Because it cannot be sold at market, male pigs are typically castrated at a young age or slaughtered before puberty. The male of the human species, under similar hormonal influence is also a large producer of skatole contributing to the enhanced offensive potency of male farts after puberty.

Of particular interest to some scientists is that androstenone, and its effect on skatole, appear to have a pheromone like effect on the human female. Much like color-blindness, there appear to be some odors that cannot be smelled by all people. Initial studies suggested that about thirty percent of human females could not sense androstenone. Further studies revealed that the majority of the non-scenters could be trained to identify it, yet there remained a small proportion of less than five percent who could not perceive the scent. The ability to sense androstenone was found to be genetic and the gene responsible was identified.

The sense of smell in the human female is intimately tied to the menstrual cycle. The height of olfactory sensitivity peaks at the time of ovulation. The androstenone and skatole scents are perceived to be less offensive or more attractive at the time of ovulation. The androstenone skatole connection also explains why the feces and flatus of males is considered more powerful or offensive than that of females.

Diet also plays a role in that the ingestion of more meat and fat also leads to more skatole production than a diet with higher fiber content. This is partly due to the diet containing more tryptophan, the amino acid precursor of skatole, as well as the diet induced change in the microbiome. Androstenone also occurs naturally in some plants, including celery, parsnip, and truffle. The celery has long had a reputation as an aphrodisiac dating from Greek and Roman times.

Thiol, Sulfhydryl, Mercaptans

The sulfur hydrogen functional group may also be referred to as a thiol group or a sulfhydryl group. Thiols are also referred to as mercaptans. The term mercaptan (Latin mercurium captans 'capturing mercury') is used because the thiolate group bonds so strongly with mercury compounds. Hydrogen sulfide is known for its characteristic odor of smelling like rotten eggs. Surprisingly women tend to produce more hydrogen sulfide then men. Diet certainly plays a role as cruciferous vegetables such as broccoli, cabbage, cauliflower, and Brussels sprouts are common offenders. Dried fruits such as apricots are often treated with sulfur products that create odiferous gasses. Red meat, beer, garlic, and aromatic spices are other significant contributors. The offensive smell of sulfur products led to religious authorities ascribing an association between the devil and sulfur.

Hydrogen sulfide is a toxic substance in high concentrations yet very valuable and beneficial on a cellular level when present in minute quantities. The human nose is exceptionally sensitive to this toxin and can identify it in minute concentrations, such as in a fart. When present in very high concentrations the olfactory cells are overwhelmed and can no longer sense it. This has led to a severe hazard for farmers and workers in animal waste manure pits and sewage treatment facilities. A worker collapses on exposure to the high concentration of hydrogen sulfide and fellow workers coming to their aid are likewise stricken because there was no olfactory warning. With a toxic potency equivalent to cyanide, workers in such hazardous occupations are urged to use self-contained breathing apparatus to avoid exposure.

Volatile thiols have distinctive and strong garlic like odor. The spray of skunks consists mainly of thiols and derivatives. These compounds are detected by the human nose at concentrations as low as ten parts per billion. Human sweat contains methyl-sulfanylhexan (MSH), found in higher concentrations in females, and has a fruity onion-like odor. Not all thiols have unpleasant odors. The aroma of roasted coffee is due to thiols as is the characteristic scent of grapefruit. Dimethyl sulfide has an aroma that is often described as sweet. Natural gas distributors were required by law to add odorants such as thiols to odorless natural gas after a tragic school explosion in New London, Texas, in 1937 due to an undetected gas leak.

Most natural odorant additives used today contain mixtures of mercaptans and sulfides. T-butyl mercaptan is often utilized as the main odorant constituent. The characteristic and pungently offensive odor of animal flesh decay is caused by the odorant additives putrescence and cadaverine. Putrescence and cadaverine are the breakdown products of the amino acids ornithine and lysine, respectively. Cadaverine and putrescence were also used as odorant additives for natural gas before improved odorants became commercially available.

Methanethiol

Methanethiol (methyl mercaptan) is a flammable, colorless compound with a powerful smell like rotten cabbage or decomposing vegetables. It is a natural substance found in certain foods such as some nuts and cheese, and is released from decaying organic matter. Methanethiol is also a byproduct produced by the metabolism of asparagus. The change in the odor of urine may be apparent within thirty minutes of eating asparagus. It is one of the main chemicals responsible for bad breath and the smell of feces and flatus.

Natural gas and propane are both colorless and odorless, and an undetected leak can lead to tragic consequences. To serve as an odorous marker that a gas leak is occurring small amount of methyl mercaptan or ethyl mercaptan may be added as an odorant. The addition of an odorant is often required by law to prevent the danger of natural gas leaks going undetected leading to death and injury.

Fatty Acids

A fatty acid is a saturated or unsaturated carboxylic acid with a long aliphatic tail or chain. Fatty acids with carbon–carbon double bonds are known as unsaturated, and those without such bonds are known as saturated. Fatty acids are derived from triglycerides or phospholipids, and when unattached to other molecules are described as "free". Fatty acids are an important cellular fuel and yield large quantities of the energy storing molecule adenosine triphosphate (ATP) when metabolized. Many cell types can use either glucose or fatty acids for this purpose. Heart and skeletal muscle prefer fatty acids, although most cells can use glucose interchangeably. The brain has the ability to use fatty acids, glucose, or ketone bodies as a fuel.

Fatty acids that must be obtained via the diet because humans cannot synthesize them are called essential fatty acids. Fatty acid chains are categorized by their length. Short-chain fatty acids (SCFA) have aliphatic tails of fewer than six carbons. Medium-chain fatty acids (MCFA) have tails of six to twelve carbons and can form medium-chain triglycerides. Long-chain fatty acids (LCFA) have tails of thirteen to twenty-one carbons, while very long chain fatty acids (VLCFA) are longer than twenty-two carbons.

Short- and medium-chain fatty acids are absorbed by the intestines directly into the blood stream. Long-chain fatty acids are absorbed into the cells of the intestinal villi and converted into a triglyceride cholesterol compound known as a chylomicron. These enter lymphatic capillaries called lacteals and are transported via the thoracic duct of the lymphatic system, eventually entering the circulatory system via the left subclavian vein. Fatty acids and chylomicrons in the blood circulation may be processed in the liver and subsequently circulate as very low-density lipoproteins (VLDL), low-density lipoproteins (LDL), and high-density lipoproteins.

Aromatic Amino Acids

Aromatic amino acids are amino acids that include an aromatic ring. Examples include phenylalanine, tryptophan, histidine, and tyrosine. Phenylalanine, histidine, and tryptophan are essential amino acids in that animals cannot synthesize them and they must be obtained from the diet. Tyrosine is semi-essential in that it can be synthesized but only if phenylalanine is ingested. The disorder phenylketonuria occurs when there is an absence of the enzyme phenylalanine hydroxylase, which is required for tyrosine synthesis.

All plants and microorganisms synthesize their aromatic amino acids, unlike animals, which obtain them through their diet. Animals have lost these energy intensive metabolic pathways, since they obtain aromatic amino acids through their diet. Herbicides and antibiotics inhibiting enzymes involved in aromatic acid synthesis, are toxic to plants and microorganisms dependent on this pathway, but not to animals which do not utilize these enzymes.

Volatile Organic Compounds

The term volatile refers to the ability of a substance to evaporate or readily vaporize at room temperature. Most instances of vaporization refer to evaporation where a liquid becomes a gas, such as liquid water boiling into gaseous steam and water vapor. Some solids vaporize from the solid state directly without entering an intermediate liquid phase, a process is known as sublimation. One example would be dry ice, frozen carbon dioxide, which leaves the solid state and is immediately transformed into a gas.

Vaporization also has another form that is not evaporation, but is the scattering or diffusing of molecules or particles through the air. The particles have so little mass that they can remain airborne for extended periods of time, and become airborne again upon being disturbed or moved even by a gentle gust of air. This is frequently noticed when a bright beam of light enters a darkened room and the dust particles circulating in the air become visible.

Mold, spores, pollens, viruses, bacteria, fecal matter of mites, volatile organic compounds and others can circulate and spread through large open spaces. Allergies, acquiring viral or bacterial infections from the sneeze or cough of others even hours earlier, occur because of this aerosolization. The ability to detect the aroma of certain compounds, and volatile organic compounds are the result of this form of vaporization, as well as their ability to enter the gaseous state by vaporizing at room temperatures.

A list of the volatile organic compounds found in strawberries includes approximately two dozen chemicals including methyl butyrate, octyl acetate, hexanol, and others. Since these compounds are volatile they may vaporize and if they reach your olfactory receptors you may detect them and identify them as coming from a strawberry.

Fart, Social Standards (see Fart Survey)

The Ontario Ministry of Health embarked on a public education campaign to curb tobacco usage. A common theme used by smokers to avoid the stigma of nicotine addiction was to describe their habit as that of being a social smoker. The public education campaign focused on that denial as being analogous to describing oneself as a social farter that enjoyed farting while in the company of others.

Fart, Sound (Acoustics, Auditory)

The physics involved in the generation of the sound of a fart is very complex. Variables of the colonic and anal components, as well as the surrounding environment when it is released are multiple. Within the colon and rectum this includes the pressure, volume, temperature, moisture content, chemical nature of the gasses within the colon, and whether it is being released concomitantly with any liquid, semisolid, or solid material.

"Yes, that was very loud, but I said
I wanted to hear your HEART!"

Within the anal canal it includes the anatomy of the sphincter including whether it is symmetrical or irregular such as with fissures, hemorrhoids, anal tags, etc., sphincter tone and pressure, elasticity and degree of relaxation, and the velocity and physical nature of the expelled material. In the immediate post expulsion state, factors include the atmospheric pressure, temperature, and volumetric constraints such as whether by clothing, sitting on a cushion, under a blanket, or voluntary social considerations.

The physics of gas and fluid dynamics allow calculations with the understanding and application of natural laws. If you have taken a course in physics you may recall with great fondness Laplace's Law, Boyle's Law, Charles' Law, Avogadro's Law, Gay-Lussac's Law that were integrated into what is called the Ideal Gas Law. This summarizes the close interrelationship between the pressure, volume, and temperature of gasses. To understand the physics of farts you need to incorporate the additional principles of physics and engineering called the "choked" compressible flow effect. The character that becomes choked or limited is the velocity, although after release the term choked may take on an entirely different meaning.

The velocity of the material increases as it is passed through a constriction. You may have experienced this if you have used a garden hose and notice that as the opening at the nozzle tip becomes smaller the velocity increases. You may also have noticed that the frequency of the sound generated also changes both by constricting the nozzle orifice or rotating the faucet leading to the garden hose. This involves recognition that the Venturi effect causes the static pressure, and therefore the density of the gasses, to decrease once released from the anus.

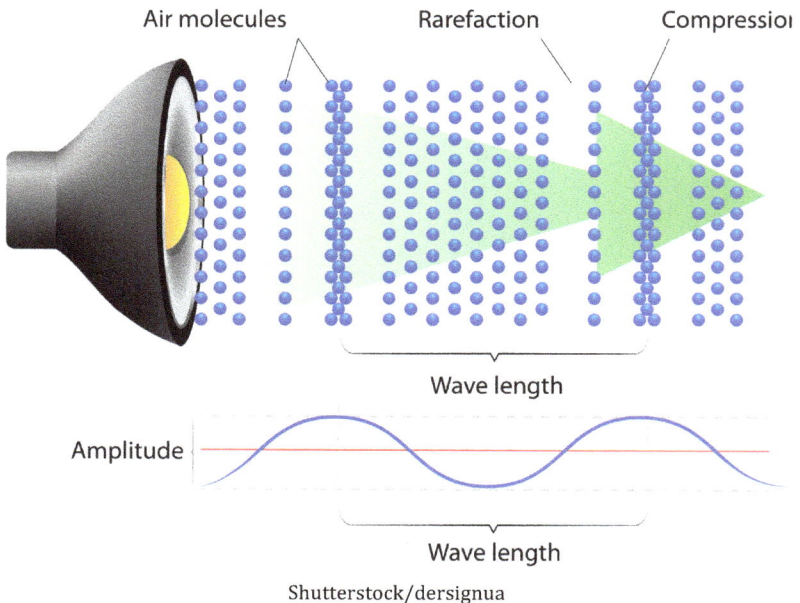

Shutterstock/dersignua

If the material passed includes a liquid component, a different type of choked flow can occur. In unusual circumstances dependent on the vapor pressure and temperature of the liquid, the liquid may partially flash into bubbles of vapor that collapse in a process called cavitation. When this occurs in a closed system of pipes such as plumbing fixtures the effect can be very noisy and sufficiently violent as to cause physical damage to valves, pipes, and associated equipment. Thankfully, humans are not a closed system but the noise and reverberations they generate may be comparable.

In general, the more tone the anal sphincter has the tighter it can hold on to the gasses to create a greater pressure gradient. The greater the pressure gradient the louder the potential sound will be. If the opposite occurs, then less noise is generated. As an example, it is said that if you blow air slowly into a trumpet without puckering your lips to generate an air pressure gradient the air will just flow through the instrument without "trumpeting".

The anal sphincter tone changes with age becoming more lax. This is also the case after childbirth, and any activities that stretch the anal opening on a regular basis, such as passing large stools with constipation, or engaging in anal receptive intercourse. With the loss of sphincter tone farts may escape involuntarily, but they also tend to be quitter as the larger the opening of the orifice the slower the velocity.

With so many variables it should come as no surprise that the sounds generated are equally variable. As the famous Greek philosopher Heraclitus (c 535 BCE- 475 BCE) said, "You could not step twice into the same river; for other waters are ever flowing on to you." It would be fair to say that no two farts are identical, much like snowflakes, although somehow pure white innocent snowflakes do not seem to be the right analogy.

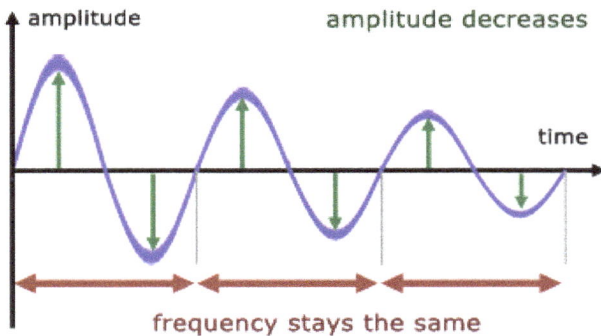

www.a-levelphysicstutor.com Creative Commons License

At the time that a fart is about to be released the variables under the control of a talented and experienced professional farter include the velocity of its release, the tension and symmetry of the sphincter, and the selection of the environmental nature of the location of its liberation. Yes, there is a significant amount of science behind the fart, but there is also an 'art to the fart'. As to the teleological question, is there an advantage to audible fart sounds, there are several theories. One is that the fart sounds are an auditory warning that noxious gasses are being released and to seek shelter or at least distance to protect oneself. A second theory suggests that these are actually primitive mating calls, especially an attempt of adolescent males to attract the female of the species. The third theory is so that people with anosmia, the loss of the sense of smell, can participate in the experience of a fart as well.

Using the principles of speed of travel of various phenomena, you may recall that you can calculate the distance of a lightning strike. The speed of light is 186,282 miles per second; the speed of sound is seven hundred and sixty-eight miles per hour in dry air at sixty-eight degrees Fahrenheit at sea level. Obviously the light will reach you first and you will see the flash, but no sound as it is lagging behind. The more distant you are from where the lightning struck, the greater the time lag. If you see the flash of lightening count the number of seconds before you hear the thunder. Now simply divide the number of seconds of lag time by the number five to adjust for the differences in speed of light and sound, and voila, you have a good approximation of the distance in miles that you are from where the lightning struck.

The lightning flash of a fart is a very special event discussed in greater detail in the section on combustible farts containing hydrogen and methane in the presence of oxygen, and the section on spontaneous human combustion. Can one use science to compare the speeds of sound and smell transmission? The answer is an unequivocal yes, but circumstances are rarely optimal. The speed of sound of a fart is the same as the speed of sound of a lightning strike, seven hundred and sixty-eight miles per hour in dry air at sixty-eight degrees Fahrenheit at sea level. The speed of smell diffusion has been measured at ten feet per second (nearly seven miles per hour) in an unventilated room with no circulating airflow.

Using the sound of the fart as a shotgun start for the stopwatch, count how many seconds it is until you smell the fart. To simplify calculations, the fart sound is about one hundred times faster than the fart smell. For a crude approximation simply take the number of seconds from the fart sound until the smell arrives as the number of feet you are distant to its source. Any circulation of air in the room, clothing that the fart has to pass through, and direction of the jet exhaust blast with which it is released can either accelerate or delay its arrival at your nose. This formula is at its most accurate in identifying the source of the fart if there are no more than two people in the room. The adage he who smelt it dealt it, is usually accurate unless the other party was in a compromised position with his own nose closer to the anus of the emanation.

The pressure generated by the abdominal muscles can be infinitely adjusted by the individual (the Valsalva maneuver generates this pressure with a bearing down motion with the breath held) and will affect the velocity and sound of a fart. Leaning to one side to deform the anal canal into an irregular shape to allow the fart to escape with less velocity is a technique learned by experience even if one does not recognize the principles of physics underlying its utility. Sitting on a cushion to muffle the sound and absorb the aroma is a common technique. With practice, some individuals have developed the remarkable musical ability to play their own human wind instrument. They have performed in public to great acclaim like Joseph Pool, known as Le Ptomaine on the Moulin Rouge of Paris. The sound of farts can be a source of entertainment and humor or offense and embarrassment, but it is a natural phenomenon that follows the laws of nature.

Scientific papers entitled "Sounds produced by herring (*Clupeid harangues*) bubble release" by Magnus Wahlberg and Haman Westerberg in the journal *Aquatic Living Resources* (2003, 16.271-275), and "Pacific and Atlantic Herring Produce Burst Pulse Sounds" by Ben Wilson, Robert S. Batty and Lawrence M. Dill in *Biology Letters* (2003, 271.S95-S97) confirm that herring communicate distress signals to the rest of the school of fish by farting. The papers are demonstrations of scholarly research and have spectrographic confirmation of the high frequency sound bursts at up to twenty-two kilohertz with visual confirmation of a stream of bubbles from the anus.

Herring communicate danger by high frequency sounds generated from bubbles escaping their anus described as F.R.T. fast repetitive ticks in published scientific papers first reported in 2003. Creative Commons License

Herring travel in enormous schools of fish that number in the billions. During the height of the cold war during the 1980's U.S. and NATO forces believed they had detected by sonar a unique sound pattern that was the signature of a new secret Soviet nuclear submarine. The new submarine appeared to be making provocative incursions into the territorial waters of Sweden and Norway, which protested vigorously through diplomatic channels. When the sound pattern was detected deep in the territorial waters of a Norwegian fjord NATO forces decided to trap the submarine and blockaded the entrance to the fjord. After days of waiting for the submarine to surrender they finally realized that the sonar sounds they were hearing were not a Soviet submarine but the sounds of a school of herring farting their way through the fjord.

AirVeda: Ancient & New Medical Wisdom

During interviews with the National Geographic Society research team leader Ben Wilson a marine biologist studying pacific herring at the Bamfield Marine Science Centre, British Columbia, Canada was quoted saying "We know [herring] have excellent hearing but little about what they actually use it for. It turns out that herring make unusual farting sounds at night." Their collaborator Robert Batty, senior research scientist at the Scottish Association for Marine Science in Oban, Scotland added "In video pictures we can see the bubbles coming out of the anal duct at the same time. It sounds very much like someone blowing a high-pitched raspberry. "They labeled the sounds generated as F.R.T. for fast repetitive tick. They were awarded the 2004 IgNobel Prize in Biology.

There is a phrase called 'holding back the helium' which refers to farting by substituting the name of another gas, in this case helium. Is there another possible connection between helium and farting? Because gases have different densities, the speed of sound in helium is nearly three times the speed of sound in air. Inhaling a small volume of helium changes the sound of the human voice into a characteristic high resonant frequency sound. The sound generated is similar to the famous cartoon character Daffy Duck. Inhaling helium gas is actually very dangerous because the human body respiratory drive is not based on low levels of oxygen, but rather by high levels of carbon dioxide. When helium is inhaled the carbon dioxide levels remain normal even though oxygen may be so low that asphyxiation occurs without the expected warning of air hunger and suffocation.

The opposite effect, with low resonant frequencies more like the Star Wars character Darth Vader, can be obtained by inhaling a gas with higher density such as xenon, sulfur hexafluoride, or tungsten hexafluoride. Helium is by far the most readily available, typically associated with access through party favor stores to fill helium balloons for parties and entertainment. Helium actually plays a major role in industry and the biomedical sciences and is critical for scientific research in the fields of quantum mechanics, super fluidity, and superconductivity.

Now to the question that is undoubtedly keeping you up at night, what happens to the sound quality of a helium fart. First question is how does the helium get into the digestive tract. Inhaling pure helium will not lead to helium farts because you would die of asphyxiation within minutes. This is why even playing with the idea of helium to make your voice sound like a cartoon character is a very foolish and dangerous idea. Those who have done so and died from oxygen deprivation are considered candidates for what is called the Darwin Awards. This is offered, usually posthumously, to those who have improved the human gene pool for future evolution by removing themselves and their substandard intelligence genes from future procreation activities.

So let's say you know better than to breathe in helium, but undertake a swallowing effort to fill your digestive tract with helium to get it to pass as a fart. Not much of an improvement as the helium is such a small molecule that it easily diffuses through most membranes, as you can tell by how quickly the helium

escapes from a rubber balloon, and over a period of a few days, even from a metallic balloon.
Which leaves only one last logical way to fill the colon with helium, yes go to a party store and ask them to 'fill it up' for you. Now that you have a colon filled with helium you don't want to waste much time, as the helium will once again diffuse through the colonic epithelium. Will you fart like a duck? The answer is yes, but not because of a high frequency sound, but because a duck fart sounds like any old fart. What went wrong with the common expectation that it would sound like fingernails scratching a chalkboard? The problem is that the anal opening does not have a structure equivalent to the vocal cords of the human larynx also so appropriately called the voice box.

Phonation, the creation of sound and voice arises from the ability of the vocal cords to open and constrict to exceptionally nuanced degrees, allowing an infinite variety and modulation of frequencies. Humans are not the sole possessors of such a talent as songbirds and other animals can generate sounds in an even greater range of frequencies, often beyond the auditory abilities of our ears to hear the sounds. You are probably familiar to dog whistles that dogs respond to but are outside of our hearing range. It is the ability of the vocal cords to generate the range of frequencies that is impacted by the density of the gasses passed through that makes the voice reach higher frequencies with helium. It also can reach much lower frequencies sounding like Darth Vader from the *Star Wars* movie franchise if you use a much denser gas like xenon, sulfur hexafluoride, or tungsten hexafluoride.

The anal opening has hemorrhoid sinusoids, the internal anal sphincter, the external anal sphincter, and the occasional skin tag and in spite of the great control of some individuals like Joseph Pujol (Le Pétomane) it does not even come close to the resonance and sensitivity of sound creation of the vocal cords. Which is too bad, as a new *Star Wars* character a very short and squat Farth Vader could have become a cult hero. Another species creates sounds in a different fashion. Many fish have a swim bladder that is inflated or deflated as needed to maintain buoyancy. Usually expelled air bladder gas exits the mouth but the sand tiger shark, *Carcharias taurus*, discharges it out the anus. The carbon dioxide produced is eliminated via the gills. Methane, hydrogen, and other gasses would typically be released as a fart.

Fart, Speed (Velocity)

The word fart in northern European languages including German and the Scandinavian languages literally means speed. In you go by a school or hospital you may go by a no farting zone. Or you might receive a police citation for exceeding the fart limit! So a title of fart speed might seem redundant. A sneeze, or sternutation, is a powerful rapid expulsion of air from the lungs through the nose and mouth. The average velocity of a sneeze is forty-two meters/second) equivalent to approximately ninety-five miles per hour. A single sneeze can disperse up to forty thousand aerosol droplets, which can transmit pathogens and disease. The sneeze is a much more effective dispersant of infectious material than a cough or peaking. The average velocity of a cough was 15.3 meters per second and the average velocity of the breath of normal speech is 4.07 meters per second.

Although the mechanism of increasing intra-abdominal pressure is similar to generating intra-thoracic pressure for a sneeze the exit orifice is a major determinant of velocity. No one has voluntarily gotten close enough to a fart blast to measure its ejection velocity or count the vapor droplets. The brave soul who does so may not get a Nobel Prize, but would certainly be worthy of nomination for an IgNobel Prize.

onpasture.com Creative Commons License

Coughing and sneezing release a large plume of aerosolized droplets impregnated with microbial pathogens. The sneeze and cough, which can easily reach a velocity of over one hundred miles per hour (one hundred and sixty kilometers per hour) and has been recorded at speeds up to five-hundred miles per hour (eight-hundred km/hour), will spread throughout a large size room. Even the flushing of a toilet will aerosolize fecal microbes that would cover a room in dimensions of twenty feet by twenty feet in a matter of seconds.

Farts have been recorded with the speed of aroma travelling at an extremely conservative ten miles per hour. It was not clear if this was from an individual wearing clothing at the time. A vigorous blast from a wet fart would probably look like the third photograph humorously labeled as Save the Whale. Perhaps science will one day answer the question about fart speed, or perhaps a watch company will sponsor a competition for the Guinness book of world records which has a number of fart categories already entered into the competitive arena. Another aspect that defines the extent of the reach of a fart besides its initial velocity and volume is the rate of diffusion. This is dependent on physical barriers such as layers of clothing or sitting on a cushion as well as air turbulence and ventilation. Please see entry on fart diffusion for more details.

Back in the 1946 a spoof recording of the International Crepitation Contest was created, and it is still commercially available today. It was apparently produced by some recording engineers for the Canadian Broadcasting Corporation and was held on February 31, 1946 as the World Championship Crepitation Contest at the

Maple Leaf Auditorium at Thunderblow, Canada between competitors Paul Boomer and Lord Windesmear.

Fart, Survey

The following Internet based survey of over one thousand three hundred male participants and an unspecified number of female participants does not qualify as scientifically or statistically valid. However for anecdotal and entertainment purposes it is as good as it gets when it comes to this subject matter.

Number of times women fart per day:

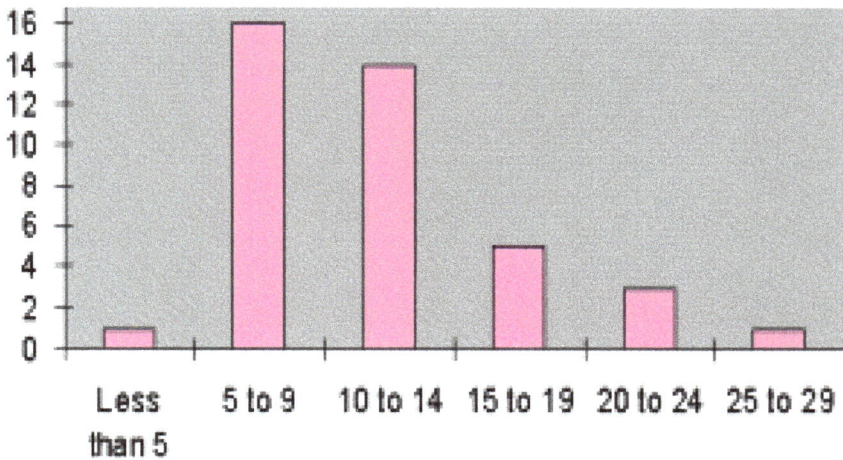

Women fart an average of eight times per day. Fifty percent of the women surveyed fart between five and ten times per day.

Women: Can you fart on command also called "Butt Breathe"?

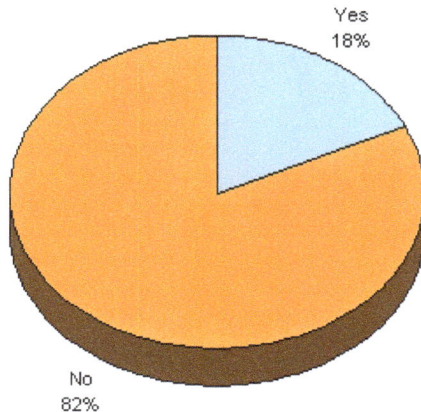

Eighteen percent of the women surveyed can fart on command by sucking air into the colon.

Women: Do you like to fart?

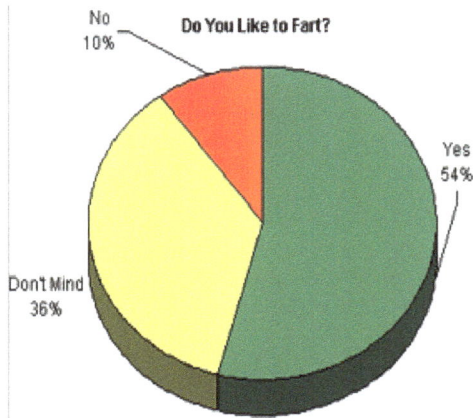

Do You Like to Fart?

No 10%

Yes 54%

Don't Mind 36%

Only half of the women surveyed admit that they like to fart. About twenty percent don't mind farting, but don't necessarily like it. Only ten percent of women are absolutely insistent that they do not like to fart, but they would certainly change their mind if they experienced the results of being unable to fart!

Women: When you were younger did you like to fart in water to make bubbles?

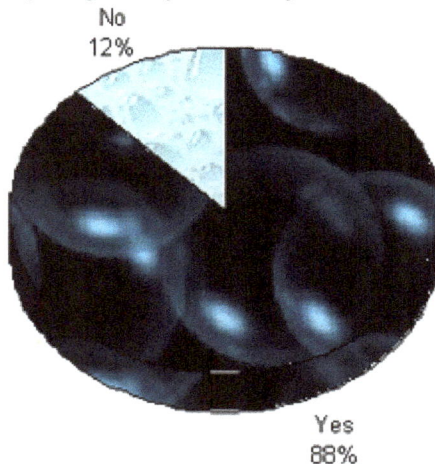

No 12%

Yes 88%

Most women liked to fart in the bathtub or pool to make bubbles.

Number of times men fart per day:

Men fart an average of fourteen times per day. Fifty percent of the men surveyed fart between five and fifteen times per day.

Men: Can you fart on command also called "Butt Breathe"?

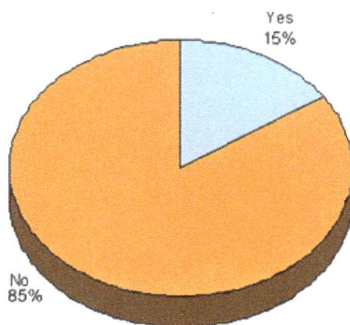

Only fifteen percent of the men surveyed can fart on command by sucking air into the colon. One third of all men did not even know that this is possible.

Men: When you were younger did you like to fart in water to make bubbles?

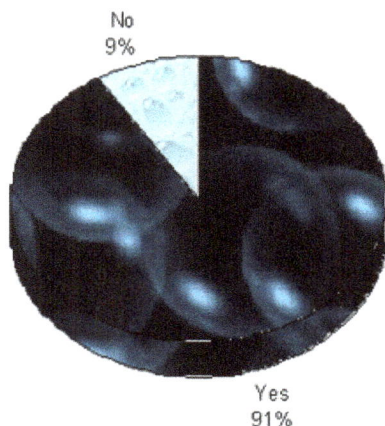

The vast majority of men liked to fart in the bathtub or pool to make bubbles.

Fart, Therapeutic Options

Many individuals have issues with unpleasant fecal odors, and unfortunately it is not as easily remedied as flushing or walking away. The fecal aroma generated by the gut microbiome that offers the characteristic smell of defecated feces is the identical aroma that may be discharged with intestinal gas, fecal incontinence, fistula, ostomies, diarrhea, inflammatory bowel disease, after gastric bypass surgery, and a host of other conditions. The numbers of individuals affected is in the millions in the United States alone. Unfortunately, the majority of the general public remains uninformed and impose a social stigma on a medical condition over which they have limited or no control.

Fortunately, there are a number of effective therapeutic options available, but too many sufferers are not aware of or have access to them. They range from external appliances and clothing, to external and internal deodorants and suppressants. Of course there are also tongue-in-cheek suggestions, such as getting a dog to blame as the source of the fart odor. The Merck Manual a few years back suggested working on perfecting one's glare, just glare at someone else as if they were the source.

More direct references to farts has been employed in the advertising campaign of air-freshener company Poo-Pourri. Although the advertising campaign received a nomination as one of the worst ads by a national newspaper, it was a major hit on social media with over thirty million views. For a holiday themed advertisement Santa Claus is farting on the toilet, while an attractive model sings a parody of a seasonal tune.

Poo-Pourri Advertising video www.ninjamarkweting.it

Shreddies advertising campaign for activated charcoal odor adsorbing underwear myshreddies.com

Beano was one of the first products to advertise a product designed to reduce intestinal gas.
Its ad first appeared in *Vegetarian Times*

Flat-D advertises and markets a wide variety of activated charcoal products to adsorb the aroma of flatus and other body odors. www.flat-d.com

*Air*Veda: Ancient & New Medical Wisdom

Flat-D advertises and markets a wide variety of activated charcoal products to adsorb the aroma of flatus and other body odors. Activated charcoal seat cushions, liners for underwear and clothing, and sleeping sack are amongst the numerous products they offer. www.flat-d.com

Flat-D offers another approach to protect the individual from offensive odors, by wearing an activated charcoal facemask covering the mouth and nose. www.flat-d.com

Surprisingly, while it can provide relief and comfort to many sufferers, some media outlets refuse to place advertisements for products dealing with flatulence and ostomy odors. Deodorants, feminine hygiene douches, tampons, sanitary napkins for menstruation, diapers for adults with incontinence, erectile dysfunction prescriptions, etcetera have been seen by the public without the downfall of social order. Devrom, an effective internal deodorant that suppresses fecal odor was not allowed to place their advertisement in *Reader's Digest* or *AARP Magazine* (Association for the Advancement of Retired People) because it contained the word stool and referred to smelling flatulence. Somehow the publications did not see the irony in that their policy did not pass the proverbial smell test of good judgment.

Devrom is an over the counter preparation of bismuth subgallate and has been marketed for over fifty years as an internal deodorant. Bismuth does have antibacterial properties it may change the microbiome by reducing the organisms that contribute to offensive flatulence. Another bismuth product that has been popular in the marketplace is Pepto-Bismol, which is a bismuth subsalicylate. Bismuth subsalicylate is related to aspirin (salicylic acid) and does not appear to provide as significant relief from the unpleasant odors as has been reported with Devrom.

It has been particularly popular for individuals who have undergone gastric bypass surgery, inflammatory bowel disease, as well as those with ostomies, and others. With advances in surgery, and the ability to preserve sphincters or create artificial sphincters, ostomies are seen less frequently. This is where the intestinal discharge exits the body through an artificial opening, the ostomy, created at surgery. Because the bowel is diverted from the colon less moisture is absorbed and the feces may be semi-formed or liquid.

The more liquid form allows for the more rapid vaporization of volatile organic compounds and gasses that give rise to the feculent odor. In spite of being in otherwise excellent health, many individuals with these issues find themselves socially restricted in their activities because of concern about embarrassment or offending others. Safe and effective products are available, but many individuals are unaware and suffer unnecessarily because of the lack of information and understanding.

Bismuth is a chemical element, number eighty-three on the periodic table, which has long history of being used in preparations designed to treat gastrointestinal complaints. It is a heavy metal with a low level of toxicity. Its various compounds have also been used historically to treat syphilis and the severe diarrhea from cholera. Bismuthinite is a mineral consisting of bismuth sulfide (Bi_2S_3) and is an important ore for bismuth.

The mechanism of action is unknown and may be related to its known antimicrobial activity, perhaps inhibiting the microbes that generate some of the more offensive gasses that usually contain sulfur as well as aromatic and volatile organic compounds. Bismuth also reacts directly with sulfur generating bismuth sulfide, a dark black insoluble compound. This can cause darkening or blackening of the tongue if sulfur is found in high concentrations in the saliva. It will also cause blackening of the stool as it binds with the sulfur that would otherwise give rise to hydrogen sulfide and other offensive sulfur gasses. The dark black color of the stool may be mistaken for melena, a sign of internal bleeding that results from the digestive process on blood cells and hemoglobin. The black coloration is not a health concern and is temporary, clearing with cessation of bismuth intake.

Activated carbon is used to treat oral poisonings by binding to and preventing the poison from being absorbed by the gastrointestinal tract. Charcoal biscuits were marketed in the early nineteenth century as an antidote to flatulence, and are still marketed today for diarrhea, indigestion, flatulence, and as a pet care product. Unfortunately, orally ingested charcoal pills are not effective in appreciably reducing intestinal gas. This may be because the adsorptive capacity of the activated charcoal is fully utilized before it finally gets to the colon where its gas adsorbing properties are most needed. Fortunately, bismuth products do provide a significant advantage by binding to the sulfur compounds and eliminating them without producing offensive gas.

Activated charcoal used as a treatment of aerophagia. Shutterstock/wasanajai

Fart, Underwater

It is to be expected that all living creatures that pass gas on land and in the air will do so underwater as well. A large number of humans find this to be a particularly pleasurable activity as confirmed on a large Internet based survey. Of course other animals will release gas underwater as a matter of nature, although they may find it entertaining as well as humans. For more information about the sounds generated by underwater farts please see entry on fart, sound (Acoustic, auditory).

The hippopotamus (Greek hippos-horse and potamus-river) is considered by many experts to be the most dangerous animal in Africa (excluding the malaria carrying mosquito) having killed many more people than lions have. The hippo is extremely aggressive with its huge canine teeth and sharp incisors, has unpredictable behavior, and is fearless of humans. Most deaths occur when the victim gets between the hippo and deep water or between a mother and her calf. Hippos weigh up to eight thousand pounds, gallop at eighteen miles per hour (twenty-nine kilometers per hour), sleep or lounge around on riverbanks and in the water most of the day, and graze on the grasslands at night. Their skin secretes sticky pinkish oil that helps protect them from the sun. They defecate generous amounts of excrement into the rivers and ponds in which they wallow all day, punctuated by voluminous farts. They also participate in marking territory by what the hippo experts refer to as "dung showering." They blow feces mixed with urine over a large area around their watering hole, twirling their relatively short tails like fans to distribute the aromatic spray.

www.home-remedies.br Creative Commons License

Marine research scientists studying the Minke whale population near Antarctica were able to capture a whale fart on film for the first time. The photograph was taken from the bow of the research vessel and the fart subsequently surfaced right under their noses. "We got away from the bow of the ship very quickly ... it does stink," said Nick Gales, a research scientist from the Australian Antarctic Division. However, the skunk like episode did not detract them from completing their mission of collecting DNA from whale dung and attaching satellite tracking devices to the whales to study their migration patterns. Many fish have a swim air bladder that is inflated or deflated as needed to maintain buoyancy. Usually expelled swim air bladder gas exits the mouth but the sand tiger shark, *Carcharias taurus*, discharges it out the anus. The carbon dioxide produced is eliminated via the gills. Methane, hydrogen, and other gasses would typically be released as a fart. Fisherman knew about herring farts and they were even written about back in 1914 by Swedish author Ludvig Runebergwrote in his masterpiece Bottenhavsfiskare (Bothnian Bay Fishermen). The section below is freely translated from the Swedish.

"In the evening they were rowing away to the barren islands, pulled up the boats, lit a fire and made coffee, opened the dinner box and ate. While they were sitting there a group of fishermen were staring out towards the sea, the sun sinking, the sky turning red, and the waves smoothing, wind dying, moon sailing out, lonely and large, the ducks moving back and forth in trains, and in all this, which no longer looked like the earth but more seemed to be an advection into the sky, a distant boiling was seen on the blank water surface. Thousands and thousands of small blisters glaring into the sea, without it being possible to say wherefrom they came, and only in one small defined place: it was the herring which was approaching them on its migration."

Fart, Vagina

Fart is also a term used for an emission or expulsion of air from the vagina. It may occur during or after sexual intercourse or during other sexual acts, stretching, exercise, getting up from a chair, etcetera. Puffs or small amounts of air passed into the vaginal cavity during cunnilingus are normally not associated with vaginal fart. However, "forcing" or purposely blowing air at force into the vaginal canal can cause an air embolism which is dangerous for the woman, and if pregnant for the fetus. The sound of flatus from the vagina is somewhat comparable to flatulence from the anus but does not have a feculent odor in the normal state. If a feculent odor is present it may be because of a colovaginal fistula, a serious condition involving a tear between the vagina and colon. A colovaginal fistula can result from surgery, childbirth, diseases such as the inflammatory bowel disease Crohn disease, trauma such as rape and sexual abuse, infections, and other causes. This condition can lead to urinary tract infection and other complications. Slang terms for vaginal flatulence include *vart*, *queef* and *fanny fart* (mostly British).

i9.photobucket.com Creative Commons License

Fart, Visual

It may sound hard to visualize a fart, but it is actually fairly simple, it's that the circumstances have to be just right. Yes, in releasing an invisible gas into invisible air you would normally not expect to see it with the limited visual spectrum of the human eye. However, if you had vision in the infrared portion of the electromagnetic spectrum it would be very visible. With the advent of infrared photography and thermographic imagery the invisible fart can be visualized. You can also see the fart if the temperature and humidity are just right. If you were in the polar zones, at very high altitude, in frigid weather, or even in a walk-in freezer, dropping a fart from exposed buttocks would look much like the steamy cloud of warm breath on a cold winter day. One should be careful about trying this when it is dangerously frigid as frostbite of this sensitive part of the anatomy may result in a new medical malady, which I hereby name 'frostbutt'.

i.telegraph.co.uk

Frostbite is a real risk for mountaineers, and for Mount Everest climbers the comforts of base camp at an altitude of 17,590 feet may be the last chance they have for a protected bowel movement without exposing their behinds to the extreme winds and weather approaching the summit. Frozen poop stays permanently frozen and does not decompose at that altitude, so there is a growing collection from earlier expeditions that is of concern. Climbers are having a more challenging timed finding ice that has not been contaminated for melting into drinking water. Drinking contaminated water and developing diarrhea at that high altitude and hostile environment would increase the exposure to frostbite dramatically. The most visible of the visual farts occur in the bathtub or when immersed in water, like a swimming pool or hot whirlpool tub. If you are sharing the water with someone else the innocent looking telltale bubbles underwater can deliver a powerful bouquet to the unsuspecting nose. The intensity of the olfactory message of the human sense of smell is modulated by the brain and limbic system. If you are in a bathroom having a bowel movement the fart odor is less noticeable and certainly less alarming then when you are in an elevator, theater, or restaurant, and you are aromatically assaulted without forewarning.

Fart, Volume (Quantity)

The fact is that all living creatures create gas from the cellular respiration, which is ubiquitous through various life forms. The bacteria in your intestinal flora generate microscopic nanofarts and microfarts, which collect into larger bubbles of gas in the bowel. They are intermixed with the atmospheric air swallowed throughout the day and particularly at meals, when chewing gum, or when chewing or smoking tobacco or other recreational products. Aerophagia is universal and we swallow on average three to five milliliters (one teaspoonful) of air with every swallow. Now add into the mixture the gasses produced during the enzymatic digestive processes as well as the neutralization of gastric hydrochloric acid and pancreatic and duodenal bicarbonate and you have a virtual windstorm of voluminous gasses transiting the bowel.

Fortunately, the vast majority of the gasses produced are absorbed by the gut, then dissolve into the bloodstream through diffusion and as a solution, finally being exhaled when they reach the alveoli of the lungs and can be exchanged with atmospheric air. The component gasses have very different properties of diffusion through the bowel wall and into the bloodstream. Carbon dioxide readily diffuses and enters solution and is exhaled, such that although it is the largest volume of gas generated by far, and temporarily is a major contributor to distension and postprandial (after meal) discomfort, it is the easiest to eliminate from the bowel and is only a minor contributor to flatulence. Nitrogen is the largest volume component of atmospheric air, and as would be expected, represents an identically high proportion of the gasses swallowed through aerophagia. Once in the body the carbon dioxide of the air is absorbed and eliminated as discussed above. The nitrogen however is a very poorly absorbed gas, and in essence will either come back up as a burp, or will sooner or later, comes out the other end as a fart.

The oxygen in the air, representing nearly twenty-one percent of the air gasses swallowed during aerophagia, is absorbed slowly, as the gut is not nearly as efficient at absorbing oxygen as the lungs are for respiration. As the carbon dioxide and oxygen are absorbed the percent of the gastrointestinal tract air that is nitrogen increases. As soon as the digestive process begins, hydrochloric acid of the stomach is neutralized by sodium bicarbonate of the duodenum and pancreas. Large volumes of carbon dioxide gas are generated, as are smaller quantities of hydrogen, methane, and other aromatic gasses discussed later. The volume of gasses in the gastrointestinal tract is dependent on the quantity and nature of foods ingested, the body's ability to synthesize and utilize specific enzymes for the various food types, the nature and quantity of the bacteria in the gut flora, the speed of gastrointestinal transit which may be influenced by drugs, hormones, food product and illness, the absorptive capacity and health of the mucosal lining, and the physical length of the individual's gastrointestinal tract.

The question of what is the average number of farts per day is similar to the question if what is an average price for a normal used car. What year, make, model, condition, diesel or gas or electric or hybrid, mileage, etc. etc. The quoted figure of eleven and one-half farts per day is a reasonable approximation from a very small sample size of male medical students, but normal has a very wide range depending on the variables. The female medical students were too smart to participate in the study so as far as science is concerned, women do not fart.

Later suggestions that they fart, but less than the guys, is just as suspect. The differences in the physical attributes between male and female of a species represent their sexual dimorphism. The theory of sexual selection advanced by Charles Darwin in 1871 is closely related to sexual dimorphism. On average adult human males are four percent taller and eight percent heavier than females. In a number of other species, it is the female that is larger, occasionally dramatically so. The triple wart sea devil, an anglerfish, exhibits extreme sexual dimorphism, with the male becoming little more than a stunted sperm-producing body that lives a parasitic existence off of the females hard work and effort in providing livelihood and producing the next generation of offspring. Some human males appear to have evolved their behavioral patterns from the anglerfish modus operandi.

In most mammals, humans included, the males are larger in size, mass, and caloric intake. In most species it is the female that is diminutive in size, sometimes dramatically so. It would only make sense that males would generate more gas, but how do the two compare if the caloric intake and composition were identical? Since there are no identically comparable cases, the studies would have to compare averages of large populations of each gender to minimize the variables as much as possible. As curious as we may be to know the answer to this question vital to gender politics and security, no studies are planned or anticipated. There have been reports of extreme flatulence in the medical literature of what may be considered the upper limits of the normal range, up to one hundred and fifty farts in a twenty-four-hour period.

As we age we produce less digestive enzymes and there is an argument to be made that there should be an adjustment and tolerance allowed for 'old farts'. Perhaps the best excuse is that you did not do anything, it's the billions of nanofarting and microfarting bacteria that are to blame. If you are told to pick on someone closer to your own size, you could blame the dog and claim it is a talented ventrilo-farter. Trying to arrive at a definition of what constitutes a discrete individual fart is a challenge. Is a staccato stutter of ten small farts completed in rapid succession to count as one or ten? Is one large long loud fart the equivalent of four small farts over thirty seconds. Should a loud tuba blast count the same as a faint toot?

Fart, Weight

As a fart is composed of atoms and molecules it has physical properties, including a mass and weight. Since it is composed of gasses and volatile molecules it is very light, yet the weight is measureable. In addition, each fart carries a sampling of the gut microbiome, aerosolized microbes the significance of which has never been evaluated in terms of potential for disease transmission. Each person's microbiome and thus fart is unique, much like fingerprints, although don't expect it to be used for personal identification on a television forensic science drama anytime soon. The total mass of the average fart is 0.0371 grams. For those wishing to lose weight every fart means you weigh just a little bit less. The constituent gasses and mass of the average fart is listed below:

Nitrogen: 0.0263 grams
Hydrogen: 0.0003 grams
Carbon Dioxide: 0.0063 grams
Methane: 0.0018 grams
Oxygen: 0.0016 grams
Odiferous Products: 0.0008 grams

Fecal Microbiota Transplant

A Fecal Microbiota Transplant (FMT) is also known as a stool transplant, fecal transplant, fecal bacteriotherapy, fecal transfusion, fecal enema, human probiotic infusion, and in its most ancient form of oral administration as coprophagia. One of the side effects of taking antibiotics is that they not only eliminate the harmful pathogenic microorganisms, but they also harm the normal commensal microbiome. When the balance of the microbiome is disrupted, an organism named *Clostridia difficile* may predominate the gut microbiome with horrific and life threatening consequences. This condition is known as antibiotic associated colitis, and is also known as pseudomembranous colitis. It results in severe and often intractable diarrhea. For many years, the treatment required multiple and prolonged course of ever stronger antibiotics, which all too often failed to eradicate the infection and led to relapses.

The alternative approach of transplanting feces from a healthy donor into the bowel of the patient with antibiotic associated colitis courses was initially perceived as counterintuitive, if not offensive to the sensibilities of modern medicine and the Western ethic of hygiene. The fact that the treatment is remarkably effective, and much safer and less expensive that intensive antibiotic therapy, surprisingly did not result in its rapid adoption. A lack of understanding on both the part of the public, as well as the medical industrial complex, brought fecal transplantation into the crosshairs of regulators and industry. Instead of recognition and accolades of the heroic status of fecal donors and establishment of national Brown Cross donation centers and stool banks, the Food and Drug Administration attempted to regulate the procedure into the realm of multi-year and multi-billion-dollar research studies within academia and industry.

Fecal transplantation is becoming more established, not only as the treatment of choice for antibiotic associated colitis from *Clostridia difficile,* but is being investigated for its reported benefits in a whole host of digestive disorders such as inflammatory bowel disease (ulcerative colitis, Crohn Disease), irritable bowel syndrome, leaky gut, constipation, and other non-digestive conditions such as arthritis, cancer, heart disease, multiple sclerosis, Parkinson Disease, autism, metabolic syndrome, diabetes, autoimmune disorders, obesity, etc. The role of the gut microbiome is an area of intense research interest, and preliminary research data suggests it will revolutionize our understanding of disease and treatment.

*Air*Veda: Ancient & New Medical Wisdom

Low-temperature electron micrograph of a cluster of E. coli bacteria, magnified ten thousand times. Each individual bacterium is oblong shaped. 2005 Photo by Eric Erbe Public Domain

With further progress in understanding the optimal gut microbiome for an individual, the future of repopulating the gut with a healthy microbiome to treat and prevent disease will advance. Rather than the relatively crude approach of transplanting the feces of a healthy donor, the gut microbiome will be repopulated (repoopulated is a popular pun in the fecal transplant world) with a scientifically designed and formulated culture with the proper mixture and proportion of desired microbes. With the nature of the biomedical industry, one can envision specific patents and branding of gut microbiome cocktails for specific diseases, conditions, and desired outcomes.

The administration of fecal transplants will also expand beyond colonics, enemas, nasogastric tubes, and high tech and expensive administration via colonoscopy or endoscopy. Freeze dried, purified, healthy microbiome probiotics in sealed odorless tasteless sterile time released capsules with reduce the less than appealing stigma of a fecal transplant. Undoubtedly, even the terminology will be adapted to appeal to modern sensibilities. Perhaps Super Microbiome Supplementation will reach the level of popularity of protein supplements in nutritious organic fruit and vegetable juice blends!

Interestingly enough, fecal transplants were part of the armamentarium of ancient medicine from the days of Ayurveda, Chinese Medicine, and beyond. Bedouins have used consumption of fresh, warm camel feces as a remedy for bacterial dysentery for ages. Its efficacy may attributable to the antibiotic subtilisin from *Bacillus subtilis* or the wholesale substitution of the gut flora. German soldiers in Africa confirmed the effectiveness of the camel feces during World War II to whom it was administered when they had dysentery. Another possibility is that a number of the 'cured' did not get better but refused to admit it in order to avoid another dose of a 'medicine' that literally tasted like shit.

Fecal Oral Contamination Route (see Pathogen)

Fecal oral route (fecal oral contamination) is the transmission of a disease pathogen via feces particles that are ingested by the now infected host. The process of transmission may be by gross contamination as described by the term coprophagia, but much more often the transmission is less visible or microscopic (although it technically remains coprophagia). Examples may include a scenario where a fly that had been feeding on feces lands and feeds on open food at a picnic, which it contaminates by the feces residue on its feet. Swimming in a pool that had an undisclosed recent toddler 'accident'. Poor hand washing after a bowel movement with less than perfect toilet paper wiping, then eating finger foods such as potato chips or popcorn from a common bowl.

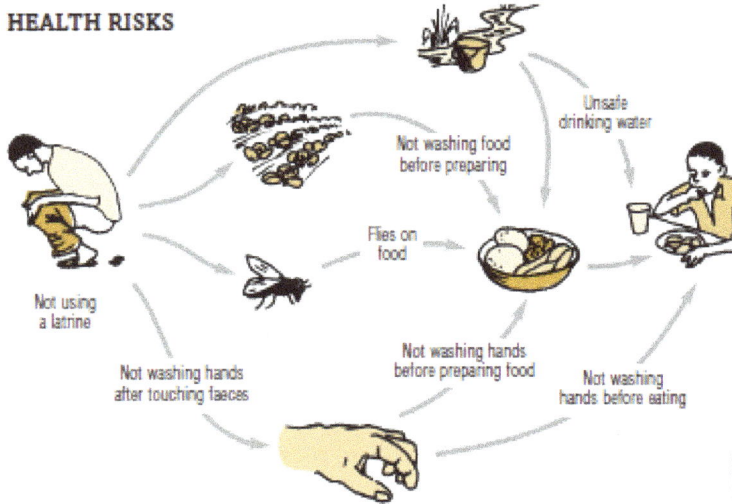

HEALTH RISKS

Unsafe drinking water

Not washing food before preparing

Flies on food

Not using a latrine

Not washing hands after touching faeces

Not washing hands before preparing food

Not washing hands before eating

The degree of fecal oral contamination that takes place on a daily basis in even the most sophisticated and highest levels of socioeconomic achievement are sobering. An illness that is easily transmitted by purely fecal oral contamination will infect nearly all members of any closely living household within a matter of days. The number of infectious particles we are exposed to each and every day is astronomical. Rotavirus is transmitted by the fecal oral route and is the most common cause of severe diarrhea among infants and young children. Nearly every child in the world has been infected with rotavirus at least once by the age of five. If is estimated to cause about forty per cent of all hospital admissions due to diarrhea among children under five years of age worldwide, leading to one hundred million episodes of acute diarrhea that result in three hundred and fifty thousand to six hundred thousand child deaths each year.

The number of infectious viral particles in one gram (less than one thirtieth of an ounce) of feces from a child with rotavirus is more than ten trillion (10,000,000,000,000). One child in a household has more than enough viral particles in a thimble of stool to infect every human on the planet Earth and another ten thousand planets with the same population. Some of the diseases that can be passed via the fecal-oral route include poliomyelitis, norovirus acute gastroenteritis, giardiasis, hepatitis A, hepatitis E, rotavirus, shigellosis (bacillary dysentery), typhoid fever, *Vibrio parahaemolyticus* infections, enteroviruses, cholera, clostridium difficile, cryptosporidiosis, ascariasis, and many others.

Disease can be transmitted from a latrine too close to the well

1 - Improperly situated pit
Privy contaminates
Water supply

2 - Water is untreated
before use

3 - Disease is transmitted

Feces

Feces (Latin fæx "dregs") (excrement, shit, turd, and dozens of other euphemisms) are the excreted waste product from the digestive tract expelled through the anus during defecation. Although the digestive tract has extracted nutrients the fecal matter often has fifty percent of its energy value remaining. This is a vital resource for organisms such as bacteria, fungi, and insects such as the fly and dung beetle. Human fecal matter varies significantly in appearance, depending on diet and health. A sticky gummy texture is often noted with substantial internal bleeding, which also often presents as black tarry stool called melena.

Brown Stool - Human feces ordinarily has a light to dark brown coloration, which results from a combination of bile and bilirubin that is derived from the breakdown products of dead red blood cells.

Yellow Stool - Stool that is yellow may suggest presence of undigested fat in the stool. The stool containing the undigested fat may appear yellowish in color, greasy, and also may smell foul. Yellowing of feces may also be caused by an infection that may also cause diarrhea, such as from *Giardia lamblia* a protozoan parasite.

Black Stool (Melena) - Feces can be black due to the presence of red blood cells that have been broken down by digestive enzymes. This is known as melena, and is typically due to bleeding in the upper digestive tract, such as from a bleeding peptic ulcer. The same color change can be observed after consuming foods that contain a substantial proportion of animal blood, such as black pudding or tiết canh.

Black feces can also be caused by a number of medications containing bismuth products (such as Pepto-Bismol and the newer formulation of Kaopectate in the United States), iron supplements, or foods such as beetroot, black liquorice (also spelled as licorice), or blueberries.

Red Stool - Hematochezia is similarly the passage of feces that are bright red due to the presence of undigested blood, either from lower in the digestive tract, or from a more active source in the upper digestive tract. Ingestion of red beets will also color the stool and can be easily misinterpreted as a sign of internal bleeding. Besides the dramatic blood red color of beets, a similar red color may also come from natural or artificial coloring such as red gelatin, popsicles, Kool-Aid, and dragon fruit.

Blue Stool - Prussian blue, used in the treatment of radiation, cesium, and thallium poisoning, can turn the feces blue. Substantial consumption of products containing blue food dye, such as blue curaçao or grape soda, can have a similar effect.

White (Acholic) Stool - Acholic stools, which are pasty white in color, are characteristic of complete biliary obstruction.

Silver Stool - Silver or aluminum feces color results when biliary obstruction of any type (acholic or white stool) combines with gastrointestinal bleeding from any source that would normally present as black stools or melena

Green Stool - Feces can be green due to having large amounts of unprocessed bile in the digestive tract. When stool passes through the intestines rapidly (diarrhea) there may be little time for bilirubin to undergo its usual chemical changes. Green feces may occasionally be the result from eating liquorice (also spelled as licorice) candy, as it is typically made with anise oil rather than liquorice herb and is predominantly sugar. Excessive sugar consumption or a sensitivity to anise oil may cause loose, green stools.

When a pediatric colleague was in medical school a professor was quizzing the medical students about the significance of different colored stools. The group was asked what question they would ask if a young lady patient told them she was passing golden stools. My friend Dick Buchta told me this story in the presence of his wife Diane so he assured us it was a different medical student, not him, who quickly responded with the question that should be asked: Will you marry me?

Feces are often used as fertilizer, both manure and guano becoming large commercial enterprises. Historically, human waste euphemistically called night soil was used as a major source of fertilizer. Animal feces, especially those of camel, bison, oxen, yak, water buffalo, and cattle can be used as fuel or building material when dried. Terms such as dung, scat, spoor, manure, castings, spraint, fewmets, guano, and droppings are used to refer to specific animal feces.

Common animal dropping (scat) names are:

cattle - tath
otter -spraints
cow - bodewash, cowpies, buffalo chips, dung, cow pats
seafowl - guano,
earthworm - wormcast
dinosaur - coprolite
Hart and deer - fewmets
hare - crotiles, crotisings
boar, bear, and wolf - lesses
fox - billitting
vermin - fuants;
hawk – mutes
dog - scumber
caterpillars and leaf beetles – frass
horse – manure, roadapple
wild carnivores - scat

Feces Waste Management

Feces waste management has been a concern from pre-Biblical times:
"And thou shalt have a paddle upon thy weapon; and it shall be, when thou wilt ease thyself abroad, thou shalt dig therewith, and shalt turn back and cover that which cometh from thee: For the LORD thy God walketh in the midst of thy camp, to deliver thee, and to give up thine enemies before thee; therefore shall they camp be holy: that he see no unclean thing in thee, and turn away from thee." (Deuteronomy 23:13-14).

Composting Toilet

A composting toilet is a dry toilet that uses managed aerobic decomposition to treat human waste. They are an alternative to flush toilets where there is a limited water supply or no waste treatment facility is available. The human excrement is normally mixed with sawdust, coconut coir, or peat moss to support aerobic processing, absorb liquids, and to reduce odor. The decomposition process is typically faster than the anaerobic decomposition used in wet sewage systems such as septic tanks.

Urine can contain ninety percent percent of the nitrogen, fifty percent of the phosphorus, and seventy percent of the potassium present in human excreta. In healthy individuals the urine is sterile and thus pathogen free. Undiluted urine may contain inorganic salts and organic compounds toxic to plants. The requirement critical for aerobic microbial action is sufficient oxygen. Some units require manual methods for periodic aeration of the solid mass. Significant reductions in the volume of waste occurs through the process with only ten percent of the inputs coming out as a humus-like material which can be used as a soil amendment.

Pit Toilet

A pit toilet is a dry toilet system which collects human excrement in a large container and can range from a simple slit trench to a more elaborate outhouse with a ventilation pipe. They are used in rural and wilderness areas as well as in much of the developing world. When the pit is improved with a small enclosed structure with a roof for shelter and a seat with a hole in it it is commonly known as an outhouse.

The ventilated improved pit latrine, or VIP, is a pit toilet outhouse with a ventilation pipe and a screen at the top outlet. VIP latrines are an improvement over simple pit latrines by reducing odors, flies, and mosquito nuisance and unpleasant odors. The ventilation pipe also removes the explosive danger of accumulated methane gas from the decomposition of the human waste in the pit.

Sewers

A sewage system may convey the wastewater by gravity, pumping, or vacuum to a sewage treatment plant. Pipelines range in size from six inches (one hundred and fifty millimeters) to tunnels of up to thirty feet (ten meters) in diameter. Although sewer systems are intended to transport only sewage and not storm runoff all sewer systems have some degree of infiltration of groundwater which can lead to sewer overflows.

The first sanitation system has been identified in prehistoric ruins near Zabol, Iran. The ancient cities of Harappa and Mohenjo-daro of the Indus Valley civilization developed networks of brick-lined sewers around 2600 BC and also had outdoor toilets that were flushed with water from reservoirs. Ancient Minoan civilization also had stone sewers that were flushed with water. Roman towns and garrisons in the United Kingdom between 46 BC and 400 AD had sewer networks sometimes constructed out of hollowed-out logs.

In the developed world sewers are usually pipelines from buildings to larger underground trunk mains, which transport the sewage to sewage treatment facilities. Vertical pipes, called manholes, connect the mains to the surface and are used for maintenance and to vent sewer gases. Sewers are generally gravity powered although pumping stations may be necessary. For decades sanitary sewer cracks or other damage could be repaired only by the expensive operation of digging up the damaged pipe and replacing it. In the mid-1950's technology advanced where a special cement mixture coated the inside of the pipe sealing all cracks and breaks.

Many cities built sewer systems to control outbreaks of disease such as typhoid fever and cholera. Initially these systems discharged sewage directly to surface waters such as rivers and lakes without treatment. As pollution of water bodies grew cities added sewage treatment plants to their systems to chlorinate and filter the water and sewage discharged. The institution of sewerage systems was a great public health advance.

Dung Beetle

Scarabaeus laticollis

Dung beetles are beetles that feed partly or exclusively on feces. "Never did adventurers hurrying from the four corners of the earth display such eagerness," the French entomologist Jean-Henri Fabre once wrote. "They are there in the hundreds, large and small, of every sort, shape and size, hastening to carve themselves a slice of the common cake." Some grab what dung they can and cram it underground on the spot. Dung beetles have been known to steal treasured dung balls from each other. Others, the ball-rollers, embark on a journey that requires the heavens to navigate.

*Air*Veda: Ancient & New Medical Wisdom

All the species belong to the superfamily Scarabaeoidea which alone comprises more than five thousand species. Many dung beetles, known as *rollers*, roll dung into round balls, which are used as a food source or brooding chambers. They can roll up to ten times their weight and some species can pull up to one thousand times their weight. Other dung beetles, known as *tunnelers*, bury the dung wherever they find it. A third group, the dwellers, neither roll nor burrow: they simply live in manure. Dung beetles are currently the only animal, other than humans, known to navigate and orient themselves using the Milky Way.

Dung beetles play an important role in agriculture by burying and consuming dung that improves nutrient recycling and soil structure. They also protect livestock, such as cattle, by removing the dung which, if left in the open could provide habitat for pests. Many countries have introduced the creatures for the benefit of animal husbandry and as an adjunct for improving standards of hygiene. Several species of the dung beetle, most notably the species *Scarabaeus sacer* often referred to as the sacred scarab, enjoyed a sacred status among the ancient Egyptians. The scarab was linked to Khepri ("he who has come into being") the god of the rising sun. The image of the scarab symbolizing transformation, renewal, and resurrection, is ubiquitous in ancient Egyptian religious and funerary art.

The ancients believed that the dung beetle was unique in that only the male gender existed, and that it reproduced by depositing semen into a dung ball. The supposed self-creation of the beetle resembles that of Khepri, who creates himself out of nothing. The dung ball rolled by a dung beetle resembles the sun. In ancient Greece Plutarch wrote: The race of beetles has no female, but all the males eject their sperm into a round pellet of material which they roll up by pushing it from the opposite side, just as the sun seems to turn the heavens in the direction opposite to its own course, which is from west to east.

The dung beetle has several appearances in the classical literature. In Aesop's fable *The Dung Beetle and the Eagle*, the eagle kills a hare despite the beetle's appeals. The beetle takes revenge by twice destroying the eagle's eggs. The eagle, in despair, flies up to Olympus and places her latest eggs in Zeus's lap, beseeching the god to protect them. When the beetle finds out what the eagle has done, it stuffs itself with dung, goes straight up to Zeus and flies right into his face. Zeus is startled at the sight of the unpleasant creature and jumps to his feet. The eggs are broken. Zeus then learns of the beetle's plea which the eagle had ignored. He scolds the eagle and urges the beetle to stay away from the bird. But his efforts to persuade the beetle fail; so he changes the breeding season of the eagles to take place at a time when the beetles are not above ground.

The ancient Greek playwright Aristophanes alluded to Aesop's fable several times in his plays. In *Peace*, the hero rides up to Olympus to free the goddess Peace from her prison. His steed is an enormous dung beetle which has been fed so much dung that it has grown to monstrous size. In Franz Kafka's *The Metamorphosis*, the transformed character of Gregor Samsa is called an "old dung beetle" (alter Mistkäfer) by the charwoman.

Chamber Pot

A chamber pot (French: pot de chambre) is a pit like receptacle for receiving human waste. It was usually kept in the same chambers and under the sleeping bed and since the sixteenth century often enclosed in a stool with a lid. Chamber pots were used in ancient Greece at least since the sixth century BC and remained in common use in any parts of the world until the mid-twentieth century. In rural areas lacking indoor plumbing they are still in use today. They have also been modified to serve as bedpans for the ill and disabled.

The affectionate term "potty" is often used with children especially during toilet (potty) training. The term potty is also used to describe child size chamber pot type toilets that are at the appropriate height and have a child size opening to sit on. Regular adult toilets have an opening that is too large and frightening for a child who could accidentally fall in if not assisted. The height of the adult toilet does not allow their feet to touch the ground to assist in the squatting maneuver that assists defecation. A foot stool to give their feet a place on which to rest can assist squatting which eases the initiation of a bowel movement and can accelerate toilet training.

Close (Night) Stool

A close stool, also called a necessary or night stool, was in popular use for nearly five hundred years from the sixteenth century until the advent of indoor plumbing. It was an enclosed cabinet at chair height with an opening in the top often covered by a lid. It contained a pewter or earthenware chamber pot. In the nineteenth century it was referred to as a night commode, and in the twentieth century the commode euphemism was extended to the flush toilet.

Gong Farmer

Gong farmer was a term used in Tudor England for the worker who removed human excrement from outhouses, privies, cesspools, and cesspits. "Gong" is derived from the Old English gang, which means "to go", and since the eleventh century has been used to refer to a toilet facility, or privy, and its contents. They were only allowed to work at night and later became known as "night soil men" or "night men". The human feces they collected was known as night soil and was used as fertilizer. The emptying of cesspits today is usually accomplished with mechanical suction, by specialized tankers or trucks referred to by the euphemism Honey Truck.

Towns usually provided public latrines, known as houses of easement. Cesspits were often placed under cellar floors some of which had wooden chutes to convey the excrement. Cesspits allowed the liquid waste to drain leaving only the solids.

*Air*Veda: Ancient & New Medical Wisdom

Besides the offensive odor cesspits were a continual problem as the accumulation of solid waste required the services of gong farmers to dig out and remove the excrement. Perhaps to avoid overfilling their cesspit it was not uncommon for the contents of chamber pots to be thrown into the streets from upstairs windows.

Despite being well paid being a gong farmer's job was not considered an enviable occupation. They were only allowed to work between nine in the morning and five in the evening and were permitted to live only in certain areas. Besides the occupational hazard of infectious diseases, the concentrations of noxious and toxic gasses sometimes led to asphyxiation. Gong farmers often employed young boys to fill and lift buckets of excrement out of the pit because of the confined spaces. The excavated solid waste was removed in large barrels which were loaded onto a horse-drawn cart called the honey cart or wagon. It was not an infrequent event to discover the corpse of an unwanted infant during the clearing of cesspits.

The job is still commonplace in India where it has estimated that up to one million and three hundred thousand Indians work with the collection of human waste. These workers are considered the lowest of the untouchable caste. They confine marriage to within its members leading to a waste collecting caste passing the profession and caste burden on to the next generation. The recent film *Slumdog Millionaire* showed a brief glimpse of their existence.

Honey Bucket & Honey Wagon

A honey bucket is a bucket that is used as a toilet in locations that do not have more advanced facilities available. It often has a frame with a toilet seat lid and may be lined with a plastic bag for ease and convenience of disposal. A cover material such as sawdust may be used to reduce the odors from collected waste. Honey buckets are common in the far northern Arctic type climates especially where permafrost makes the installation of septic systems or outhouses impractical. They are seen throughout the world, especially in rural and undeveloped areas.

A honey wagon is a cart, wagon or truck for collecting and carrying excrement or manure. The term is often applied to the trucks that service septic tank systems as well as the bathroom on commercial aircraft. A recent news incident of a motor home bungled burglary of the siphoning of gasoline was reminiscent of a honeywagon. The police were called to investigate what was presumed to be an attempt to steal the gasoline from a parked vacation motor home. They found several empty gasoline transport containers, a length of rubber tubing, a pool of fecal material and vomited food.

The nighttime would be fuel thieves opened the flap door, removed the cap, and put the siphon hose in an applied oral suction to start the flow of what they assume would be gasoline. The thieves opened the cap and valve to the septic system by mistake, got a mouthful of sewage which they vomited up and fled the scene leaving their paraphernalia behind.

AirVeda: Ancient & New Medical Wisdom

Night Soil

Night soil is the common name used for human fecal waste collected at night from cesspools and outhouses. It is often used as a fertilizer in developing countries where it contributes to risk of acquiring parasites because the feces may contain eggs, such as is commonly seen in the roundworm *Ascaris lumbricoides*. Rarely, diseases have been transmitted into developed countries by the importation of vegetables with contaminated soil.

The use of night soil as fertilizer was common in Japan. The feces of rich people were sold at higher prices because their diet was better and it was thought that there would be more nutrients remaining in their waste. It brings a new level of understanding to the common phrases "filthy rich" and the "rich get richer". It could also serve as a learning and teaching model for salespeople in a competitive business to recognize that the salesperson who sold the shit of the rich at a higher price was the ultimate salesperson and marketer who could sell anything and would be a valuable addition to any company's sales force.

Selling night soil as fertilizers became less common after World War II for sanitary reasons as well as the increased availability of chemical fertilizers. Modern Japan still has some areas with ongoing traditional night soil collection and disposal. The Japanese name for the 'outhouse within the house' style toilet, with the night soil collected, is Kumitori Benjo (汲み取り便所). China, Singapore, and Hong Kong also had extensive use of night soil collection, especially from urbanized areas where open honey buckets were carried through the streets. Hong Kong has a euphemism called 倒夜香, which literally means "pour night fragrant".

Septage

The partially treated waste in a septic tank that does not drain into the soil or is decomposed by the bacteria in the tank is called septage. This term should not be confused by a septuagenarian who in their seventies may occasionally feel like a septagegenarian. It can be transported to local waste water treatment centers or stored to be used as fertilizer.

The septage in a septic tank is usually considered in one of three categories. Scum which floats to the top generally harbors the greatest concentration of bacteria. The layer below is called the effluent and is a semi-treated liquid. The layer of solids at the bottom of the tank is called sludge, or more descriptively as fecal sludge. The sludge accumulates over time and dependent on the number and volume of deposits and usage as well as the septic tank capacity, may function for many years of use before requiring emptying or service. An overflowing or backed up septage system is not a pleasant experience. A septage pump truck removes the septage material from septic tanks, portable toilets, recreational vehicles such as motor homes, and boats. In commercial aviation and other industries, this type of vehicle may also be called a honey wagon.

Outhouse

Many outhouses are simply holes in the ground, once the capacity is reached a new site selected and the outhouse structure moved. Keeping the waste site away from the source of drinking water important from a disease prevention and hygiene perspective. Many of the deaths attributed to military campaigns were actually caused by poor sanitation and waste management. The lack of hygiene and contaminated drinking water frequently led to more death and incapacitation of soldiers than those injured or killed in battles.

A two story outhouse with a political satire message.

I have been in locations with primitive toilet facilities, but had the most unusual experience in a very old three story building in Egypt. Much like in modern times the bathrooms were stacked directly over each other for ease of plumbing and drains. When this building was built the bathroom was a simple room with a hole in the ground, with lined up holes in the floors of the levels above. If you were using the ground floor hole as bathroom you had to make sure that you could see skylight through the holes above. If any of the floor holes above was eclipsed by a human moon, better get out of the way because sewage is about to be deposited!

Deities associated with defecation and elimination have an ancient history preceding Babylonian times. They were worshipped in Roman times and still have a role in folk beliefs of indigenous peoples of Japan, China, New Zealand and other parts of the world. Such deities have been associated with bowel health, general well-being, and fertility because of the use of human waste as a fertilizer for agriculture.

245

Ancient Rome had three gods involved in the passage of human waste. The sewer goddess Cloacina (Latin sewer) had her origins in Etruscan beliefs and was the protectors of the Cloaca Maxima, Rome's sewage system. Titus Tatius, who ruled early Rome with Romulus, built a shrine to her in his toilet and she was appealed to if sewers backed up. She was also the Goddess protector of sexual intercourse in marriage and her worship was later combined with that of Venus. Her image was placed on Roman coins.

Crepitus was described as the Roman god of flatulence but probably was a fiction created to denigrate Roman theology. He appears as a god in several works of French literature by Voltaire, Baudelaire, and Flaubert as well as material promoting Roman Catholicism as the true faith. Stercutius (Latin stercus 'excrement') was the god of dung who was particularly important to farmers when fertilizing their fields with manure. Worshipping the porcelain god, or ceramic throne, is a jocular reference to past toilet worship when heaving into the toilet bowl during vomiting.

only 5% of fecal bacteria in water is of human origin*

Fiber

Dietary fiber, also referred to as roughage is the indigestible component of plants consumed as food. There are two main types, differentiated by their solubility in water. Soluble fiber, which dissolves in water, is readily fermented in the intestinal tract producing gases and byproducts. It us further divided into viscous fiber and prebiotic fiber and is commonly found in oat bran, beans, peas, and most fruits. Although the fiber is not directly digestible by the human or animal ingesting it, it is of vital importance to the microbes living within its digestive tract. Fiber is the mainstay of nutrition for the microbiome, and as has become increasingly clear with further research advances, the microbiome is critically important for the health of the host organism. The microbes produce metabolites which are otherwise not found in the diet, and many of these are critical for function and health of the host.

The microbes also possess the ability to digest the fiber which the host cannot, releasing nutrients that can then be absorbed by the host. In ruminant and other animals, the fiber is processed by microbial fermentation. The fermentation process releases abundant quantities of gas, which the ruminant animal releases as eructation or flatulence. The contribution of a grazing ruminants to global warming has been attributed to their large populations and prodigious gas production.

Insoluble fiber does not dissolve in water. It is further divided into fiber that is metabolically inert and simply provides added bulk and fluid retention, or prebiotic which is metabolically fermented by the gut flora. The bulk enhancing fibers ease defecation both by adding moisture to the stool as well as stimulating gut peristalsis and colonic mass movements.

Soluble fiber can be found in foods such as oatbran, barley, nuts, seeds, beans, lentils, fruits (citrus, apples), strawberries and many vegetables

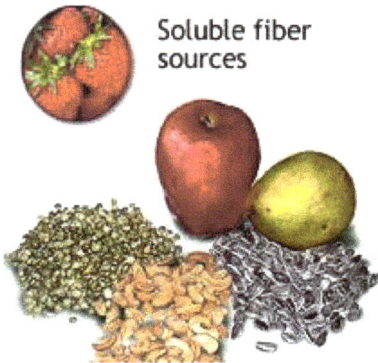

Insoluble fiber is found in foods such as whole wheat and whole grain products, vegetables, and wheat bran

Soluble fiber sources

Insoluble fiber sources

The added bulk also reduces the incidence of spasmodic contractions of the bowel, which may contribute to the pain, and discomfort of irritable bowel syndrome, previously known as a spastic colon or spastic colitis. This is the type of fiber found in wheat bran and some vegetables. Dietary fiber is comprised of non-starch polysaccharides such as arabinoxylans, cellulose, resistant starch, resistant dextrins, inulin, lignin, waxes, chitins, pectins, beta-glucans, and oligosaccharides.

Lignin, a major dietary insoluble fiber source, may alter the rate and metabolism of soluble fibers. Lignin is found in high concentrations in tree bark and its difficulty in being digested and decomposed played a major role in the

AirVeda: Ancient & New Medical Wisdom

Carboniferous era when tree bark was a multiple of the thickness it is today. On the other hand, insoluble fibers like the resistant starches are fully fermented. The main disadvantage of a diet high in fiber is the increased intestinal gas production with bloating and being a social outcast as a possible consequence.

The original definition of fiber was the components of plants that were not affected by digestive enzymes, a definition that includes lignin and polysaccharides. The definition was later expanded to include resistant starches, polysaccharides, lignin, and inulin with other oligosaccharides. While dietary fiber is present in nearly all fruits and vegetables, the type and quantity of fiber varies widely. Persimmons have safety issues and if eaten unripen the soluble tannin shiboul can lead to gastric phytobezoars a condition where a hardened wood like mass of fiber remains within the stomach for years or a lifetime.

Fiber Content Of Popular Foods			
Food Source	Soluble Fiber (g)	Insoluble Fiber (g)	Total Fiber (g)
Apple (1 med)	0.9g	2.0g	2.9g
Banana (1 med)	0.6g	1.4g	2.0g
Orange (1 med)	1.3g	0.7g	2.0g
Broccoli (1 stalk)	1.3g	1.4g	2.7g
Carrots (1 large)	1.3g	1.6g	2.9g
Tomato (1 small)	0.1g	0.7g	0.8g
Potato (1 medium)	1.0g	0.8g	1.8g
All Bran (1/2 cup)	1.4g	7.6g	9.0g
Oat Bran (1/2 cup)	2.2g	2.2g	4.4g
Corn Flakes (1 cup)	0g	0.5g	0.5g
Rolled Oats (3/4 cup)	1.3g	1.7g	3.0g
Wheat Bread (1 slice)	0.3g	1.1g	1.4g
White Bread (1 slice)	0.3g	0.1g	0.4g
Green Peas (2/3 cup)	0.6g	3.3g	3.9g
Kidney Beans (1/2 cup)	1.6g	4.9g	6.5g
Lentils (2/3 cup)	0.6g	3.9g	4.5g

source: USDA/ARS Nutrient Data Laboratory

Public Domain

Soluble fiber is present, in variable quantities, in plant food including legumes (peas, soybeans, lupins, beans), oats, rye, chia, and barley, some fruits and fruit juices (including prune juice, plums, berries, ripe bananas, apples, and pears), certain vegetables such as broccoli, carrots, Jerusalem artichokes, root tubers and root vegetables such as sweet potatoes and onions (skins of these are sources of insoluble fiber also), psyllium seed husk (a mucilage soluble fiber) and flax seeds, and nuts, with almonds being the highest in dietary fiber. Sources of insoluble fiber include, whole grain foods, wheat and corn bran, legumes such as beans and peas, nuts and seeds, potato skins, lignins, vegetables such as green beans, cauliflower, zucchini (courgette), celery, nopal, some fruits including avocado, and unripe bananas, the skins of some fruits, including kiwifruit, grapes and tomatoes. Vegetable gum fiber, such as guar gum and acacia Senegal gum, dissolve easily and have no aftertaste making them a popular fiber supplement additive.

Dietary fibers have three primary mechanisms: bulking, viscosity and fermentation. As they can change the nature and transit of the intestinal contents they may impact how other nutrients and materials are absorbed. Some soluble fibers bind to bile acids preventing their normal reabsorption in the small intestine. This interruption in the normal enterohepatic circulation of the bile from the small intestine to the liver results in the loss of cholesterol in the form of bile acids via the stool. The cholesterol levels in the blood are subsequently lowered since the liver removes cholesterol from the circulation to synthesize replacement bile salts. Viscous soluble fibers may also inhibit the absorption of sugar thus reducing the sugar insulin response after meals.

Fatty foods and hypertonic solutions delay gastric emptying and gut transit time. The intestinal contents are called chyme once they leave the stomach. Chyme consists of food compounds, digestive enzymes, stomach acid and pancreatic and duodenal bicarbonate, bile acids, complex lipids in changing micellar, aqueous, hydrocolloid, hydrophobic, and hydrophilic phases all in a mixture of solid, liquid, colloidal and gas bubble phases. In other words, it is one chaotic churning, digesting, fermenting mass with selective absorption and secretion occurring throughout the process. Non-absorbed carbohydrates such as pectin, gum Arabic, oligosaccharides and resistant starch, are fermented by the gut flora to short-chain fatty acids (mainly acetic, propionic and n-butyric), carbon dioxide, hydrogen and methane. The colon will absorb nearly all of the short-chain fatty acids, with the butyric acid being utilized as the main source of energy for colonic cells.

Soluble and insoluble fiber both increases food volume without additional caloric content. The increased volume can provide greater satiety, which may eat to decreased food intake and weight loss. Intestinal fermentation can increase the production of beneficial short chain fatty acids. Soluble fiber absorbs water and forms a viscous gel, known as a hydrophilic mucilloid that slows gastric emptying and intestinal transit. The increase bulk may shield carbohydrates from enzymes, delay the absorption of glucose, and reduce the fluctuations of blood sugar levels that result. On the other and the delayed transit allows more time for enzymatic activity as well as fermentation by the gut flora.

Insoluble fiber enhances gut motility and speeds transit time, as well as adding bulk and moisture to the stool promoting defecation and preventing constipation. Current recommendations for daily dietary fiber intake are thirty grams for the average adults. The average American consumes about half of that amount. Sugars and starches provide four Calories per gram as the digestive system has enzymes to break them down into the simple absorbable sugars of glucose, fructose, and galactose. Insoluble fiber cannot be digested so no calories are absorbed. Soluble fiber is partially fermented, and the caloric intake is determined by the degree that it is broken down into absorbable nutrients. As a result of the variability in calories generated there is controversy on their calorie count. Two calories per gram of soluble fiber is a reasonable compromise. Fibers with partial or low ferment ability include cellulose, hemicellulose, lignans, plant waxes, and resistant starches. Fibers with high ferment ability include beta-glucans, pectins, natural gums, inulins, oligosaccharides, and resistant dextrins.

Flatology

The scientific study of flatulence is termed flatology. Flatulence is defined as flatus (Latin blowing) expelled through the anus, as well as the state of being affected with gases in the intestinal tract. The noises commonly associated with flatulence ("Blowing a raspberry") are caused by the vibration of the anal sphincter and occasionally by the buttocks. Both the noise and smell associated with flatus leaving the anus can be sources of embarrassment or comedy in many cultures. There are five general symptoms related to intestinal gas: pain, bloating and abdominal distension, excessive flatus volume, excessive flatus smell and gas incontinence.

Flatulence

Flatulence is defined as flatus (Latin blowing) expelled through the anus as well as the state of being affected with gases in the intestinal tract. The scientific study of flatulence is termed flatology. The noises commonly associated with flatulence are caused by the vibration of the anal sphincter and occasionally by the buttocks. Both the noise and smell associated with flatus leaving the anus can be sources of embarrassment or comedy in many cultures. Further characterizations of the nature of flatulence are found under the topics of fart, flatus, and intestinal gas, which are commonly used, interchangeably in the English language.

⚠ CAUTION

THIS HOME IS OCCUPIED BY AT LEAST ONE PERSON WITH CHRONIC FLATULENCE

FODMAP Diet

FODMAP is an acronym that stands for Fermentable Oligosaccharides, Disaccharides, Monosaccharides, And Polyols. These short chain carbohydrates and related sugar alcohols are poorly absorbed in the small intestine. Many of the sugar alcohols including sorbitol, mannitol, xylitol, isomalt, and maltitol are added to commercial food products as non-nutritive bulk sweeteners. Originally developed at Monash University in Melbourne, Australia it has become popular worldwide as a means of reducing the symptoms of irritable bowel syndrome, functional gastrointestinal disorders, and excess intestinal gas

FODMAP foods to avoid or limit

FRUIT	VEGETABLES	LEGUMES	LACTOSE-CONTAINING FOODS
Apples, apricots, cherries, mango, pears, nectarines, peaches, pears, plums, prunes, watermelon and high concentrations of fructose from canned fruit, dried fruit or fruit juice	Artichokes, asparagus, avocado, beets, broccoli, brussel sprouts, cabbage, cauliflower, garlic (in large quantity), fennel, leeks, mushrooms, okra, onions, peas, radiccio, lettuce, scallions (white parts), shallots, sugar snap peas, snow peas	Baked beans, chickpeas, lentils, kidney beans, soy beans **SWEETENERS** Honey, fructose, high fructose corn syrup, isomalt, maltitol, mannitol, sorbitol, xylitol	Custard, ice cream, margarine, milk (cow, goat, sheep), soft cheese (including cottage cheese and ricotta), yogurt **GRAINS** wheat or rye in large amounts, eg. bread, crackers, cookies, cous cous, pasta

Suitable foods for a Low-FODMAP diet

FRUIT	VEGETABLES	STAPLES	LACTOSE ALTERNATIVES
Banana, blueberry, grapefruit, grapes, honeydew melon, kiwi, lemon, lime, mandarin oranges, orange, raspberry, strawberry	Bell peppers, bok choy, carrots, celery, corn, eggplant, green beans, lettuce, parsnips, scallions (green parts only) spinach, sweet potato, white potato, tomato	Meats, fats, eggs **SWEETENERS** Artificial sweeteners that do not end in "ol," glucose, maple syrup, sugar (sucrose)	Butter, hard cheese, brie and camembert, lactose-free products, such as lactose-free ice cream and yogurt, gelato, rice milk & sorbet **GRAINS** Oats, gluten-free products & spelt products

Food Intolerance

Food intolerance is often very individualized and is not the same as food allergy. In food allergy the food that triggers the reaction is known as the antigen, and the allergic reaction is mediated by the body's immune and inflammatory response systems. The chart following identifies several of the other differences.

Allergy	Intolerance
Obvious symptoms	Subtle symptoms
Immediate reaction - within one hour	Delayed reaction - 12 to 72 hours
Rapid onset of symptoms and often reaction magnifies with each exposure	Slow onset and often slow magnification of symptoms, even after the often long delay
Often triggered by minute amount of food	Not predominantly affected by food quantity
Affects Immunoglobulin E (IgE)	Affects Immunoglobulin G (IgG) and/or other mechanisms (prostaglandins, leukotrienes, etc.)
Allergies are uncommon	Intolerances are very common
Generally non-reversible	Reversible
Well recognised by medicine	Just beginning to be recognised by medicine
Test : Prick or RAST (Radio-immunodiffusion Test)	Test : Electro-Dermal Screening (EDS) or Blood Immunoglobulin G (IgG)

lunar.thegamez.net Creative Commons License

In a number of cases of food intolerance, the sensitivity is the result of lower levels of the necessary enzymes to digest specific foods. For example, the milk sugar lactose requires the specific enzyme called lactase, to properly digest this complex sugar into absorbable simple sugars. If insufficient lactase is present the gut flora, which is comprised of various microorganisms, ferments the residual undigested sugar. This process leads to the release of various gases that may accumulate within the digestive tract and are eliminated as a series of farts. A portion of the gases produced such as carbon dioxide are readily absorbed by the digestive tract and transported by the circulatory system to the lungs where they are eliminated through respiration.

The ability of the individual to produce the necessary lactase enzyme is often hereditary. Many populations have limited lactase production, which results in the common occurrence of lactose intolerance. If the intake of lactose is restricted the limited amount of lactase present may be sufficient to prevent the development of the symptoms of lactose intolerance. These symptoms such as excess intestinal gas, diarrhea, and abdominal cramps are often dependent on the quantity of lactose ingested that exceeds the available lactase enzyme necessary for its digestion.

A number of the digestive enzymes, which are lacking in individual populations, can be supplemented either by purchased enzyme products, or by the production of the enzymes by the individual's gut flora. The flora may be supplemented with commensal organisms such as lactobacillus, which aid in the digestion of dairy products. Other commonly malabsorbed complex sugars include fructose, mannitol, sorbitol, and a variety of sugar substitutes.

Food Intolerance and Common Symptoms

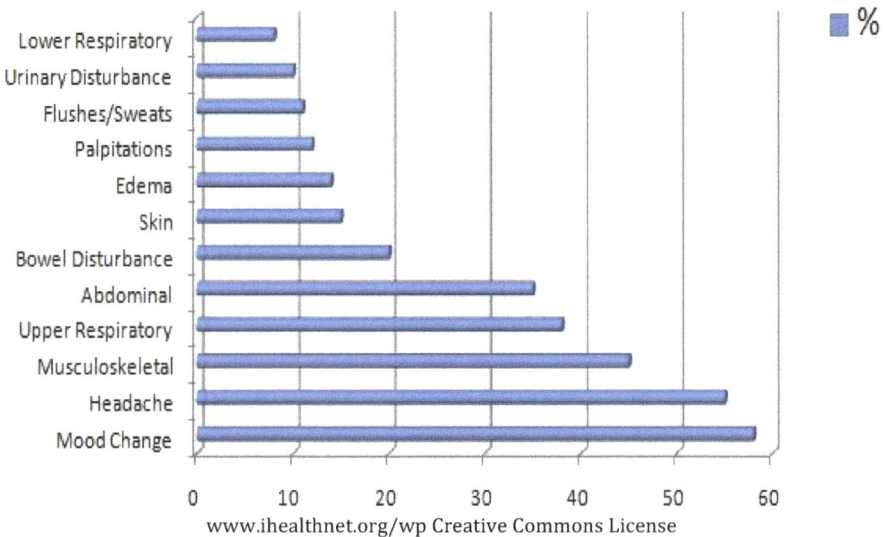

www.ihealthnet.org/wp Creative Commons License

Fructose in particular has limited enzyme available for its digestion and frequently leads to intolerance when ingested beyond the enzyme capacity. In some cases, the necessary enzyme for digestion of the complex sugar or starch does not naturally occur in humans. One example is the enzyme cellulase, which is required for the digestion of cellulose, a sugar commonly found in plants. This enzyme is naturally found in herbivorous animals that consume grasses and cellulose containing food products.

The complex sugars found in legumes are in the raffinose class, which includes the trisaccharide raffinose (consisting of one unit each of glucose, galactose, and fructose), the tetrasaccharide stachyose (consisting of two units of galactose, one unit of glucose, and one unit of fructose), and the pentasaccharide verbascose (consisting of three units of galactose, one unit of glucose, and one unit of fructose). The enzyme required for their digestion is called alphagalactosidase. This enzyme is not naturally occurring in humans and must be obtained from external sources. Without the availability of this enzyme the gut flora metabolism releases large quantities of gases, which are often most often released as a series of farts. The enzyme is found naturally in beans and legumes once the seed is germinated. The enzyme is also available commercially as over-the-counter products such as Beano, Say Yes to Beans, and other products.

Many individuals also have difficulty digesting the cereal grains, especially those that contain gluten. Gluten intolerance may range from mild excess gas production to true inflammation and damage of the intestinal lining. When the villi, which are the fingerlike projections of the bowel lining, are damaged malabsorption occurs. This condition known as gluten sensitive enteropathy (also known as celiac disease, celiac sprue, nontropical sprue, and sprue) is a serious health concern. Adherence to a strict gluten-free diet is required to prevent further injury and complications from the malabsorption of nutrients and other features of the disorder.

A number of the food intolerances may be addressed easily by avoiding the inciting foods in the diet. A number of food intolerances are more challenging to control by diet alone, as the commercial food products in the marketplace may contain small quantities. It is necessary to carefully read the ingredient labels of all commercial food products purchased or consumed if one has specific food intolerance. With further understanding of the gut microbiome, prebiotics and probiotics may be used to have commensals, microbes that are beneficial to the host, supplement the natural enzymes of the human host. There are a wide variety of food intolerances and enzyme deficiencies that can be major contributors to gastrointestinal and other symptoms. Enzyme deficiencies are not uncommon and there are many possible enzymes to investigate including proteases such as pepsin, pepsinogen, trypsin, trypsinogen, chymotrypsin, and chymotrypsinogen. Other enzymes include amylase, lipase, invertase, sucrose, maltase, lactase, and about one thousand six-hundred others.

Taking a Sherlock Holmes approach and trying an elimination diet is certainly reasonable. Enzyme supplements are commercially available and are another approach for an empiric trial if the suspect foods are not well defined. It is important to take the appropriate enzyme with the appropriate food. The right enzyme for the wrong food, or the wrong enzyme for the right food, will not make a bit of difference in helping your digestion. The most common enzyme deficiency is lactase resulting in lactose intolerance. Medications can also interfere with enzyme activity and give rise to digestive symptoms.

The most widely distributed naturally occurring non-enzyme food chemical capable of provoking reactions is salicylate, with tartrazine and benzoic acid sensitivity seen less often. Benzoates and salicylates occur naturally in many different foods, including fruits, juices, vegetables, tomatoes, spices, herbs, nuts, tea, wines, and coffee. Other natural chemicals, which commonly cause reactions and cross reactivity, include amines, nitrates, sulphites, and some antioxidants. Reactions to chocolate, cheese, bananas, avocado, tomato, or wine suggest that bioactive amines may be a likely candidate as a food chemical that triggers sensitivities.

Franklin, Benjamin

Benjamin Franklin (1706-1790) was a polymath scientist, author, statesman, philosopher, publisher, diplomat, inventor, and humorist. In 1781 he was serving as the United States ambassador to France and with his scientific background kept in close communication with the European community of scientists. As is typical for a scientific congress, an announcement from the Royal Academy of Brussels was made calling for the presentation of scientific papers on a host of subjects.

Portrait of Benjamin Franklin by Joseph Siffrein Duplessis c. 1785 National Portrait Gallery Washington D.C. Public Domain

Franklin found some of the proposals so pretentious that his "bawdy, scurrilous nature" was stirred to compose a satirical response in the form of a proposal for research. As an illustrious statesman and scientist his proposal would demand serious attention. His proposal to the Royal Academy of Brussels is reprinted in its entirety in the companion volume to this book *Artsy Fartsy, Cultural History of the Fart*.

"Let every fart count as a peal of thunder for liberty. Let every fart remind the nation of how much it has let pass out of its control. So fart, and if you must, fart often. But always fart without apology. Fart for freedom, fart for liberty... and fart proudly!"

"He that lives upon Hope, dies farting." is another of his famous quotes.

His proposal to the Royal Academy called for scientific research to discover food additives that would provide a variety of attractive aromas to produce good smelling farts that would be socially welcomed.

Fructose

Fructose, fruit sugar, is a simple monosaccharide found in many fruits, berries, flowers, honey, artichokes, wheat, onions, and root vegetables. Fructose was discovered in 1847 by the French chemist Augustin-Pierre Dubrunfaut. It is prepared commercially from sugar cane, sugar beets, and corn. High-fructose corn syrup (HFCS) is made from the enzymatic conversion of corn starch and is often added as a sweetener to soft drinks and other foods.

Apples and pears contain more than twice as much free fructose as glucose. High concentrations of free fructose in these fruits and their juices can cause diarrhea in children, as they are unable to absorb fructose as well as glucose and sucrose. The fructose creates higher osmolality in the small intestine drawing water into the gastrointestinal tract resulting in diarrhea. It is because of the fructose that apple juice; raisins, grape juice, and bananas will increase flatulence.

Crystalline fructose Creative Commons License

Fructose exists in foods either as a monosaccharide (free fructose) or as a unit of a disaccharide (sucrose). Fructose is seventy-three percent sweeter than sucrose. The enzyme sucrase catalyzes sucrose into glucose and fructose, both of which are absorbed by the small intestine, as is the other monosaccharide galactose. Fructose has a very low glycemic index of nineteen, compared with one hundred for glucose, and sixty-eight for sucrose.

Fructose Intolerance, Hereditary

Dietary fructose intolerance is the decreased capacity to absorb fructose because of deficient fructose carriers in the small intestine's enterocytes. Hereditary fructose intolerance is a more serious liver enzyme deficiency that requires total abstinence from fructose. Hereditary fructose intolerance is a defect of fructose metabolism caused by an autosomal recessive gene mutation resulting in a deficiency of the enzyme aldolase B. Hereditary fructose intolerance individuals are asymptomatic until they ingest fructose, sucrose, or sorbitol. Symptoms can include vomiting, hypoglycemia, jaundice, hemorrhage, hepatomegaly, hyperuricemia, and kidney failure.

The pathways of fructose in HFI & Fructose Malabsorption

(Fructose - a sugar found in fruit & vegetables)

Fructose

Fructose should normally be absorbed in the small intestine before moving onto the liver

Stomach

In the case of HFI...

... fructose is not metabolised by the liver and this causes a toxic accumulation in the liver, kidneys and intestines

In the case of fructose malabsorption...

... if fructose is not absorbed by the small intestine it moves into the large intestine

Liver **Small intestine**

In the large intestine bacteria can use it as a food source, resulting in excess hydrogen (excess wind = bloating, pain, flatulence)

Large intestine

It can cause either constipation or, by attracting fluid back into the colon, diarrhea.

Creative Commons License

Diagnosis of hereditary fructose intolerance is suspected in infants who become symptomatic when fructose-containing foods are introduced into their diet.

Affected individuals are asymptomatic and healthy, provided they do not ingest foods containing fructose or its precursors sucrose and sorbitol. Fructose is absorbed in the small intestine without the need for digestive enzymes. About twenty-five to fifty grams of fructose per intake can be properly absorbed in healthy people. People with fructose malabsorption cannot absorb more than twenty-five grams per intake. In the large intestine the fructose is metabolized into short chain fatty acids, producing hydrogen, carbon dioxide and methane. The increased osmotic load can cause diarrhea. The abnormal increase in hydrogen is detectable with the hydrogen breath test.

Foods that contain more glucose than fructose are usually well tolerated since glucose enhances absorption of fructose. Foods with a high fructose to glucose ratio like apples and pears can be difficult to process and so should be avoided. Additional foods to be avoided include those rich in fructans such as artichokes, asparagus, leeks, onions, wheat, sorbitol, xylitol, erythritol, inulin, fructo-oligosaccharide, and mannitol.

Fructose Malabsorption

Fructose malabsorption, formerly named hereditary fructose intolerance or dietary fructose intolerance, is the decreased capacity to absorb fructose because of deficient fructose carriers in the small intestine's enterocytes. This condition is common in patients with irritable bowel syndrome. It is not synonymous with the more serious hereditary fructose intolerance, a liver enzyme deficiency that requires total abstinence from fructose.

How Much Fructose Can I Eat Per Day?

We can only absorb 20 grams of Fructose per day. That's 4 ⅓ teaspoons or two apples.

Any more is harmful to the liver, causing fat deposits, obesity, and insulin resistance.

Fructose in fresh fruit

Fruit portion	Grams of Fructose
1 Lime	0.0
1 Lemon	0.6
1 cup cranberries	0.7
1 date	2.6
1/8 cantaloupe	2.8
1 cup raspberries	3.0
1 kiwi	3.4
1 slice pineapple	4.0
1 grapefruit	4.3
1 tangerine	4.8
1 peach/nectarine	5.8
1 orange	6.1
1/2 papaya	6.3
1 banana	7.1
1 cup blueberries	7.4
1 apple	9.5
1 pear	11.8
¾ cup raisins	12.3
1 cup grapes	12.4
1/2 mango	16.2
1 cup dry apricots	16.4
1 cup dry figs	23.0

Gas, Therapy (see Intestinal Gas Therapy)

Gastric Acid (Stomach Acid)

Gastric acid is hydrochloric acid produced by the stomach to aid in the digestive process. Once the gastric acid leaves the stomach via the pyloric channel it is neutralized by the sodium bicarbonate secreted by the duodenum (first portion of the small intestine) and pancreas. The neutralization releases large quantities of carbon dioxide gas which may result in temporary distension and bloating.

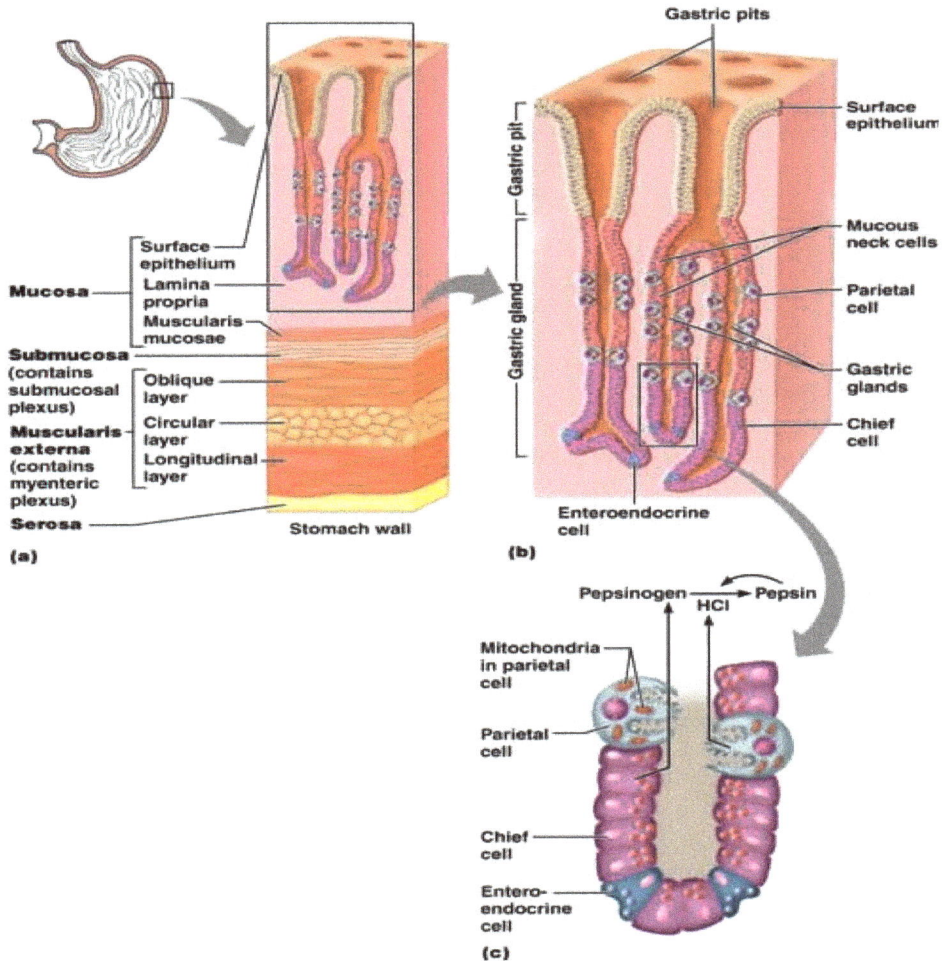

Gastric parietal cell secretion of hydrochloric acid (HCl) is stimulated by acetylcholine (ACh), histamine, gastrin through secondary messenger systems. The release of HCl is low if only one of above ligands binds to parietal cell The release of HCl is high if all three ligands bind to parietal cells. Antihistamines block H_2 receptors and decrease HCl release. Public Domain.

When a piece of meat was placed in simulated gastric juices and heated to body temperature only the mixture containing pepsin and HCl broke down the meat fully.

Gastric acid is a digestive fluid, formed in the stomach. It has a pH of 1.5 to 3.5 and is composed of hydrochloric acid (HCl) (around 0.5%, or five thousand parts per million) as high as 0.1 M and large quantities of potassium chloride (KCl) and sodium chloride (NaCl). There are about twenty thousand gastric pits per square centimeter of gastric mucosa. Each pit receives secretions from three to seven gastric glands. Previous information that gastric acid was diminished with age has been proven to be incorrect. Both the autonomic nervous system and several hormones regulate gastric acid production. The parasympathetic nervous system, via the vagus nerve, and the hormone gastrin stimulate the parietal cell to produce gastric acid, both directly acting on parietal cells and indirectly, through the stimulation of the secretion of the hormone histamine from enterochromaffin-like cells (ECL). When gastric chyme is at a pH above three gastric acid is stimulated, when the pH of chyme falls below a pH of two the gastric secretion is inhibited.

During the intestinal phase gastric secretion is stimulated by the presence of peptides and amino acids in the distended duodenum, which stimulate the G cells in the duodenum and upper jejunum to release gastrin. This gastrin is released into the blood and can stimulate parietal cells of the stomach to secrete gastric acid. The enzyme carbonic anhydrase catalyzes the reaction between carbon dioxide and water to form carbonic acid. This acid dissociates into hydrogen and bicarbonate ions. The hydrogen ions leave the cell through H+/K+ ATPase transport pumps and enter the gastric lumen as hydrochloric acid. The proton pump enzyme is the target of proton pump inhibitors, used to decrease gastric acid secretion and increase gastric pH. Histamine H_2 antagonist mechanism of action is through the histamine two receptor, which is not as efficient in decreasing gastric acid production as the proton pump inhibitor. Antacids neutralize existing acid but do not decrease gastric acid production. Calcium based antacids may cause an increase in gastric acid secretion by the stimulating effect of the absorbed calcium.

In the duodenum, gastric acid is neutralized by sodium bicarbonate, summarized by the chemical reaction $HCl + NaHCO_3 \rightarrow NaCl + H_2CO_3.$ The carbonic acid equilibrates with carbon dioxide and water through catalysis by the enzyme carbonic anhydrase found in the gut epithelial lining. In the absorptive upper intestine, such as the duodenum, both the dissolved carbon dioxide and carbonic acid will tend to equilibrate with the blood, leading to most of the carbon dioxide gas produced on neutralization being exhaled through the lungs.

Gastroenterology

Gastroenterology is the scientific study of the digestive system and digestive diseases. In the United States it is a field of medicine considered a subspecialty of internal medicine. A physician who specializes in gastrointestinal diseases is referred to as a gastroenterologist. Most of the practicing specialists have completed a three-year residency in internal medicine followed by a two or three-year fellowship in gastroenterology. Individuals who have excessive gas complaints frequently see a gastroenterologist in consultation.

Gastroenterologists frequently perform a variety of endoscopy and colonoscopy examinations that are expanding in therapeutic and diagnostic capabilities with technological advances. Board certification is voluntary, and in a number of the state medical licensing jurisdictions physicians and surgeons may self-designate an area of specialty practice without necessarily completing advance training. Surgical specialist in the field of colon and rectal surgery are often referred to as a proctologist or colon and rectal surgeon. They may also perform endoscopy and colonoscopy examinations.

Gastroesophageal Reflux Disease (GERD, Reflux, Heartburn)

Gastroesophageal reflux disease (GERD) is mucosal damage of the esophagus caused by the reflux of gastric acid, bile, and digestive enzymes. In Western populations GERD affects approximately ten to twenty percent of the population. The most common symptom is heartburn, formally known as pyrosis, from the Greek word πῦρ (pyro, fire). In the United States twenty percent of people have symptoms in a given week, and seven percent every day.

GERD is usually caused by abnormal relaxation of the lower esophageal sphincter or hiatal hernia with contributing factors such as obesity, Zollinger-Ellison hypergastrinemia, hypercalcemia, scleroderma, and esophageal dysmotility. Carminatives, drugs, hormones, alcohol, tobacco, fried or fatty foods, and chocolate all of which can reduce the lower esophageal sphincter pressure can aggravate it. Treatment is typically via lifestyle changes and medications such as proton pump inhibitors, H_2 receptor blockers or antacids. Some antacids can be absorbed leading to an alkalosis syndrome. Antacids also generate large volumes of carbon dioxide as they neutralize the gastric hydrochloric acid, Magnesium containing antacids can cause diarrhea, aluminum containing antacids can cause constipation, and often a combination of the two is used to minimize the impact on bowel movements, Calcium based antacids can lead to a rebound of acid secretion as calcium is a stimulant of gastric acid production.

Healthy   **GERD**

Gastroesophageal Reflux Disease Shutterstock/designua

Surgery treatment with tightening of the lower esophageal sphincter has a similar response rate as medications. If inadequately treated GERD may progress to Barrett esophagus with intestinal metaplasia where the epithelial cells transition from the normal esophageal squamous epithelium to intestinal columnar epithelium. With the development of atypia and dysplasia this can progress to the development of adenocarcinoma of the esophagus. If Barrett esophagus has developed a screening endoscopy with biopsies to evaluate for dysplasia is suggested to allow more aggressive treatment if premalignant changes are noted.

The diagnosis of GERD is usually by history with typical symptoms of heartburn and reflux. Atypical manifestations of GERD include laryngitis, unexplained chest pain, chronic cough, sinusitis, pulmonary fibrosis, earache, recurrent ear infections, asthma, and obstructive sleep apnea. Another unusual symptom is called water brash, which is a rush of salivary secretions after an episode of regurgitation to dilute and clear the acid in the esophagus. A possible cardiac cause of atypical chest should be excluded before ascribing the source to GERD. Approximately forty percent of GERD patients have a *Helicobacter pylori* infection. The eradication of *Helicobacter pylori* can lead to a worsening of the GERD symptoms since the resolving gastritis leads to an increase in gastric acid secretion.

The current gold standard for diagnosis of GERD is esophageal pH monitoring. Endoscopy is advised if any alarm symptoms are present including dysphagia, anemia, blood in the stool, wheezing, weight loss, respiratory or laryngeal symptoms. Long-standing or severe symptoms would also prompt endoscopic evaluation for Barrett esophagus and dysplasia.

The treatments for GERD include lifestyle modifications, medications, and possibly surgery. Initial treatment is typically with a proton-pump inhibitor or histamine two blocker that usually provides prompt and significant relief. Weight loss, avoiding large heavy meals, not lying down, bending over, or doing headstands immediately after meals, decreasing or discontinuing tobacco, alcohol, and carminatives can be helpful. Elevation of the head of the bed, not with pillows but with wood blocks under the legs at the head of bed as long as it is not a waterbed can be useful.

Antacids and mucosal protectants such as alginic acid or sucralfate can also be helpful but have a more frequent dosing schedule. Prokinetic agents to enhance esophageal motility and tighten the lower esophageal sphincter can also be used. The oldest generic prokinetic metoclopramide has a high incidence of central nervous system side effects and is now rarely used. Newer prokinetics have a safer profile.

A variety of endoscopic therapies have been developed, including procedures designed to reduce the lumen diameter to reduce reflux. Laparoscopic procedures using magnets and other implantable devices have also been utilized to create a physical barrier to the reflux of gastric contents into the esophagus. The standard surgical treatment for severe GERD is the Nissen fundoplication, where the upper part of the stomach is wrapped around the lower esophageal sphincter (LES). This corrects the hiatal hernia by keeping the stomach and LES below the diaphragm preventing reflux. Medical therapy and surgical therapies appear to be equally effective for this often chronic condition.

Gastrointestinal Motility

Motilin

Motilin is a hormone secreted by endocrine M cells in the small intestine, especially in the duodenum and jejunum. It was named motilin because of its ability to stimulate gastric activity. Erythromycin and related antibiotics act as motilin agonists, and are sometimes used for their ability to stimulate gastrointestinal motility. Another hormone ghrelin can also induce motilin like effects.

Motilin triggers the migrating myoelectric complex component of gastrointestinal motility, which induces brief episodes of peristaltic activity several times an hour in between meals. Contractions of the gastric fundus and antrum triggered by motilin can cause stomach rumble or growls, borborygmi, and cramp like discomfort often described as hunger pains since they occur during a fasting period. The gastric emptying and peristaltic sweeping action clearing the stomach and small bowel of food residue or chyme has earned motilin the moniker 'housekeeper of the gut'.

Gastrointestinal Pacemaker Cells

Interstitial cells of Cajal are pacemaker cells similar to the pacemaker cells of the heart, which cause the heart to beat regularly. They are present in the wall of the gut and communicate between the nervous system and the smooth muscle of the gut wall. When the signal arrives from the nervous system to the interstitial cells of Cajal that a person has eaten they begin their pacemaker function. This results in a coordinated and rhythmic set of contractions of the gut known as peristalsis, which propels food along the entire length of the digestive tract. The interstitial cells of Cajal were studied in relative obscurity for over one hundred years until the discovery that gastrointestinal stromal tumors (GIST) arise from interstitial cells of Cajal or an interstitial cell of Cajal-like precursor cell.

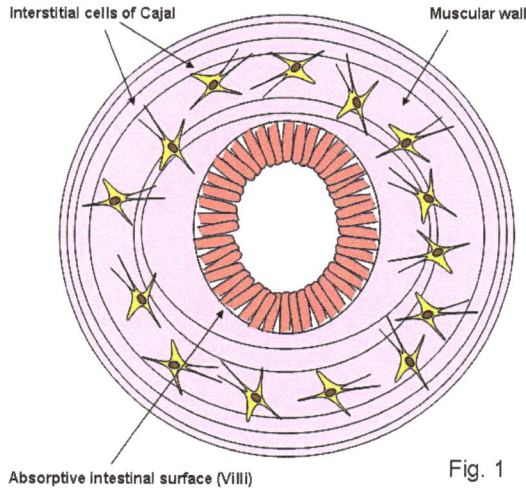

Fig. 1

liferaftgroup.org/wp Creative Commons License

The interstitial cells of Cajal are derived from the mesoderm of the gastrointestinal tract and serves as a pacemaker for the peristaltic contractions of the smooth muscle. The interstitial cells of Cajal are named after Santiago Ramón y Cajal (1852-1934) a Spanish pathologist and Nobel laureate who was considered by many as the father of neuroscience.

The frequency of interstitial cell of Cajal pacemaker activity differs in different regions of the gastrointestinal tract, three per minute in the stomach, twelve per minute in the duodenum, ten per minute in the ileum, and three per minute again in the colon. The loss of interstitial cells of Cajal may interrupt normal neural control of gastrointestinal contractions and lead to functional GI disorders, such as irritable bowel syndrome and chronic intestinal pseudo-obstruction. Diabetes mellitus often leads to gastrointestinal motility disorders.

Gastrointestinal motility disorders are a major source of morbidity and can have a profound influence on the quality of life. Irritable bowel syndrome is one of the most common of gastrointestinal disorders. Its prevalence in various countries around the world is between six and forty-six percent of the population. In the United States an estimated forty million people have the condition

Rapid Gastric Emptying

Rapid gastric emptying, also called dumping syndrome, occurs when undigested food empties too quickly into the small intestine. Early rapid gastric emptying begins during or right after a meal. Symptoms include nausea, vomiting, bloating, cramping, diarrhea, dizziness, and fatigue. Late rapid gastric emptying occurs one to three hours after eating. Symptoms include hypoglycemia (low blood sugar), weakness, sweating, and dizziness.

DUMPING SYNDROME

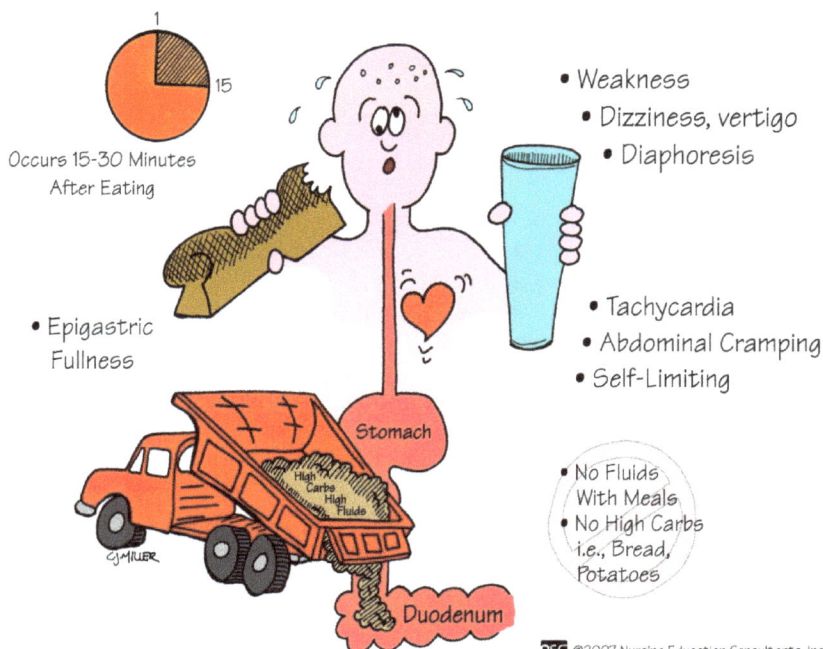

Occurs 15-30 Minutes After Eating

- Weakness
  - Dizziness, vertigo
    - Diaphoresis

- Epigastric Fullness

- Tachycardia
- Abdominal Cramping
- Self-Limiting

Stomach

- No Fluids With Meals
- No High Carbs i.e., Bread, Potatoes

High Carbs High Fluids

CJMILLER

Duodenum

@2007 Nursing Education Consultants, Inc.

Dumping syndrome arabnurses.com Creative Commons License

Rapid gastric emptying is usually the result of stomach surgery such as fundoplication or gastric bypass. The condition is also seen in people with Zollinger-Ellison syndrome, a rare disorder involving a gastrin hormone secreting tumor in the pancreas. Treatment of rapid gastric emptying focuses on the underlying cause and may include changes in eating habits and medication. People who have the condition should eat several small meals a day that are low in carbohydrates. They should also drink liquids between meals and not with them. Prescription medications may also be utilized, with surgery as a last resort.

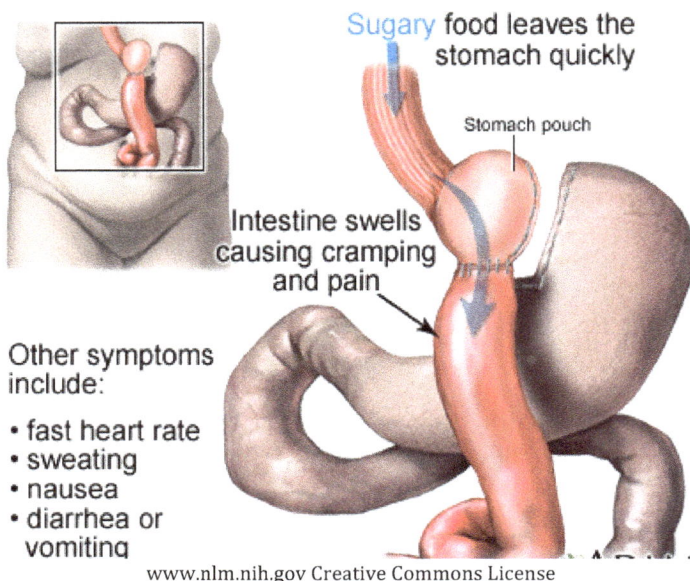

Sugary food leaves the stomach quickly

Stomach pouch

Intestine swells causing cramping and pain

Other symptoms include:

• fast heart rate
• sweating
• nausea
• diarrhea or vomiting

www.nlm.nih.gov Creative Commons License

Gastrointestinal Transit Time

Gastrointestinal transit time is the time period from ingestion of food or a biomarker until its elimination and exit from the digestive tract. The time period is highly variable, usually between twenty and forty-eight hours, and can be influenced by many factors including diet, physical activity, infection, inflammation, pharmaceuticals, etc. The gastrointestinal transit time can also be divided into the three subsets of gastric emptying, small intestinal transit, and colonic transit.

The transit time is the general period of time it takes, from the swallow of ingestion to the elimination at defecation, for food to pass through the gastrointestinal track. Normal ranges are from half a day to two days but individuals vary. Certain conditions especially those with diarrhea may have a more rapid transit time, while those with neurologic conditions or diabetes may have a slow transit time.

In general, it takes about one hour for half of the gastric contents to be processed and advanced into the duodenum, and the stomach is usually empty two hours after ingestion. Approximately two to four hours is involved in digestion and absorption before the chyme is released into the colon for water absorption and packaging as feces. The material is eliminated approximately twelve to forty-eight hours after ingestion. Diabetics are particularly prone to a condition called gastroparesis, where the delay is primarily in gastric emptying. Although it is not uncommon to see certain undigested foods passed, like kernels of corn, more undigested foods may be seen with a rapid gut transit time.

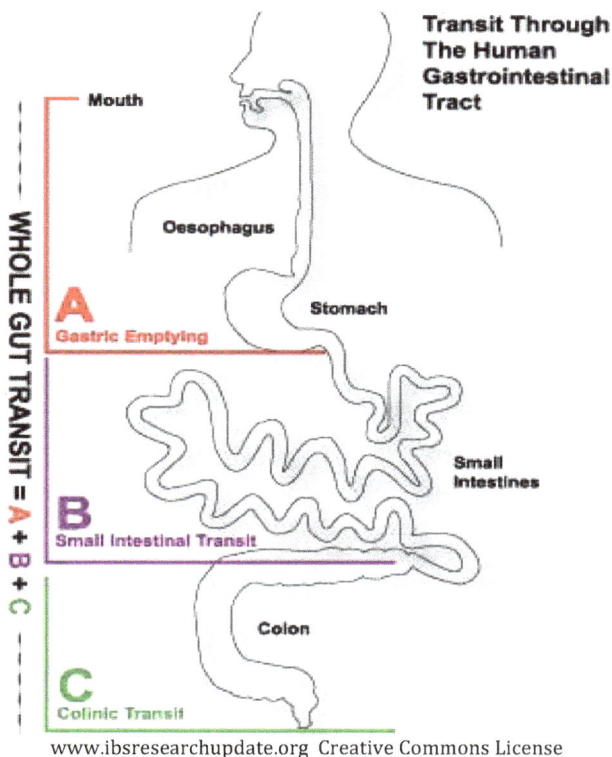

Transit Through The Human Gastrointestinal Tract

Mouth

Oesophagus

A
Gastric Emptying

Stomach

WHOLE GUT TRANSIT = A + B + C

Small Intestines

B
Small Intestinal Transit

Colon

C
Colinic Transit

www.ibsresearchupdate.org Creative Commons License

Gastroparesis

Diabetes mellitus is one of the most common causes of delayed gastric emptying known as gastroparesis diabeticorum. It can also lead to generalized gastrointestinal motility disorder with delayed total gut transit times. Irritable bowel syndrome is also associated with gastrointestinal motility disorder.

This disorder of delayed gastric emptying is most often seen as a consequence of neuropathy secondary to diabetes mellitus. The delayed gastric emptying prevents both the nutritional intake as well as swallowed gasses from leaving the stomach. Meals that are high in fat cause the release of hormones that slows down gut motility and delays gastric emptying.

This can lead to increased burping and belching as well as distension. Side effects from medications, especially narcotic analgesics, and antidepressants are well-recognized causes of delayed gastrointestinal peristalsis and bloating. There are a number of pharmacological agents that have prokinetic actions that may be of value in treating delayed gastric emptying.

Peristalsis & Segmental Contractions

Peristalsis (Greek peri-, "around" and stallein, "to place") is the propulsive wave of muscular contraction and relaxation, which advances digestive material through the intestinal tract. Earthworms use a similar mechanism in their movement. The process of peristalsis is controlled by the medulla oblongata of the brainstem. Segmental contractions are used to mix the chime with digestive juices and enzymes and to bring additional nutrient material in contact with the villi and microvilli of the small bowel mucosa.

Digestive material in the esophagus and stomach is called a bolus, while material upon entering the duodenum of the small intestine is called chyme. The peristaltic wave in the esophagus advances the bolus in a wave lasting less than ten seconds. In the small intestine peristaltic waves lasts for a few seconds and the chyme is advanced a few centimeters. It serves to mix the chyme as digestion and absorption of nutrients occurs during the transit through the small intestine.

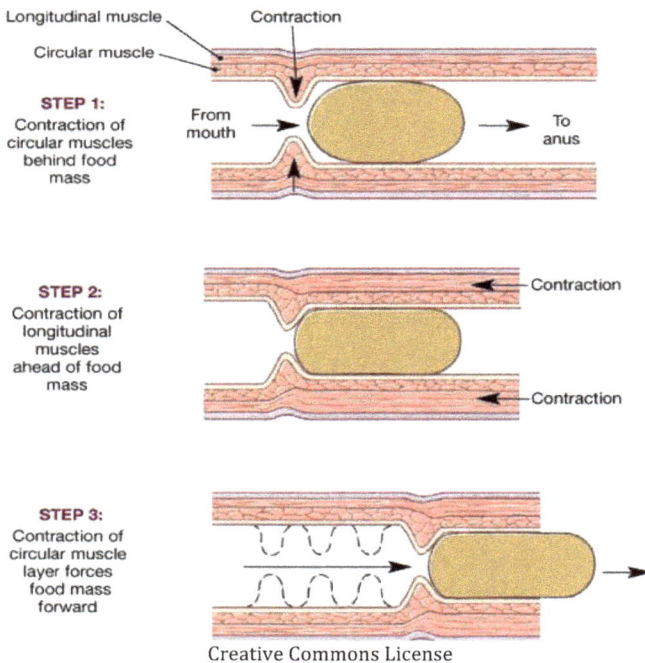

Creative Commons License

Migrating motor complexes (MMC) are waves of gastric emptying followed by peristaltic activity that sweep through the stomach and small intestines in between meals. They each last for a moment or two and occur in a cyclic pattern several times an hour, advancing any remaining food residue or chyme through the small intestine into the colon. The maintenance of regular peristaltic activity during meals and intermittently during fasting is also thought to prevent the migration of colonic bacteria into the terminal Ileum.

The hormone motilin triggers the MMC, as can motilin like agonists such as the antibiotic erythromycin. The at times audible borborygmi from the MMC are also referred to as stomach rumbles or growls and are also commonly thought of as hunger pains since the cramps occur during a fasting state.

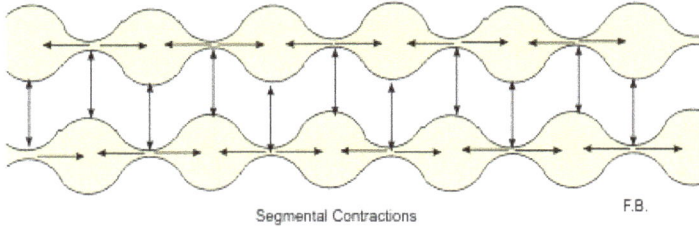

Segmental Contractions

F.B.

Segmental contractions in the gut. Author Boumphreyfr Creative Commons License

Gastrointestinal motility is also under the control of local enteric neurons that coordinate intestinal motility. Cholinergic neurons cause contraction and shortening of the circular muscle layer, shortening of longitudinal muscle, and distension of the intestine. As chyme enters the duodenum, carbohydrates and proteins are only partially digested, no fat digestion has taken place. Digestion continues in the small intestine where hypertonic chyme has a low acidic pH and mixing is required for the enzymes and substrates to interact.

The most common motion of the small intestine is the motility action called segmentation. It is initiated by intrinsic pacemaker cells (Cajal cells) with the segmentation mixing the contents while peristaltic activity moves the bolus distally towards the ileocecal valve. After the bulk of the nutrients have been absorbed the gastroileal reflex and gastrin relax the ileocecal valve (sphincter) and allow chyme to pass into the large intestine. The colon absorbs the water and electrolytes from the still liquid chyme that is increasingly solidified by water absorption as it transits the large intestine.

Mass Movement

The large intestine (colon) does not have peristaltic activity like the small intestine illustrated above. Feces are propelled through the large intestine by mass movements, which occur one to three times per day. The stool stored in the rectum is expelled via the anus by defecation. Haustral contractions are slow segmenting movements that move the contents of the colon by peristaltic activity towards the rectum. The haustra sequentially contract as they are stimulated by distension.

The defecation reflex is triggered by distension of rectal walls by feces. When stimulated the defecation reflex contracts the rectal walls and relaxes the internal anal sphincter. Voluntary signals stimulate relaxation of the external anal sphincter and defecation occurs.

Gastrointestinal Tract (Alimentary Tract, Digestive Tract, Gut)

The gastrointestinal tract is also known as the alimentary tract or alimentary canal. It consists of the esophagus, stomach, small intestine and large intestine. It may be considered to be the continuous passageway of the hollow viscous organs, from the mouth to the anus. It is also known as the digestive, intestinal, gastrointestinal, or GI tract. The gastrointestinal system is an expanded entity that includes structures other than the hollow viscus.

The gastrointestinal system includes the accessory organs necessary for digestion, such as the salivary glands, pancreas, liver, gallbladder, and their associated ducts. In an adult male human, the alimentary tract is twenty feet (five meters) long in a living subject. If the alimentary tract is measured at autopsy its length may be increased up to thirty feet (nine meters) because of the loss of the muscular tone and peristaltic contractions

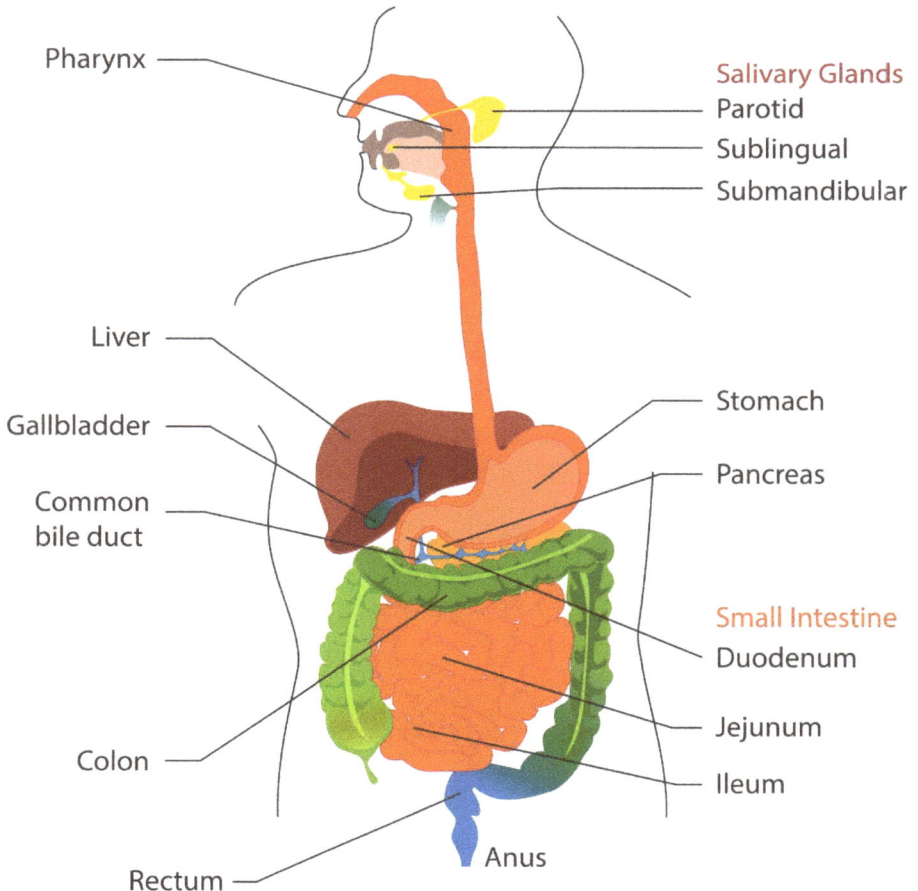

Digestive System. Shutterstock/yaruna

AirVeda: Ancient & New Medical Wisdom

The alimentary tract may also be delineated as three distinct regions, the foregut, midgut, and hindgut. This terminology reflects the embryological origin of each segment of the tract. The tissue of the gut actively secretes and releases hormones that help to regulate the digestive process. The long recognized gastrointestinal hormones, including gastrin, secretin, cholecystokinin, have now been joined by more recently discovered hormones. These include leptin, ghrelin, bombesin, neuropeptide Y and others that are mediated through either intracrine or autocrine mechanisms. The multiple hormones may have individual effects, as well as acting with their counterparts in both positive and negative feedback loops. They have powerful effects not only on the digestive tract, but also on the brain and enteric nervous system. They have a profound influence on the satiety center, the area of the brain that plays a vital function in the control of appetite and weight.

The upper alimentary tract consists of the esophagus, stomach, and duodenum. The ligament of Treitz is considered the anatomical landmark that serves as the dividing line between the upper and lower alimentary tracts. The lower alimentary tract includes most of the small intestine, including the jejunum and ileum. The lower alimentary tract also includes all of the large intestine, consisting of the appendix, cecum, ascending colon, transverse colon, descending colon, sigmoid colon, rectum, and anus. The intestines may also commonly be referred to as the alimentary tract, alimentary canal, digestive tract, gastrointestinal (GI) tract, bowels, small bowel, large bowel, hollow viscus, gut, entrails, viscera, or innards. The lumen is the hollow distensible cavity where digestion and absorption take place.

The swallowed food is described as a bolus as it leaves the mouth. When the bolus leaves the stomach and exits through the pyloric sphincter and enters into the duodenum it is now known as chime. The chime has already been partially digested by salivary and gastric enzymes and acids, as well as having gone through a churning and mixing process in the stomach. When the chime leaves the last portion of the small intestine, known as the ileum, it passes through the ileocecal valve. Once it has passed through the ileocecal valve it has entered the cecum, the first portion of the colon, also known as the large intestine or large bowel. The material, which was known as chime on the small intestine side of the ileocecal valve, is now described as feces as it has entered into the colon. The major function of the colon is the absorption of water from the liquid feces that enters the cecum.

As the water is absorbed through the colonic epithelium the feces is solidified and finally stored in the rectum until defecation and elimination take place. The absorption of water is important to conserve the body's fluid balance and maintain adequate hydration. If too little water is absorbed from the feces it may remain liquid or loose and contribute to diarrhea. If excess water removal takes place the feces can become firm and difficult to eliminate resulting in constipation.

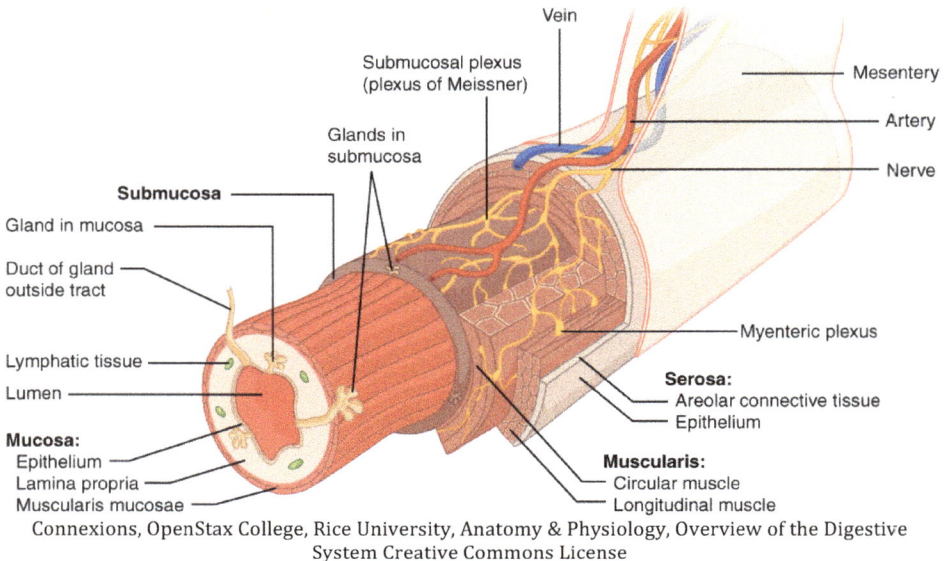

Connexions, OpenStax College, Rice University, Anatomy & Physiology, Overview of the Digestive System Creative Commons License

Going from the inside of the lumen towards the outer wall, there are several layers of tissue found in the anatomy of the gastrointestinal organs. The layers of the intestine, starting from the lumen, includes the mucosa (glandular epithelium and muscularis mucosa), submucosa, muscularis externa (made up of inner circular and outer longitudinal muscles), and the covering serosa. The sensory nerve fibers of the small intestine and colon can sense distension and spasm, but not other pain sensations such as those that would normally be felt by the skin if cut or burned.

The small intestine is divided into three anatomical segments. The short first portion is immediately distal to the pyloric sphincter, the valve that empties the stomach. This first portion of the duodenum following the stomach is called the duodenum. The term duodenum comes from the middle Latin phrase, duodenum digitorium "space of twelve digits,". A translation of the Greek dodekadaktylon, literally "twelve fingers long," was described by the Greek physician Herophilus (c 353-280).

The first portion of the duodenum has the critical function of receiving the highly acidic gastric contents. It secretes sodium bicarbonate to neutralize the potent stomach acid. Without its natural ability to neutralize gastric acid, the duodenal mucosa may become injured or inflamed, possibly resulting in an ulcer and internal bleeding. Brunner glands (duodenal glands) are secretory compound tubular submucosal glands. They are commonly found in the proximal duodenum. The main function of Brunner glands is to produce mucus and an alkaline solution containing sodium bicarbonate. It protects the duodenal mucosa from the potent gastric acid and neutralizes the chyme leaving the stomach and entering the duodenum.

Brunner glands also secrete the polypeptide hormone urogastrone. Urogastrone inhibits the gastric parietal and chief cells from secreting hydrochloric acid as well as their digestive enzymes. The hormone was given the name urogastrone because it can be identified and isolated from the urine as a fluorescent pigment. The hormonal structure is derived from epidermal growth factor.

Additional quantities of sodium bicarbonate enter into the second portion of the duodenum after being secreted by the pancreas. The pancreatic duct, as well as the bile duct, typically enter the second portion of the duodenum together. They enter the duodenum via an anatomical structure called the Ampulla of Vater. Within the Ampulla of Vater is a muscular valve known as the Sphincter of Oddi. The Sphincter of Oddi controls the flow of bile and pancreatic juice into the duodenum. The bile is produced in the liver and may be stored in the gallbladder for later release as needed. The pancreas also produces and secretes digestive enzymes, in addition to the sodium bicarbonate it secretes to neutralize gastric acid. The pancreas is also an important endocrine organ that manages blood glucose levels through insulin and glucagon, as well as secreting other hormones

The neutralized chime is mixed with the potent digestive enzymes and bile furthering the digestive process and preparing nutrients for absorption. The jejunum, the middle portion of the small intestine between the duodenum and the ileum, was given its name after the Latin word jējūnus, which means empty or poor, so called because it was always thought to be empty after death. The ileum, from the Latin ilium meaning flank or groin, is the final segment of the small intestine and enters the cecum of the colon close to the appendix at the ileocecal valve. The small intestine is described as small because the lumen is narrower than the lumen of the large intestine. The average length of the small intestine is twenty-three feet (seven meters) and is approximately one inch (two and one half centimeters) in diameter. It is substantially longer than the approximately five-foot length of the large intestine, also called the colon.

(a) Histological organization of the digestive tract

In spite of the relatively long length of the small intestine, its absorptive capacity would not be sufficient to maintain nutrition for an organism the size of humans, if it were a simple hollow tube. Without modifications to increase its surface area, the nutritional needs of a large mammal such as humans would exceed its absorptive ability. The small intestine has several remarkable features that dramatically increase its absorptive capacity. These consist of deep circular folds of the mucosa and submucosa known as plica circulares or plica. These folds work in conjunction with millions of fingerlike extensions of the mucosa called villi.

Villi increase the surface area for absorption. Creative Commons License

These villi are provided with additional microscopic projections of the mucosal cell plasma membranes called microvilli. Each of these modifications dramatically increases the surface area available to meet the nutritional needs of larger animals such as humans.. The surface area available to the average human adult for digestive processes, enzymatic activity, and absorption exceeds that of a championship tennis court.

wellcomeimages.org Close up of intestinal villi Creative Commons License

Diagrammatic anatomy of a villous. Wikibooks Gastrointestinal Physiology Frank Boumphrey, MD
Creative Commons License

The small intestinal mucosal epithelial cells consist of absorptive cells, mucus secreting goblet cells, entero-endocrine cells that secrete gastrointestinal hormones, and interspersed intraepithelial lymphocytes and T cells. The lymphocytes and T cells are important in the immune response, as the gut is exposed to the vast majority of foreign pathogens introduced into the body.

Each villous has thousands of microvilli, as demonstrated on this scanning Transmission electron microscope image of a human jejunal epithelial cell. Image shows absorptive cell with the densely packed microvilli that make up the absorptive border. Eac Louisa Howard, Katherine Connolly
Creative Commons License

There is growing evidence that exposure to microorganisms during a normal childbirth leads to a healthy gut flora. Those who were delivered via a Caesarian section are more prone to a number of gastrointestinal disturbances as well as other systemic conditions. The microbiome are the microorganisms that live within our digestive tracts, on our skin, and in several regions on and in our body. The vast majority of these organisms are beneficial. They may provide active benefits, including supplying nutritional metabolic products that humans cannot manufacture. In addition, these beneficial organisms, known as commensals, prevent pathogens from establishing colonies, which could lead to illness.

The cells of the intestinal crypts also secrete an intestinal juice in response to irritation of the mucosal lining. This solution is slightly alkaline and isotonic with blood plasma. It is predominantly water, with some mucus, and with very little enzymatic activity. A number of intestinal infections, toxins, or inflammatory processes may stimulate the release of intestinal juice, which may lead to diarrhea. The liquid chyme has over ninety percent of its nutritional value digested and absorbed by the small intestine. The chyme exits the small intestine via the ileocecal valve, entering into the cecum of the large intestine, also called the colon. The lumen of the gastrointestinal tract, although commonly thought of as being deep within the body, is actually contiguous with and exposed to the external environment. It is a potential pathway for pathogenic microorganisms. Peyer patches are lymphoid nodules located in the laminae propria layer of the mucosa and submucosa of the ileum. They are located only in the ileum and are not present in the duodenum or jejunum of the small intestine

There are approximately thirty Peyer patches, each a few centimeters long. They are involved in the immune surveillance of the gastrointestinal tract and have a response and defense mechanism Peyer patches are covered by specialized epithelial cells called microfold cells (M cells). They contain B and T lymphocytes and are an important feature of the gastrointestinal immune response. The cells of Peyer patches allow the sampling of antigens in the gut lumen. The antigen may stimulate a response from the Peyer patches T cells, B cell lymphocytes, and memory cells. Activated lymphocytes may stimulate and magnify the immune response. They can pass into the mesenteric lymph nodes and travel via the lymphatic thoracic duct into the blood stream. From there, they may circulate throughout the gastrointestinal tract as a defense.

Pathogenic microorganisms and other antigens that enter the intestinal tract may encounter several layers of the body's immune defense. Besides the B-lymphocytes, and T-lymphocytes from Peyer patches, the antigen may also encounter macrophages, and dendritic cells. The Mucosa Associated Lymphoid Tissue (MALT) also provides immunological defenses. If injured, the ability of the small bowel to digest and absorb nutrients may be compromised. A condition that temporarily damages the small intestine, like diarrhea from a viral or bacterial gastroenteritis, often called a stomach flu, can cause a blunting or shortening of the villi. This decreases the absorptive capacity of the small intestine and may lead to diarrhea.

The damage to the villi will also lead to the loss of digestive enzymes that reside on the villi. This is one of the reasons people are often advised to avoid dairy products for a week or so after stomach flu. The villi need time to recover and return enzyme levels to normal. If you eat or drink lactose without waiting until the recovery is complete, you may end up with symptoms of lactose intolerance such as gas and diarrhea.

When the liquid chyme leaves the jejunum and ileum of the small intestine, it goes through the ileocecal valve and becomes feces. In the cecum of the colon lies the infamous appendix, which for thousands of years was a mystery as to its purpose. Its function has only very recently been identified. It serves as a reservoir of intestinal bacteria, representing the healthy gut microbiome, from which the gut flora can be replenished after a bout of intestinal dysentery. The gut microbiome is much more important than most people, including physicians and research scientists, have given it credit for. The microbes of the body far outnumber the number of human cells. The vast majority are commensals, and are engaged with us in a symbiotic relationship from which we both benefit.

The colon, unlike the small intestine, is less involved in the digestion of foods and nutrients. It is primarily involved in the absorption of water and sodium. The colon also serves to absorb nutrients, vitamins, and metabolites produced by the gut microbiome, including Vitamin K, Vitamin B_{12}, thiamine, and riboflavin. The colon removes the excess moisture from the watery chyme, and the stool solidifies as it transits the gut. It is stored in the rectum and sigmoid colon, awaiting the right opportunity to be eliminated through defecation. A process or illness that impairs the colon's absorption of water will lead to more fluid stool and diarrhea. If the elimination is delayed moisture continues to be absorbed and the stools can become harder resulting in constipation. The colon is not a vital organ, and people can live a normal life span without it, in spite of the challenges of avoiding dehydration.

Global Warming

Global warming due to greenhouse gas production from human activity is mainly due to deforestation, the combustion of fossil fuels, livestock enteric fermentation and manure management, and landfill emissions. In terms of biomass bacteria would be the main contributors to global warming by their methane production. Other contenders nominated have been termites, which have over two thousand species and are prolific methane producers (initial reports suggested that they produce forty percent of global methane), livestock such as cows, sheep, and pigs, and lastly dinosaurs, which are no longer around to defend their reputations.

A ruminant (Latin *ruminare* - to chew over again) is a mammal that digests plants in a multi compartment stomach through bacterial fermentation. It regurgitates the semi-digested mass, called cud, and chews it again and repeats the swallow. The process of re-chewing the cud is called "ruminating". There are about one hundred and fifty species of ruminants, which include both domestic and wild species. Ruminating mammals include cattle, goats, sheep, giraffes, yaks, deer, camels, llamas, and antelope. Ruminant bacterial fermentation is a significant contributor to global methane production, which is over twenty times as potent a greenhouse gas as carbon dioxide. To incentivize efforts to reduce livestock methane production a number of countries have proposed taxes on the release of greenhouse gasses.

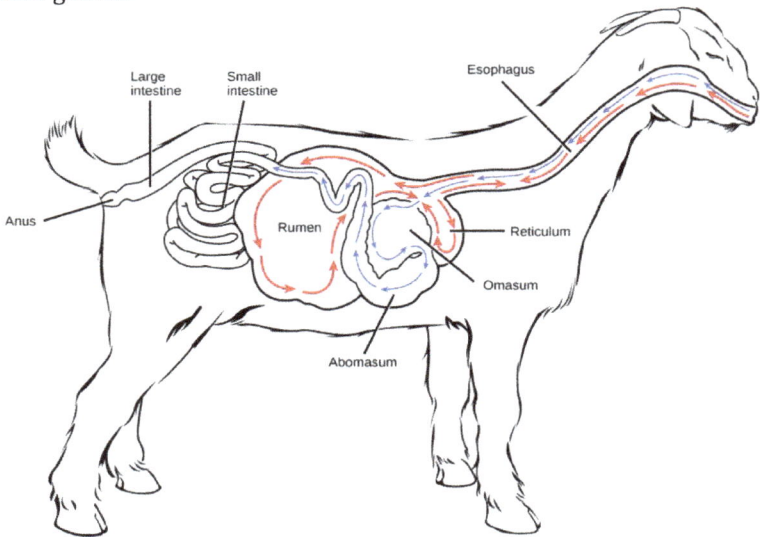

www.rice.edu Creative Commons License

It took extensive scientific experimentation to collect the intestinal gasses of herds of cattle before it was discovered that the methane production was not coming from their rear ends, but from the other end of the cows and other ruminants. It is the burps and belches from the multi compartment ruminant stomach that is the primary source of methane. The Great Chicago Fire, which destroyed the city in 1871, has traditionally been blamed on Mrs. O'Leary's cow kicking over a kerosene lamp. With the large volume of methane produced it is just as likely to have been caused by her cow farting and belching near the open flame. But that would not have been considered an acceptable cause in Victorian times.

Kangaroos are herbivores and as marsupial their burps and farts contain little or no methane, a potent greenhouse gas. It appears that the reduced methane emissions are due to the microbes in the kangaroos' gut flora. Australian researchers hope that introducing a similar gut flora to other methane producing herbivores such as cattle and sheep will contribute to a reduction in greenhouse gasses and the resultant global warming. Methane can cause about twenty times as much atmospheric warming as an equivalent volume of carbon dioxide.

Kangaroos, like cattle and sheep, are ruminants that re-chew their cud with the assistance of the gut flora to digest the and metabolize their cellulose based grazing diet. In the foregut the meal is broken down by fermentation with carbon dioxide and hydrogen released. In cows and other ruminants, microbes called methanogens transform these gases into methane. But in the kangaroos' guts the same hydrogen and carbon dioxide may be utilized by bacteria called acetogens to produce acetate, a volatile fatty acid.

These microbes compete with methanogens to use the carbon dioxide and hydrogen, so the more acetogens the less methane production. The odds are generally in favor of methanogens, since the process of methane production is generally more energy efficient than producing acetate. One of the acetogen microbes, *Blautia coccoides,* live in cows as well as in kangaroos. Further research is being undertaken to understand why the organism is more successful in competing with the methanogens in kangaroos than in other herbivores.

Carbon dioxide, methane, nitrous oxide, and three groups of fluorinated gases (sulfur hexafluoride, hydro fluorocarbons, and per fluorocarbons) are the major greenhouse gases impacted by human activity. These are regulated under the Kyoto Protocol an international treaty that was adopted in 2005. Nitrogen dioxide (NO_2) warms the atmosphere three hundred and ten times more than carbon dioxide, and methane twenty-one times more than carbon dioxide. Although CFCs are greenhouse gases, regulations were initiated because CFCs' cause ozone depletion, not because of their contribution to global warming. Ozone depletion itself has a relatively minor effect on greenhouse warming.

Dinosaurs are no longer around to defend themselves and have been accused of contributing to global warming. We do not know if they were ruminants and contributed by belching up gasses as well, but there should be no doubt that they were big time farters. Their nickname "thunder lizards" may have more to do with their farts than their footsteps.

Gluten

Gluten (Latin gluten, "glue") is a protein composite of gliadin and glutenin found conjoined with starch in the endosperm of various grass grains related to wheat, and some forms of oats. In barley the gluten component is known as hordein, in rye it is known as secalin. Corn, maize, and rice do not contain gluten. Gluten gives elasticity to dough and gives the final product a chewy texture. Bread flours are high in gluten (hard wheat); pastry flours have a lower gluten content. Kneading promotes the chewiness of a product by the formation of gluten strands and cross-links. In wheat, alpha-gliadins are not only seed storage proteins, but also act as inhibitors of alpha-amylase activity. About one in one hundred and thirty-three people in developed nations have sensitivity reactions to gluten, which can damage the villi and microvilli of the small intestine. This condition is known by a number of different names including Gluten Sensitive Enteropathy, Celiac Disease, Celiac Sprue, Nontropical Sprue, and Sprue. This disorder can lead to malabsorption, gas, diarrhea, and a variety of metabolic disorders, physical ailments, and associated conditions. The treatment is a strict gluten free diet.

Buddhist monks discovered gluten in the seventh century. The monks, who were vegetarians, were trying to find a substitute for meat. They discovered that when they submerged dough in water, the starch washed off and all that was left was a meat-like, textured, gummy mass, the gluten. Gluten sensitivity as the cause of Celiac Disease was discovered during the World War Two occupation of the Netherlands where celiac patients actually improved when all of the wheat was confiscated by Nazi Germany for consumption by their military.

Gluten, a substance in wheat and other grains, may be found in a variety of foods including breads, cakes, cereals, pasta, commercial dairy products and alcoholic beverages

digestivedisease.uthscsa.edu Creative Commons License

Gluten Sensitive Enteropathy (Celiac Disease, Celiac Sprue, Sprue)

Gluten Sensitive Enteropathy is also known by a number of other names, including, Celiac Sprue, Celiac Disease, Sprue, and Non-Tropical Sprue. It is not synonymous with gluten intolerance although it may be considered a more severe form of intolerance leading to physical and physiological changes in the gut and other areas of the body. Celiac (Greek κοιλιακός (koiliakós, "abdominal") disease is an autoimmune disorder of the small intestine that occurs in genetically predisposed people and is thought to occur in up to one percent of United States population. It is caused by a reaction to gliadin, a prolamin protein of gluten, found in wheat, rye, barley, and sometimes oats.

Humans first started to cultivate grains in the Fertile Crescent of Western Asia about 9500 BCE) it is probable that celiac disease did not occur before this time. Aretaeus of Cappadocia, living in the second century described a malabsorptive syndrome presumed to be celiac disease with pain, flatulence, and a malodorous intractable diarrhea. While a role for carbohydrates had been suspected, the link with wheat was not made until the 1940's by the Dutch pediatrician Dr. Willem Karel Dicke. He noticed that during the Dutch famine of 1944 the scarcity of wheat and bread led the rate among children affected by CD to drop to essentially zero, but returned to over thirty-five percent once wheat was again available after the war. On exposure to gliadin the enzyme tissue transglutaminase modifies the protein triggering an immune response causes an inflammatory reaction in the small bowel. This leads to damage and atrophy of the villous lining of the small intestine that is critical for digestion and absorption of nutrients. Treatment requires a lifelong gluten free diet to avoid the offending protein.

CELIAC DISEASE

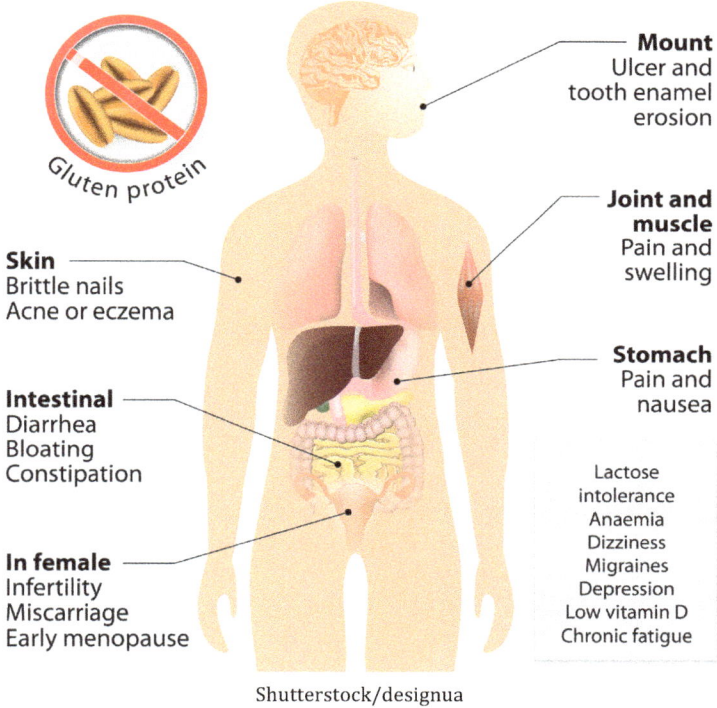

Gluten protein

Mount
Ulcer and
tooth enamel
erosion

Joint and muscle
Pain and
swelling

Skin
Brittle nails
Acne or eczema

Stomach
Pain and
nausea

Intestinal
Diarrhea
Bloating
Constipation

Lactose
intolerance
Anaemia
Dizziness
Migraines
Depression
Low vitamin D
Chronic fatigue

In female
Infertility
Miscarriage
Early menopause

Shutterstock/designua

Celiac disease can present with malabsorption, steatorrhea, weight loss, anemia, fatigue, and other symptoms related to the nutritional deficiencies. Milder or subclinical cases may present without symptoms, often discovered by abnormal results on a routine blood test. When chronic diarrhea is present in celiac disease it is often pale, voluminous, and malodorous because of fat absorption leading to steatorrhea. Abdominal pain, cramping, bloating, distension, and gaseousness with mouth ulcers may also be present. It is not unusual for patients to be seen and treated for irritable bowel or other conditions for several years before the correct diagnosis becomes apparent.

Untreated celiac disease has an increased risk of adenocarcinoma and lymphoma of the small bowel. Malabsorption may lead to nutritional deficiencies such as minerals and the fat-soluble vitamins A, D, E, and K. Anemia may develop from iron insufficiency as well as from deficiencies of folic acid and vitamin B_{12} which may give rise to megaloblastic anemia and neuropathy. Calcium and vitamin D malabsorption (and secondary hyperparathyroidism) may cause osteopenia (decreased mineral content of the bone) or osteoporosis. Vitamin K deficiency interferes with to the bloods ability to clot and can present as abnormal bleeding. Bacterial overgrowth of the small intestine can occur aggravating malabsorption or preventing the resolution of malabsorption with a gluten free diet.

THE CONTENT OF GLUTEN IN FOODS

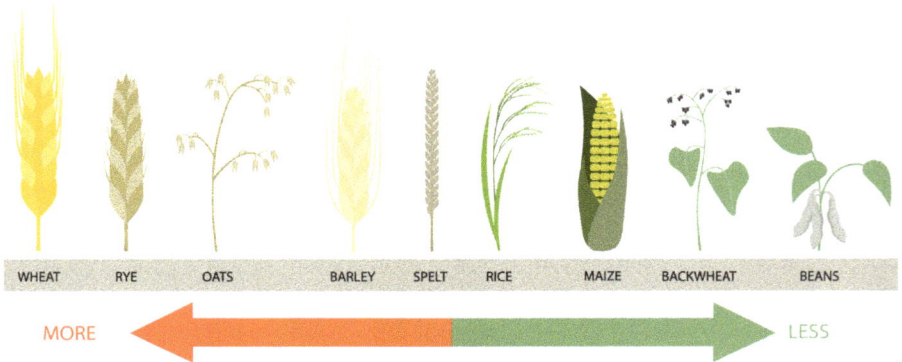

| WHEAT | RYE | OATS | BARLEY | SPELT | RICE | MAIZE | BACKWHEAT | BEANS |

MORE — LESS

Shutterstock/Moremar

A variety of other conditions, especially autoimmune disorders are more common in those with celiac disease. These include those IgA deficiency, dermatitis herpetiformis, diabetes mellitus, autoimmune thyroiditis, primary biliary cirrhosis, hyposplenism, and microscopic colitis, abnormal liver function tests, delayed growth and development, Addison disease (adrenal insufficiency), alopecia areata, Down syndrome (trisomy 21), osteoporosis, Sjögren Syndrome, systemic lupus erythematosis, and Turner syndrome.

Celiac Disease

Normal

Damaged

Intestinal villi in celiac disease are atrophic ih.constantcontact.com Creative Commons License

There are several tests that can be used to assist in diagnosis. The level of symptoms may determine the order of the tests, but all tests lose their usefulness if the person is already eating a gluten-free diet. Intestinal damage begins to heal within weeks of gluten being removed from the diet, and antibody levels decline over months. For those who have already started on a gluten-free diet, it may be necessary to perform a challenge with some gluten-containing food in one meal a day over six weeks before repeating the investigations.

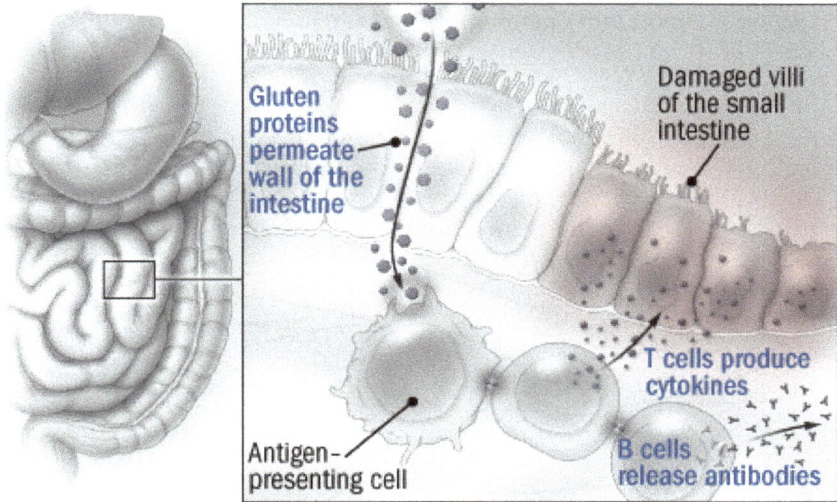

www.health.harvard.edu Creative Commons License

Diagnostic tests are very accurate unless a gluten free diet was instituted before testing. The tests accuracy is diminished with longer time periods from the last gluten exposure. Serological blood tests have high sensitivity and specificity for celiac disease but endoscopy and small bowel biopsy is usually necessary for a definitive diagnosis of celiac disease. Anti-endomysial immunoglobulin A (IgA) antibodies and IgA tissue anti-transglutaminase (tTG) have over ninety percent sensitivity and nearly ninety-nine percent specificity.

Gut-Brain-Microbiome-Food Axis

A relatively recent discovery has been that the gut brain axis has a very important third component, the microbiome. The gut microbiome is also known as the gut flora and consists of the multitude of other life forms residing within the gut. These include bacteria, viruses, protist, Archaea, parasites, prions, fungi, and probably other undiscovered or unidentified organisms. By number of cells, the human cells of our body are outnumbered ten to one by the over one hundred trillion microbes living on and within the average human.

If instead of cell population the comparison were based on genes that can be expressed and control biological functions, the human genes are outnumbered one hundred to one. In addition to the gut microbiome, there are unique microbiomes on all aspects of the human body exposed to the external environment. Research activities are studying all areas of the human microbiome including, skin, oral, nasal, genitourinary, etcetera. The research findings to date are so dramatic that many scientists describe the microbiome as if a new major organ system of the body has just been discovered. The hundreds of trillions of microorganisms that make up the gut flora are a major source of the intestinal gasses produced during digestion and fermentation. The interaction between these organisms, food, and the human gut and brain are just beginning to be uncovered. More important than their major contribution to intestinal gas, is their even more important contribution to human health and vitality.

The brain gut axis has been recognized for over a century. It has also been well recognized that information and influence travels in both directions. The brain can trigger digestive system symptoms and disorders including the common functional conditions such as irritable bowel syndrome. Digestive disorders frequently send signals to the brain and may lead to systemic anxiety, fear, depression, and distress. The brain, central, and autonomic nervous systems are intimately connected with the enteric nervous system of the gastrointestinal tract.

Healthy status

Healthy CNS function

Normal gut physiology

Physiological levels of inflammatory cells/mediators Normal gut microbiota

Stress/disease

Alterations in behaviour, cognition, emotion, nociception

Abnormal gut function

Increased levels of inflammatory cells/mediators Intestinal dysbiosis

Gut intuition, know it in your gut, gut wrenching experience, gut wrong, gut check, butterflies in the stomach, gut instinct, gut reaction, listen to your gut, go with your gut, are all common expressions to describe the common experiences of intuition most commonly known as gut feelings. The gastrointestinal tract is sensitive to stress and emotion. Anger, anxiety, sadness, fear, elation are all among the many feelings that can trigger symptoms in the gut ranging from mild spasm to intense nausea, vomiting, cramps, diarrhea, and fecal incontinence.

c431376.r76.cf2.rackcdn.com Creative Commons License

The brain has a direct effect on the digestive tract. As demonstrated by Ivan Pavlov, dogs accustomed to hearing a bell before being fed begin to salivate with just the sound of the bell even if no food is offered. The release of saliva, digestive enzymes, hormones, and gut motility can all be stimulated by thoughts generated by the brain alone. Ninety-five percent of the body's supply of the well-recognized and critically important neurotransmitter serotonin is found in the gut. The brain and its serotonin receptors, representing only five percent of the body's serotonin, is a frequent target of prescription medications such as Prozac (fluoxetine). These pharmaceuticals are known as a selective serotonin re-uptake inhibitor (SSRI). The gut and the brain each have fifty percent of another important neurotransmitter, dopamine.

Gut Feeling (Gut Instinct)

Gut intuition, know it in your gut, gut wrenching experience, gut wrong, gut check, butterflies in the stomach, gut instinct, gut reaction, listen to your gut, go with your gut, are all common expressions to describe the common experiences of intuition most commonly known as gut feelings. The gastrointestinal tract is sensitive to stress and emotion. Anger, anxiety, sadness, fear, elation are all among the many feelings that can trigger symptoms in the gut ranging from mild spasm to intense nausea, vomiting, cramps, diarrhea, and fecal incontinence.

The brain has a direct effect on the digestive tract. As demonstrated by Ivan Pavlov (1849-1936), dogs accustomed to hearing a bell before being fed begin to salivate with just the sound of the bell even if no food is offered. The release of saliva, digestive enzymes, hormones, and gut motility can all be stimulated by thoughts generated by the brain alone. The brain-gut axis has been recognized for over a century. It has also been well recognized that information and influence travels in both directions. The brain can trigger digestive system symptoms and disorders including the common functional conditions such as irritable bowel syndrome. Digestive disorders frequently send signals to the brain and may lead to systemic anxiety, fear, depression, and distress. The brain central and autonomic nervous systems are intimately connected with the enteric nervous system of the gastrointestinal tract.

Ninety-five percent of the body's supply of the well-recognized and critically important neurotransmitter serotonin is found in the gut. The brain and its serotonin receptors, representing only five percent of the body's serotonin, is a frequent target of prescription medications such as Prozac (fluoxetine). These pharmaceuticals are known as a selective serotonin re-uptake inhibitor (SSRI). The gut and the brain each have fifty percent of another important neurotransmitter, dopamine. A relatively recent discovery has been that the gut-brain-axis has a very important third component, the microbiome. The gut microbiome is also known as the gut flora and consists of the multitude of other life forms residing within the gut. These include bacteria, viruses, protozoans, archaea, parasites, prions, fungi, and probably other undiscovered or unidentified organisms. By number of cells, the human cells of our body are outnumbered ten to one by the over one hundred trillion microbes living on and within the average human.

If instead of cell population the comparison were based on genes that can be expressed and control biological functions, the human genes are outnumbered one hundred to one. In addition to the gut microbiome, there are unique microbiomes on all aspects of the human body exposed to the external environment. Research activities are studying all areas of the human microbiome including, skin, oral, nasal, genitourinary, etcetera. The research findings to date are so dramatic that many scientists describe the microbiome as if a new major organ system of the body has just been discovered! The microbiome has an important role in the production and utilization of the neurotransmitters serotonin and dopamine. Additional metabolites also produced by the microbiome include the principal excitatory neurotransmitter amino acid glutamic acid (glutamate), and its derivative the principal inhibitory neurotransmitter gamma amino butyric acid (GABA). A wide variety of other neurotransmitters and metabolites with hormone like activity are intimately associated with the gut microbiome.

We are all aware that certain microbes are pathogenic, and can lead to disease, disability, and even death. Most of us were taught to believe that microbes are harmful, dangerous, and should be avoided at all possible costs. Personal hygiene including hand washing, mouthwash, frequent bathing, showering, and use of anti-microbial soaps and cleansers has become the routine system advocated for protecting one's health. The benefits of cleanliness may well have been overrated. Advances in public health and a safe drinking water supply has markedly reduced the incidence of parasites. One of the paradoxical results was an increase in autoimmune diseases in countries with improved public hygiene. It appears that those infected with chronic parasites such as hookworms have an improved immune system. They have a much lower incidence of autoimmune disease than do parasite-free humans. Research involving the purposeful infection with hookworm and pig whipworm eggs in autoimmune conditions is underway.

The premise that microbes are harmful and pathogenic has been incorrectly expanded from known pathogens to the whole world of microbes. The vast majority of microbes are beneficial, both in their own right by metabolic functions that support human health and by their large populations preventing pathogenic organisms from becoming established. These beneficial microbes are known by the biological term as commensal organisms. The commensal organisms in the gut interact with the human host through a wide variety of mechanisms. They influence hormonal levels and activities, including reducing the stress response. They provide nutritional support and produce vitamins, metabolites, neurotransmitters, immune modulators, and other beneficial products. The population of various organisms in the microbiome also undergoes rapid changes in response to environmental factors. These include changes in the diet as well as exposure to new organisms from other humans, pets, travel, use of antibiotics, supplements, artificial sweeteners, etcetera.

The physiology and population growth of microbes rely on many of the same basic metabolic pathways as human cells. They also share the same mechanisms of ion transport, which plays a critical role in cellular communications. The genes of microbes control and express bioactive metabolites that are often identical to those from human cells. Neurotransmitters, hormones, and other metabolites generated by the microbes within the gastrointestinal tract can be absorbed and are active within the human host. Approximately twenty percent of the bioactive metabolites circulating in human blood are of microbial origin.

The profound implication is that the microbiome may be playing an important role in influencing or controlling human physiology. This in turn leads to the conclusion that the enteric and central nervous system and ultimately, the brain may likewise be influenced by the microbiome. The rapidly accumulating scientific evidence is that this is indeed the case. The understanding of the critical importance of the microbiome is leading to major advances in a wide variety of disease processes well beyond digestive disorders. One of the most exciting areas of investigation suggests that a number of psychiatric and neurological disorders may be due to alterations in the gut microbiome. Likewise, manipulation of the gut microbiome may be effective as preventive or therapeutic measures. Probiotic approaches that have such benefits are now described as a new class of psychobiotics.

Researchers have found that the microbiome can modulate a part of the brain involved in emotion and mood. This includes increases in a chemical called brain-derived neurotrophic factor (BDNF), which plays a role in learning and memory. Low levels of BDNF have been associated with clinical depression, chronic anxiety syndromes, and other psychiatric disorders. The field is rapidly advancing with the recognition that the microbiome profoundly influences the immune, endocrine, and neurological function of their host. Novel neurochemicals and hormones are defining a new field best described at this time as microbiome neuroimmunoendocrinology. In addition to communication between microbes and their host, it is now recognized that the microbes are also communicating with each other. Another critically important factor that expands the brain-gut-microbiome axis is the role of diet and food. The food and diet not only profoundly influence the gut microbiome, but they also may have direct bioactive and epigenetic effects on the whole organism. To the degree that the diet may contain residue of pesticides, herbicides, fertilizers, genetically modified organisms (GMO) otter factors may also be playing a role in the expanded brain-gut-food-microbiome axis.

The ability of the brain to influence the intestinal microbiota

Perturbation of normal habitat via stress-induced changes in gastrointestinal:
- Physiology
- Epithelial function
- Mucin production
- EE cell function
- Motility

Release of neurotransmitters

GBA

Microbiota-gut interplay

The ability of the microbiota to influence brain and behavior

Activation of neural afferent circuits to the brain

Activation of mucosal immune responses

Production of metabolites that directly influence the CNS

While we may like to believe that our brains are in total control of our minds and body, studies of the brain-gut-food-microbiome axis suggest that we may have to reconsider this assumption. The volume of information being sent from the brain to the gut is just a fraction of the amount traveling in the opposite direction. The torrents of information come in a variety of forms including metabolites, neurotransmitters, hormones, immune modulators, epigenetic factors, endocrine disruptors, chemicals, etcetera.

Some of the most intriguing findings are that the billions of humans infected with the ubiquitous cat-harbored protist parasite *Toxoplasma gondii* are often thought to be symptom free until they develop evidence of the disease state called toxoplasmosis, which has severe complications during pregnancy. The

*Air*Veda: Ancient & New Medical Wisdom

Toxoplasma gondii cysts are often ingested by farm animals and frequently passed to humans through poorly cooked foods, usually pork, lamb, and venison. In many parts of the world over ninety-five percent of the human population is infected. In the United States over twenty-two percent of the population over the age of twelve is infected. The most recent scientific evidence shows that the parasite is harbored in the human brain where it can affect mood, anger, hostility, depression, risk taking behavior, and is associated with a have a higher risk of developing schizophrenia.

Not only do they develop this psychiatric disorder but they are also influenced to engage in unusual behaviors known as a pica, such as eating dirt. This induced behavior has specific benefits for the parasite but not for the human host. In essence, the parasite is controlling the human to do its bidding, suggesting a scene taken from the pages of science fiction. While the role of the microbiome in the pathogenesis of disease is being aggressively explored, the possibility of altering the microbiome for therapeutic purposes is also being investigated. Over the last few years the use of fecal microbiota transplants has become the treatment of choice for pseudomembranous colitis, also known as antibiotic associated colitis. Preliminary findings suggest that modifying the gut microbiome may also be beneficial in inflammatory bowel disease and irritable bowel syndrome.

Élie Metchnikoff (1845–1916) was a Nobel laureate who proposed over a century ago that the gut microbiome may play a major role in health and longevity. His research prompted a keen interest in using the live microbes of yogurt cultures to improve the gut flora. He influenced physician John Harvey Kellogg (1852-1943) to develop prebiotic dietary fiber additives leading to the creation of Kellogg's cereals. Kellogg's other approach to bowel health, using yogurt as a colonic to implant a healthy microbiome, was not as palatable or commercially successful as his Kellogg's Corn Flakes. Alteration of the gut microbiome is under investigation for a wide variety of conditions ranging from common digestive disorders to autism. The eagerness to treat many of these conditions may be premature as the organisms that may be the cause of disease has yet to be identified. In addition, what organisms constitute an optimal therapeutic microbiome is still an open question, but will be clarified with further study.

At birth our gut is sterile, but we rapidly become colonized beginning with exposure to microbes at birth. The microbiome of those who are born via the normal route of a vaginal delivery have a microbiome different from those born by Cesarean section. There are health differences with advantages to the children who arrived via a vaginal delivery. There is growing evidence that the gut bacteria are closely tied to immunity as well as early brain development and subsequent behavior. The absence or presence of gut microorganisms during infancy may permanently alter gene expression. The advantages of a vaginal delivery are so striking that many infants delivered by Cesarean section are being purposefully exposed to the vaginal microbiome of their birth mother. Further research will hopefully identify the optimal microbiome for infant health and welfare.

The mechanism of the transmission of information in the brain-gut-microbiome axis is under intense investigation. One of the intriguing research findings in mice was that the microbiome was very different in mice that were anxious versus mice that were fearless. When their microbiomes were exchanged their behaviors reversed. If the vagus nerve, the major nerve connecting the brain and the gut, is surgically severed the changes in behavior do not occur. In addition to information transfer via the vagus nerve, it is clear that the microbes produce neurotransmitters and metabolites, which can influence brain chemistry and behavior.

Further research will identify the illnesses and conditions associated with specific microbes and combinations of microbes. In systems biology, the causation of an illness or symptom may be due to a single agent, or multiple agents acting in concert. For example, it is known that most cancers do not arise as a result of as single genetic mutation, but rather as the consequence of a combination of random mutations. Other than the limited number of infectious diseases known to be caused by a single pathogen, causation of disease may be difficult to identify with certainty. The more variables that are involved, the more challenging it is to identify the combination of agents and actions that are the true causation of an illness. The microbiome by its very nature includes near infinite variations of possible combinations of organisms and their genomic and metabolomic activity. The megadata generated from studies requires supercomputers for analysis.

Specific organisms that act as commensals may be also be considered as therapeutic when administered to modify the microbiome. Probiotics are the name given to beneficial and commensal strains of microbes. Prebiotics are dietary supplements, which encourage commensals to predominate. Certain strains of probiotics increase the bioavailability of tryptophan, the amino acid that is a key precursor in the neurotransmitter serotonin. Other strains play a role in a variety of neurotransmitters that may play an important role in psychiatric and neurological diseases. Strains of microbes that affect the brain or behavior are called psychobiotics. The concept of the brain-gut-food-microbiome axis has become the forefront of research across the fields of medicine and psychiatry.

Gut Fermentation Syndrome (Auto Brewery Syndrome)

Gut fermentation syndrome is also known as the auto-brewery syndrome and is a rare medical condition in which not only gas but alcohol is produced within the gastrointestinal tract through endogenous fermentation. The alcohol produced is absorbed and can lead to intoxication if sufficient substrate is ingested into the digestive system. Numerous cases have been documented in the medical literature with isolation of the fermenting organism *Saccharomyces cerevisiae*. Interestingly enough many people use *Saccharomyces* and Brewer's yeast as a probiotic supplement. It has also been investigated, but eliminated, as a possible cause of sudden infant death syndrome. Claims of endogenous fermentation of this type have also been used as a defense against drunk driving charges. Often the defendant is required to submit to medical isolation and documentation that their blood alcohol level will rise spontaneously if given a fermentable carbohydrate rich meal. If the blood levels do not confirm the existence of the extremely rare disorder they are convicted of the driving while intoxicated charge and have additional medical expenses added to their penalty.

www.egotastic.com Creative Commons License

Alcoholic beverages typically contain less than one percent to up to forty percent ethanol (alcohol) by volume. They have been produced and consumed by humans since pre-historic times. Ethanol is obtained via fermentation using glucose that is produced from the hydrolysis of starch in the presence of yeast. Several of the benign bacteria in the intestine use fermentation as a form of anaerobic metabolism, which produces ethanol as a waste product. Human bodies contain some quantity of alcohol produced by these bacteria. In rare cases, this can be sufficient to cause "auto-brewery syndrome" in which intoxicating quantities of alcohol are produced by the bacterial flora of the gastrointestinal tract. Ethanol is further metabolized by the liver.

Hiatus Hernia (Hiatal Hernia)

A hiatus hernia is a defect in the large flat muscle called the diaphragm that separates the chest (thorax) from the abdomen. Below the diaphragm is the intra-abdominal (peritoneal) cavity holding the stomach, liver, gall bladder, pancreas, small intestine, and large intestine. Above the diaphragm are the lungs and the heart, and the esophagus. The lower esophageal sphincter is located at the opening in the diaphragm that allows the esophagus and stomach to connect. This opening is called the diaphragmatic hiatus (Latin Hiatus opening, gap). Hiatal hernias occur when the opening through the diaphragm allows the stomach to protrude from the abdomen into the chest. This common condition increases with age and may lead to burping and belching, heartburn and gastroesophageal reflux disease (GERD).

By the age of fifty approximately sixty percent of individuals have a hiatal hernia. Less than ten percent are symptomatic if the lower esophageal sphincter maintains its competence. The vast majority (ninety-five percent) is of the sliding hiatus hernia variety where the gastroesophageal junction moves above the diaphragm together with a portion of the stomach. The other and more dangerous variety is a paraesophageal hiatus hernia (five percent) where the stomach herniates through the esophageal hiatus and lies parallel to the esophagus with the gastroesophageal junction remaining at the level of the diaphragm.

Reflux

Hiatal hernia

Esophageal damage
from reflux

Risk factors that may increase the likelihood of developing a hiatus hernia include increased intra-abdominal pressure caused by heavy lifting, bending over, frequent or vigorous coughing, vigorous sneezing, pregnancy and delivery, forceful vomiting, straining with bowel movements, obesity. Heredity and tobacco usage are associated with a higher incidence as well. In most cases, sufferers experience no discomfort and no treatment is required. The most frequent symptoms are those of gastroesophageal reflux disease (GERD), which is usually managed with lifestyle changes, avoidance of products that relax the lower esophageal sphincter, and acid suppressing medications. The less frequent paraesophageal type of hiatal hernia has a higher risk of gastric torsion and surgical repair is often required.

Diaphragm — Esophagus

Stomach

**Normal Esophagus
and Stomach**

**Sliding
Hiatus Hernia**

**Paraesophageal
Hiatus Hernia**

Hiatus tightened

Stomach and lower esophagus replaced

The stomach is placed back below the diaphragm in a hiatal hernia repair with the diaphragmatic hiatus tightened and the stomach wrapped around the esophagus below the hiatus to act as an anchor. After a hiatus hernia repair, commonly a procedure known as a Nissen fundoplication, the lower esophageal sphincter may be so tight that individuals complain of an inability to burp or belch. The inability to release distending gasses may be so uncomfortable that an esophageal dilation procedure is advised to stretch the now too tight sphincter.

The lower esophageal sphincter is the key safety valve between the durable gastric lining with acid contents and the smooth mild mannered passageway of the esophagus. If the sphincter allows excess acid material into the lower esophagus heartburn and mucosal damage can occur. In the case of a hiatal hernia the upper portion of the stomach begins to slip through the opening, the diaphragmatic hiatus, and now has entered into the thorax, the chest cavity. The mechanism that allows the lungs to inflate is dependent on the intercostal (rib cage) muscles and the diaphragm. When the diaphragm contracts it pushes down on the abdominal contents and creates in essence a vacuum (referred to as negative intra-thoracic pressure) in the chest that causes the lungs to draw in air and inflate.

This vacuum effect is present through the chest cavity, so it influences the esophagus as well. Now that a part of the stomach, and the critical lower esophageal sphincter have migrated through the diaphragmatic hiatus into the chest cavity it is now subject to the negative intra-thoracic pressure. Acting like a vacuum it creates the opposite effect on the sphincter pulling it open rather than allowing it to stay closed. As acid and gastric contents are drawn into the esophagus its limited defenses can be overwhelmed and symptoms can arise and damage to the lining can occur. Unfortunately, there is a danger than the damage may lead to conditions such as Barrett Esophagus where the esophageal lining is at higher risk of developing cancer of the esophagus. So although heartburn may be a minor annoyance, it could also be serious warning sign.

The hiatal hernia working against the lower esophageal sphincter may allow reflux and GERD. It also allows the easier escape of air in the stomach, including swallowed air. Belching or burping may be impaired after surgery or procedures to tighten the Lower Esophageal Sphincter or correct a hiatal hernia. That is a surprisingly uncomfortable situation that can usually be corrected with a relatively quick and simple procedure of endoscopic esophageal dilation.

High Altitude Flatus Expulsion (HAFE)

The higher the altitude the lower the atmospheric pressure. Gasses expand with the decreasing pressure of higher altitudes.

High-altitude flatus expulsion (HAFE) is a gastrointestinal syndrome, popularly referred to by its military abbreviated acronym, which involves the spontaneous passage of increased quantities of rectal gases at high altitudes. As the atmospheric pressure decreases with an increase in altitude, the volume of gas in the intestine increases consistent with the principles of physics (Boyle's Law). Military pilots and astronauts have repeatedly verified the sensation of distention and the need to expel the expanding intestinal gasses.

Intestinal gasses, like gasses everywhere, must comply with the laws of physics and the laws of nature. Boyle's law states that at a constant temperature the product of a gasses volume and pressure must remain constant. This requires that they move in opposite directions so that an increase in pressure will result in the decrease of the gases volume and vice versa. The atmospheric pressure on earth is set at a standard of one atmosphere at sea level. As you go deeper into the earth or oceans the atmospheric pressure increases. As you go higher in elevation whether in a building on a mountain or in a hot air balloon the atmospheric pressure drops. Using Boyle's law, you can calculate how much the volume will compress as you go deeper underground or underwater and can likewise calculate how much a gas will expand as you go higher in altitude and the atmospheric pressure is declining.

If you have ever gone diving into a swimming pool, or snorkeling, or scuba diving you can feel the increasing atmospheric pressure on your eardrums, sometimes to such a degree that the pressure can be painful. To relieve the discomfort, you have to equalize the pressure on both sides of your eardrums, usually by performing the Valsalva maneuver of attempting to exhale against a closed epiglottis, much like straining during a bowel movement. As you go up an elevator in a high-rise building, or drive up a mountain road, or fly in an airplane you may feel or hear your ears 'pop' as they adjust to the decreasing atmospheric pressure. Once again to relieve the discomfort you need to equalize pressure on both sides of the eardrum. Since you are not underwater you can use the more comfortable maneuver of yawning instead of the Valsalva maneuver.

The changes in atmospheric pressure in aerospace are more dramatic than in mountain climbers, both in intensity and rapidity. With commercial aircraft commonly flying at over thirty thousand feet in elevation the atmospheric pressure outside of the plane is a fraction of atmospheric pressure at sea level. The pressure loss at that altitude would not be tolerable to passengers so the aircraft is pressurized to simulate what the atmospheric pressure would be at approximately eight thousand feet above sea level. That is still a significant reduction in pressure, which means a proportional increase in volume. Any pockets of air in your gut will expand quickly, distend the gut to uncomfortable levels, and want to be released.

Second World War pilots flying unpressurized aircraft at altitudes over thirty thousand feet above sea level described disabling abdominal pain from gas distension that could not be readily evacuated. At that altitude the atmospheric pressure was a fraction of that at sea level allowing intestinal gas to balloon to nearly four times its original volume. Pressurized aircraft have a more modest but still noticeable effect on intestinal gas volume. Pilots and flight attendants are well aware of this effect but do not offer you any explanation for your discomfort, either from your own gas or the person sitting directly in front of you. In fact, it is typical that there is much more turbulence inside an aircraft than outside.

If you would like another visual example of the differences in atmospheric pressure between being on the ground and at an atmospheric pressure equivalent to an altitude of eight thousand feet look at what happens to carbonated beverages served at high altitude. Have you ever noticed that the release of the bubbles of carbon dioxide is more dramatic when flying? Flight attendants have to spend more time pouring the drinks letting the bubbles release themselves or you would be handed a container of fizz and foam instead of the beverage you wanted.

For those involved in space travel, including the growing population of space tourists, the pressure changes are unparalleled. Nitrogen also dissolves in the bloodstream and body fats. Rapid decompression of astronauts decompressing too quickly can lead to life threatening decompression sickness formerly known as caisson sickness or the bends when nitrogen bubbles form in the bloodstream, nerves, joints. As you are above and no longer in the atmosphere you basically have a carte blanche to blame Boyle's Law for any and all flatulence you may wish to release. Alan Shepard, Jr. (1923–1998) was an American naval aviator, test pilot, NASA astronaut, who in 1961 became the second person, and the first American, to travel into space. When reporters asked Shepard what he thought about as he sat atop the Redstone rocket waiting for liftoff he replied "The fact that every part of this ship was built by the low bidder".

Ten years later Shepard commanded the Apollo 14 mission to the moon. Despite thick gloves and a stiff spacesuit Shepard struck two golf balls on the lunar surface driving the second "miles and miles and miles." As director of astronaut program Shepard received the following memorandum from astronaut John Young. "RE: Safety Issues. No less than six times have I had to listen to Borman complain about his lactose intolerance when someone stole his weird not-milk milk stuff. Additionally, when Borman drinks regular milk, he gets the farts. That's all I'm going to say about that."

Benjamin Franklin was quoted as saying "Instead of cursing the darkness, light a candle." Alan Shepard created another memorable quote while waiting for interminable delays to end. The quote became the title of his biography, *Light This Candle*. NASA engineers had delayed his first flight so many times the Soviets were able to send the first man into orbit. On the day of his voyage Shepard sat on the launchpad, waiting inside his rocket for over four hours while engineers tackled one problem and then another. The wait was longer than anyone expected and Shepard ended up having to urinate inside his spacesuit. They had to turn off his monitoring equipment so that he did not create a short circuit. When one more problem cropped up, Shepard exclaimed, "Why don't you fix your little problem and light this candle!"

The NASA space program was concerned about intestinal gas during space flight. Their concern is well placed because excessive distention of the gut with gas can lead to barotrauma, perforation, peritonitis, and death. It would be beyond a tragic irony if an astronaut were to die of an explosion during space travel, and it was his own combustible fuel that led to his demise. After liftoff while experiencing weightlessness he also experienced this other anticipated consequence of virtually zero atmospheric pressure. His internal gas bubbles expanded with production of continuous farting, which he graphically described over the radio communications with mission control. If you listen closely to the recording of the communications not all of the background noise is static! Gus Grissom was scheduled to go into space two months after Shepard's inaugural flight on Friendship Seven. He insisted that the "pottie" problem had to be solved and a naval flight surgeon was assigned to the task. He sent one of the nurses into town to buy a women's panty girdle, which was layered with absorbent pads. Grissom was the first astronaut to go into space wearing women's lingerie.

Astronauts, cosmonauts, and taikonauts have to deal with bodily functions in space, and modifications have been required. The Hamilton Standard Company was the maker of the astronaut spacesuits and male astronauts used a condom catheter under the spacesuits for space-walks and moonwalks. Ingenuity was required to come up with a comparable solution for female astronauts. In the microgravity environment of space, farting results in the body being propelled when the 'digestive gas thruster is fired'. On the space station Mir restraining seat belt devices were installed on the toilet so the user would not be thrust off the seat with a fart.

When the Gemini program began the astronauts graduated to urine and fecal bags and special diapers for spacewalks. They disposed of the urine by an overboard dump valve. The solid waste was handled differently with a germicide placed in the storage bag, which was sealed in a locker. Since the lunar model itself had no overboard dump or storage locker astronauts left very personal mementos of their visits behind. More than the US flag was deposited on the moon surface and remain there to this day. When the Space Shuttle program was initiated a space toilet called the "Waste Collection Facility" or WCF for short was developed. It was budgeted to cost three million dollars to develop but with cost over-runs it ended up being the world most expensive toilet by far, costing more than thirty million dollars.

For those living in high altitude communities such as Mexico City at over seven thousand feet above sea level, the atmospheric pressure is much lower than at sea level. Commercial aircraft are pressurized to an equivalent of nine thousand feet above sea level. With the atmospheric pressure at just over two thirds of sea level the gas volume expands by about forty percent. That is more than enough to cause a person to notice a significant increase in their flatulence and that of everyone else as well.

High Altitude Living (see Atmospheric Pressure, Ideal Gas Laws)

The majority of the world's population lives close to the seashore and have the standard atmospheric pressure of one atmosphere found at sea level. A significant percentage of the world's population lives at higher altitudes with atmospheric pressures less than one atmosphere. One hundred and forty million people live at altitudes above two thousand five hundred meters (eight thousand two-hundred ft.). The higher above sea level you are, the lower is the atmospheric pressure you are subjected to. As a consequence, although the number of molecules of gas produced is identical, it will require a larger volume of space to contain it.

Those who travel to higher altitudes, whether by climbing a mountain, driving up a mountain road, or traveling by air, experience an increase in flatulence. The underlying principle is the same, according to the gas laws of physics a reduction in atmospheric pressure results in an increase in the volume of intestinal gas. Those who reside in high altitude communities become used to this degree of flatulence as normal for their elevation.

The Potala Palace, Lhasa, Tibet is higher yet at 11,450 feet altitude. Photo by Antoine Taveneaux
Creative Commons License

If you live in Denver Colorado, the mile-high city with an elevation of five thousand one hundred and eighty-three feet (one thousand six hundred and nine meters) feet above sea level, the volume of an identical number of gas molecules will be larger than residing in Los Angeles or New York City. It is all relative, as residing in Mexico City, which is at seven thousand three hundred and fifty feet (two thousand two hundred and forty meters), will produce a much larger volume than Denver. Working or living in high-rise buildings may also give rise to changes in atmospheric pressure. This is most readily demonstrated by taking a high-speed elevator in a high-rise building. The rapid decrease in atmospheric pressure traveling from the lower to the higher floors often results in pressure changes on the eardrum (tympanic membrane). The equalization of pressure on both sides of the tympanic membrane may give rise to an ear popping sensation. The rapid ascent in the elevator may give rise to other popping noises from expanding intestinal gas.

Another important consideration for those engaged in high altitude activities is the recognition that the oxygen content of air decreases with an increase in altitude. The percentage saturation of hemoglobin with oxygen determines the oxygen content of the blood. Atmospheric pressure decreases exponentially with altitude, so while the O_2 fraction remains relatively constant the absolute amount of oxygen in a given volume of air decreases exponentially as well. At an altitude around two thousand one hundred meters (seven thousand feet) above sea level, the oxygen saturation of hemoglobin begins to decrease dramatically.

Many air travelers are under the false impression that pressurization of the aircraft means the oxygen content of the air is the same as that on the ground at sea level. The aircraft is typically pressurized to maintain a cabin pressure equivalent to an altitude of approximately eight thousand feet. This leads to a reduction in the oxygen content of the air on the aircraft. Some normal individuals find this reduction in oxygen uncomfortable and develop headaches and other symptoms. Others are more sensitive, or recognize that their underlying medical condition requires that they have access to supplemental oxygen for their safe travel.

At an altitude of five thousand meters (sixteen thousand feet), the altitude of the Mount Everest base camp, hemoglobin oxygen saturation is reduced by fifty per cent. At the summit of Mount Everest, at an altitude of 8,848 m (29,029 ft.) above sea level, the oxygen saturation is reduced by two thirds. Travel to high altitude regions can lead to medical problems, from the mild symptoms of acute mountain sickness to life threatening high altitude pulmonary edema and cerebral edema. The higher the altitude, the greater the risk. For those with underlying circulatory or lung conditions the additional stress of even mildly lower oxygen content of the air can be potentially life threatening. Altitude sickness can develop rapidly and is a life-threatening condition requiring an immediate descent in altitude.

Hydrogen

Hydrogen and methane are two explosive gasses produced by the gut microbes. Their presence in farts make the fart ignitable and flammable, used to the amusement of some and the chagrin and painful burns of others. These same microorganisms continue their gas production in the feces after it exits the host digestive tract. Both hydrogen and methane are odorless. Hydrogen sulfide and other aromatic and volatile substances are also produced by the microorganisms in feces that produces its characteristic odor even though they only comprise a fraction of one percent of the fart gasses.

Hydrogen is lighter than air and lighter than helium. Unfortunately, it is also explosively flammable. Hydrogen fires are less destructive to immediate surroundings because of the buoyancy of H_2, which causes heat of combustion to be released upwards as it ascends in the atmosphere. On May 6, 1937, the hydrogen filled German airship Hindenburg burst into flames while attempting to land at Lakehurst, New Jersey. In little more than thirty seconds, the largest object ever to soar through the air was incinerated.

Public Domain

Hydrogen is a chemical element the symbol H and atomic number one. It is the lightest element and in its single atom form it is by far the most abundant element in the universe, comprising approximately seventy-five percent of its total identified mass. Present in the earth's atmosphere as the diatomic H_2 molecule it is a colorless, odorless, tasteless, non-toxic, highly explosive gas. Most of the hydrogen on Earth is in molecules such as water and organic compounds because hydrogen readily forms covalent bonds. In 1766 Henry Cavendish was the first to identify hydrogen gas. In 1783 Antoine Lavoisier gave the element the name hydrogen (Greek ὕδρω hydro water and γενῆς genes creator) when he and Laplace confirmed Cavendish's finding that water is produced when hydrogen is burned.

Moment of ignition of a fart, video is at youtu.be/Zt9rvaijpPY

Hydrogen and methane are the two flammable gasses that may be found in a fart making them flammable. Lighting a fart to see if one produces these gasses is actually a dangerous activity. Significant burns to the anogenital area have occurred as a result, especially when ignited without a clothing barrier. The popular television show *Mythbusters* filmed an episode confirming that many farts are indeed flammable. It appears that the network found the episode too provocative, and perhaps for liability concerns that children watching might attempt their own demonstrations decided to not 'air' the episode.

Hydrogen, The Big Bang

For those entertained by the lighting of the hydrogen or methane of farts, there is another 'big bang' associated with hydrogen gas. According to the Big Bang theory of the origin of the universe, atoms were created as the super-heated and compressed dense mass of the universe expanded and cooled. It is virtually beyond our ability to comprehend the astronomical numbers of atoms in the universe. All the more remarkable is that after billions of years the cooling and expansion continues yet ninety percent plus of the energy and matter in the universe remains invisible to our scientific instruments and exploration to date.

Big Bang Theory illustrated Time Magazine graphic

Through the process of nuclear fusion within stars two atoms of hydrogen combined into one atom of helium. The process of fusion continued to create the heavier elements through stars and supernova. In spite of the billions of years that have passed since the Big Bang the development of the heavier elements is still in its infancy. Ninety-eight percent of all known matter in the universe is the simplest element hydrogen. Another one percent is the next earliest element helium. All of the other elements that populate our universe and that were created from stardust are less than one percent of the known elements.

The known universe is ninety-nine percent hydrogen and helium, the two lightest elements and nearly always found as gases if not in combination with other elements. Planets are the extreme oddity of being comprised of heaver elements of liquids and solids as well as gasses. Our planet Earth is a remarkable find with heavier elements as well as the primary element hydrogen. Most of Earth's hydrogen has been oxidized in a ratio of two hydrogen atoms to one oxygen atom into H_2O, liquid water, frozen ice, or water vapor depending on its local environment. The primary elements are gasses but as compounds they form other states of matter as liquids or solids. If you think of the human body, we are primarily and predominantly hydrogen and oxygen gasses that have formed a liquid compound water.

When we observe an object with our vision what we are seeing are the photons of light energy being reflected back to us. The object is absorbing all of the wavelengths of light except those that are reflected back. So we are not actually seeing the object, what we are seeing is a reflection of what it did not absorb. Likewise, we know that there are vast areas of empty space between the nuclei of atoms and their electron clouds. The impression of an object being solid, yet consisting of atoms with enormous volumes of empty space, is just one of the many mysteries we experience every day. The Buddhist philosophers who believed that everything we experience is an illusion find that quantum physicists and scientists are validating their beliefs.

Hydrogen Sulfide

Hydrogen sulfide with the formula H_2S is a colorless gas with the characteristic foul odor of rotten eggs. It is heavier than air, poisonous, corrosive, flammable, and explosive and often results from the bacterial fermentation of organic material in anaerobic environments such as in swamps and sewers. H_2S also occurs in volcanic gases, natural gas, and well water.

WARNING
HAZARDOUS
AREA

HYDROGEN SULFIDE

EXTREME HEALTH
HAZARD

FATAL OR HARMFUL
IF INHALED

Public Domain

Hydrogen sulfide (HS) is also produced by some cells and has biologically active signaling functions. Nitric oxide (NO) and carbon monoxide (CO) are the only other gases known to have this property. It acts as a relaxant of smooth muscle and as a vasodilator. It is also active in the brain where it may play a role in memory as well as Alzheimer Disease, where the brains hydrogen sulfide concentration is markedly decreased. Hydrogen sulfide's ability to act as a vasodilator may be protective against cardiovascular disease. The sulfur group in allicin, garlic's bioactive component, is catabolized to hydrogen sulfide and may explain garlics reported cardio protective properties. Like nitric oxide, hydrogen sulfide is involved in the relaxation of the smooth muscle that causes vasodilation and erection of the penis. Nitric oxide and hydrogen sulfide appear to work via different mechanisms suggesting that new therapeutic options for erectile dysfunction and a variety of medical conditions may be possible.

An excess of hydrogen sulfide can also be detrimental. The overproduction of HS is involved in the pathogenesis of type 1 diabetes and leads to the injury and death of the insulin producing beta cells. The injurious effects of hydrogen sulfide have been implicated in mass extinctions that have occurred in the Earth's past. Buildup of hydrogen sulfide in the atmosphere, perhaps from major volcanic eruptions, may have caused the Permian-Triassic extinction event two hundred and fifty-two million years ago.

Hydrogen sulfide (H_2S) is found in high concentrations in the calderas of volcanoes, which is also where significant mining activity for sulfur takes place. In spite of the harsh conditions and dangerous gasses, active mining for sulfur takes place in the crater of Kawah Ijen volcano in Java, Indonesia. Next to a sulfuric acid lake with a measured pH as low as 0.5 a number of vents in the caldera emit volcanic gasses like sulfur dioxide (SO_2) and hydrogen sulfide (H_2S). These gasses are channeled through ceramic pipes where the gasses are condensed into liquid sulfur as the gas cools. Deep red molten sulfur pours out of the pipes, further cools to the yellow mineral, which forms solid yellow cakes of sulfur, and are then carried out of the area in baskets by miners. The miners work without protective equipment and have to hike up and down out of the high altitude volcanoes caldera twice a day. Typical miners earn the equivalent of thirteen U.S. dollars per day.

Sulfur mine. Shutterstock/Zephyr_p

A number of Archaea organisms utilize hydrogen sulfide, and even elemental sulfur as an energy source. The relatively recent discovery of Archaea, and the organisms that are considered extremophiles, has revolutionized our understanding of life itself. These organisms can exist, and thrive in environments previously considered incompatible with life.

Stanley Miller and Harold Urey became famous for their pioneering studies of what the early earth's atmosphere was like and what might have been brewing there millions of years ago. Using discharges of electricity as a substitute for lightning they used a few basic chemicals, water, methane, hydrogen, and ammonia, to simulate the atmospheric conditions on Earth before life began. They demonstrated that some of the early building blocks of life were spontaneously created in this environment. Early experiments showed five to ten different amino acids, the building blocks for plants, animals, and fungi were generated.

Harold Urey (inset) and Stanley Miller devised an experiment that revealed the earliest building blocks of life may have been generated in the early planetary atmosphere of the Earth. Creative Commons License

In 1958 they added hydrogen sulfide to the mix and the long forgotten vials from their primordial-soup-in-a-bottle experiments were rediscovered just a few years ago. Using much more sophisticated analysis than was available over fifty years ago, restudy showed that the volcanic activity seeping hydrogen sulfide helped create the rich environment from which early life evolved. The recent analysis showed that by adding hydrogen sulfide the number of amino acids generated increased up to twenty-three, with additional compounds and amines generated as well. Included in the new amino acids was methionine, which is a required building block for many life forms.

Ideal Gas Law

Many aspects of the human body deal with gasses, in particular the respiratory system and the gastrointestinal systems both deal with large volumes of gas. Unlike solids and liquids, the gasses in nature are dramatically impacted by changes in temperature, pressure, and volume. For example, when the temperature of a gas increases its volume increases or if its volume cannot increase because it is contained than its pressure increases. The individual laws of physics discovered and named after Avogadro, Boyle, Charles, and Gay-Lussac deal with gas at different temperature, volume, and pressure and have been combined into the ideal gas law: $PV = nRT$. The symbols represent the properties of the gas, P is pressure, V is volume, n is the amount of mass measured as moles, R is the ideal gas law constant, and T is temperature.

Ideal Gas Law

```
Boyle's Law    Charles' Law    Avogradro's Law


              Ideal Gas
                Law
```

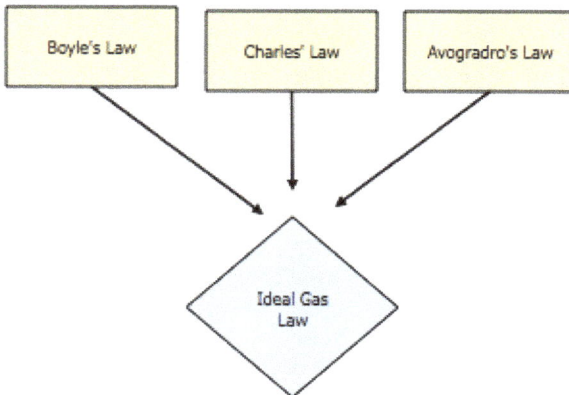

http://chemwiki.ucdavis.edu Creative Commons License

Farts are no exception and obey the ideal gas laws. The volume of a fart is related to its temperature and pressure. As an example, if you happen to have a fever and your body temperature is elevated the pocket of gas in your intestines will expand or the pressure will increase, or you will release a fart with more power, volume, and sound than usual. The laws of physics are the basis for the changing behavior of intestinal gas in scuba diving, mountain climbing, airplanes, and a wide variety of situations you may or may not have thought about. Because there is a real risk of injury or even death with internal gas expanding to the point of inducing barotrauma and rupturing a gas containing internal organ such as the bowel leading to peritonitis or the lungs leading to pneumothorax, this is a very serious concern.

Hot air balloons are an example of hotter temperature leading to volume expansion. Creative Commons License.

Indole

Indole is an organic compound known as an aromatic heterocyclic because it consists of a six-membered benzene ring fused to a five-membered nitrogen-containing pyrrole ring. Indole is often used as a component of fragrances and is used in the production of a number of pharmaceutical products. The amino acid tryptophan is the precursor of the neurotransmitter serotonin and is an example of an indole derivative.

Tryptophan is one of the twenty-two amino acids, and is also considered an essential amino acid. Essential amino acids are those amino acids that cannot be synthesized by humans, and therefore must be obtained through the diet. Because of its importance as an essential amino acid, tryptophan is a common constituent of most protein foods and supplements. A diet rich in tryptophan can contribute to the fecal aroma of intestinal gas. Indole occurs naturally in human feces and contributes to the characteristic fecal odor. Surprisingly, at very low concentrations it has a flowery smell and is a constituent of many perfumes. The name indole is a portmanteau created from the words indigo and oleum. Indole was first isolated by the dye industry in treatment of the deep blue indigo dye with oleum.

Indole is widely distributed in the natural environment and can be produced by a variety of bacteria as a degradation product of the amino acid tryptophan. Tryptophan is an indole derivative and the precursor of the hormone melatonin, the neurotransmitter serotonin, and the plant hormone auxin. Indole serves as an intercellular signal molecule. Indole regulates various aspects of bacterial physiology, including spore formation, plasmid stability, resistance to drugs, biofilm formation, and virulence. It takes several million jasmine blossoms to make one pound of natural jasmine oil, which is two-point-five percent indole. It is priced over one thousand times as much as synthetic jasmine, which takes advantage of the commercial production of indole.

Intestinal Gas, Therapy

When it comes to therapy for intestinal gas the first attempt is to identify foods or products that exacerbate the gas problem and avoid them. One can try an elimination diet, where one food or food group at a time is abstained from. If there is no improvement in the degree or symptoms related to intestinal gas a different food or food group is substituted for an elimination period.

One of the most common foods to which people are sensitive, which results in an excess of gaseousness, is lactose intolerance. Lactose is the complex sugar found in milk and requires the enzyme lactase for its conversion to the two simple sugars, glucose and galactose, to allow its absorption. Most individuals have some degree of lactose intolerance, and can adequately digest small amounts of dairy product without symptoms. The symptoms of lactose intolerance become manifest when the amount of lactose consumed exceeds the individual's ability to produce lactase. The ability of the digestive tract cells to produce lactase diminishes with age especially after infancy and childhood.

The avoidance of dairy products, particularly in excess of the individual's lactase production, results in symptom resolution. The most common symptoms are those of excessive gaseousness including distension and flatulence, and diarrhea. There are many dairy substitute products in the marketplace including those manufactured from rice, soy, various nuts such as almonds and cashews, coconuts, and others. Another approach is the commercial availability of the enzyme lactase itself. It may have already been added to the dairy product and is commonly found in the marketplace, now labeled as lactose free. Lactase supplements, which are taken orally with dairy products, are also available and effective. Some dairy products such as various yogurts and cheeses are already lactose free because the lactose sugars have been digested in the fermentation process generating the end product.

Another common source of excessive gaseous is a diet high in legumes and cruciferous vegetables. A number of vegetables have a high content of complex sugars known as raffinose, verbascose, and stachyose. The enzyme required to metabolize and digest these complex sugars is known as alpha-galactosidase. Humans as well as other animals do not have this enzyme, which is found only in plants. When the undigested complex sugar reaches the gut flora the microbes ferment and metabolize it releasing gases in the process. One approach is to reduce the quantity of these food products in the diet. In the case of beans soaking them for several hours, and in particular allowing them to sprout, starts the process of alpha-galactosidase production within the bean itself. Another approach is taking an alpha-galactosidase supplement such as Beano just prior to the meal. Alpha-galactosidase is destroyed by heating, and thus should not be added to foods prior to cooking or preparation.

Other food sensitivities such as to gluten are controversial. There is a known condition of gluten sensitive enteropathy also known as celiac disease, sprue, and nontropical sprue. In this condition a portion of the gluten known as gliadin damages the villi of the intestinal tract. As the damage continues the villi are blunted and shortened, eventually resulting in malabsorption. The inability to digest and process foods provides material for the gut microbiome to metabolize and release gases as well as causing diarrhea. A much larger portion of the population has reported sensitivity to gluten, and indeed a significant number do have difficulty digesting wheat and the other cereal grains that do contain gluten including rye, barley, and oats.

The sugar fructose most commonly found in fruits is a frequent source of intestinal gas and diarrhea if consumed in excess. All humans have a limited capacity to process the fruit sugar fructose. Nonnutritive sugars such as mannitol sorbitol and other food additives such as polysorbate-80 may cause excessive gaseousness as well. The most common foods related to belching and burping, known as eructation, are those which contain gases in solution such as carbonated beverages, beer, and champagne. Many foods also have very high air content. This includes whipped foods, baked goods including bread, fruit, ice cream, and others.

Some individuals are also prone to aerophagia. Everyone swallows air but those prone to aerophagia gulp down more than the average amount of air. The activities that can result in excess of aerophagia include rapid eating, drinking with a straw or from a bottle, tilting the head and neck back while swallowing, poorly fitting dentures, chewing gum or tobacco products, sucking or chewing on hard candies, as well as smoking. Talking while eating will also result in excessive swallowing of air. Individuals with sinus condition or postnasal drip tend to swallow their secretions frequently, every swallow also including about one teaspoonful of air.

Most of the individuals who have excessive burping and belching also have a hiatal hernia and gastroesophageal reflux disease, commonly known by the acronym GERD. In this condition the most common problem is inappropriate relaxation of the lower esophageal sphincter, when it should be closed tight after each swallow to prevent regurgitation. The gastric contents are usually very acidic from the addition of hydrochloric acid produced by the gastric glands. When this acidic material is refluxed into the esophagus irritation and damage of the esophageal lining may occur. If it occurs on a chronic basis the development of a change in the mucosal lining, known as a Barrett esophagus, may arise with an increased risk of the development of esophageal cancer.

The usual treatment for gastroesophageal reflux disease includes conservative measures such as reducing excess body weight, avoidance of foods and social habits that relax the lower esophageal sphincter. This includes fried foods, fatty foods, alcohol, tobacco, chocolate, and peppermint. Other measures may include elevating the head of the bed and avoiding any recumbent position until at least one hour after mealtime. Over-the-counter antacids and gastric acid suppressants are frequently used. If symptoms persist stronger prescription medication may be required to suppress the stomach's hydrochloric acid production. Fortunately, conservative treatment or acid suppressants are very effective. In some individuals the symptoms of heartburn are not present or minimal, and other more atypical symptoms result including cough, laryngitis, sleep apnea, asthma, sinusitis, earache, ear infections, chest pain, dental caries, and others.

The gas symptomatology of bloating and distension is most frequently seen in irritable bowel syndrome. It is considered a functional gastrointestinal disorder most probably related to altered motility and heightened sensitivity to intraluminal pressure. Recent evidence suggests that alterations in the gut microbiome may be playing a very important role in this condition. Some individuals benefit from introduction of the FODMAP dietary modification. Other conditions may also cause such symptoms including inflammatory bowel disease, bacterial infections, parasites, and others. One condition in particular that causes great concern in women is the possibility of ovarian cancer. This is typically a silent disease and bloating may be one of its first manifestations because of fluid buildup within the abdomen known as ascites. Early diagnosis is critically important in the management of this aggressive cancer.

Chronic pancreatitis and pancreatic insufficiency can result in enzyme deficiencies leading to malabsorption of fats, proteins, and carbohydrates. Fat malabsorption often leads to a form of diarrhea known as steatorrhea. In this condition the gas as well as the oily floating stool have a particularly characteristic offensive odor. Fortunately, pancreatic enzyme replacement supplements are commercially available and effective.

The approach to the intestinal gas problem of flatulence is addressed in the same manner as those above, as any unresolved burping, belching, and distension will nearly always eventually result in the gas passing down below. Because flatulence is of great social concern various treatment approaches have been attempted. One of the most important issues is to exclude significant underlying disease such as inflammatory bowel disease, bacterial overgrowth, parasites, and others.

Dietary modification or the usage of enzyme supplements can be very helpful. If this approach does not provide symptomatic improvement there are several over-the-counter safe products designed to be internal deodorants. The use of bismuth subgallate as well as chlorophyll products have been particularly successful. The use of prebiotics, probiotics, and changes in the gut microbiome may be attempted. The use of antibiotics is usually limited to proven small intestinal bacterial overgrowth. Individuals who have undergone bariatric surgery, particularly with a gastric bypass, are especially prone to gas issues.

The use of activated charcoal has a long history of adsorbing toxins and gases. It has been used in chair cushions and other external modalities with some degree of effectiveness. Oral ingestion of activated charcoal has been less successful, presumably because the absorptive capacity of activated charcoal is markedly diminished by the time it reaches the colon. The addition of activated charcoal pads, as well as impregnating fabric with activated charcoal, have the potential to provide a significant benefit. To be effective all of the gas released has to pass through the activated charcoal. Form fitting underwear made with activated charcoal impregnated fabric has been very successful, albeit more expensive. The successful use of activated charcoal pads is dependent on the consumer placement of the pad in a manner that does not allow gas to escape. New product development including the use of other adsorbent material and metal ions hold promise for the availability of additional approaches.

Many individuals have issues with unpleasant fecal odors, and unfortunately it is not as easily remedied as flushing or walking away. The fecal aroma generated by the gut microbiome that gives the characteristic smell of defecated feces is the identical aroma that may be discharged with intestinal gas, fecal incontinence, fistula, ostomies, diarrhea, inflammatory bowel disease, after gastric bypass surgery, and a host of other conditions. The numbers of individuals affected is in the millions in the United States alone. Unfortunately, the majority of the general public remains uninformed and impose a social stigma on a medical condition over which the sufferers have limited or no control.

Fortunately, there are a number of effective therapeutic options available, but too many sufferers are not aware of or have access to them. They range from external appliances and clothing, to external and internal deodorants and suppressants. Of course there are also tongue-in-cheek suggestions, such as getting a dog to blame as the source of the fart odor. The Merck Manual a few years back suggested working on perfecting one's glare, just glare at someone else as if they were the source.

More direct references to farts have been employed in the advertising campaign of air-freshener company Poo-Pourri. Although the advertising campaign received a nomination as one of the worst ads by a national newspaper, it was a major hit on social media with over thirty million views. For a holiday themed marketing advertisement Santa Claus is farting on the toilet while an attractive model sings a parody of a seasonal tune.

Surprisingly where it can provide relief and comfort to many sufferers, some media outlets refuse to place advertisements for products dealing with flatulence and ostomy odors. Deodorants, feminine hygiene douches, tampons, sanitary napkins for menstruation, diapers for adults with incontinence, erectile dysfunction prescriptions, etcetera have been seen by the public and the social order has not collapsed. Devrom, an effective internal deodorant that suppresses fecal odor was not allowed to place their advertisement in *Reader's Digest* or *AARP Magazine* (Association for the Advancement of Retired People) because it contained the word stool and dealt with flatulence. Somehow the publications did not see the irony in that their policy did not pass the proverbial smell test for basic fairness.

Devrom is an over the counter preparation of bismuth subgallate and has been marketed for over fifty years as an internal deodorant. Bismuth does have antibacterial properties and it may change the microbiome by reducing the organisms that contribute to offensive flatulence. Another bismuth product that has been popular in the marketplace is Pepto-Bismol, which is a bismuth subsalicylate. Bismuth subsalicylate is related to aspirin (salicylic acid) and does not appear to provide as significant relief from the unpleasant odors as has been reported with Devrom.

Bismuth is a chemical element, number eighty-three on the periodic table, which has a long history of being used in preparations designed to treat gastrointestinal complaints. It is a heavy metal with a low level of toxicity. Its various compounds have also been used historically to treat syphilis and the severe diarrhea from cholera. Bismuthinite is a mineral consisting of bismuth sulfide (Bi_2S_3) and is an important ore for bismuth. Bismuth has been particularly popular for individuals who have undergone gastric bypass surgery, inflammatory bowel disease, as well as those with ostomies, and others. With advances in surgery, and the ability to preserve sphincters or create artificial sphincters, ostomies are seen less frequently. This is where the intestinal discharge exits the body through an artificial opening, the ostomy, created at surgery. Because the bowel is diverted from the colon less moisture is absorbed, and the feces may be semi-formed or liquid. The more liquid form allows for the more rapid vaporization of volatile organic compounds and gasses that give rise to the feculent odor. In spite of being in otherwise excellent health, many individuals with these issues find themselves socially restricted in their activities because of concern about embarrassment or offending others. Safe and effective products are available, but many individuals are unaware and suffer unnecessarily because of the lack of information and understanding.

The mechanism of action is unknown and may be related to its known antimicrobial activity, perhaps inhibiting the microbes that generate some of the more offensive gasses that are usually contain sulfur as well as aromatic and volatile organic compounds. Bismuth also reacts directly with sulfur generating bismuth sulfide, a dark black insoluble compound. This can cause darkening or blackening of the tongue if sulfur is found in high concentrations in the saliva. It will also cause blackening of the stool as it binds with the sulfur that would otherwise give rise to hydrogen sulfide and other offensive sulfur gasses. The dark black color of the stool may be mistaken for melena, a sign of internal bleeding that results from the digestive process on blood cells and hemoglobin. The black coloration is not a health concern and is temporary, clearing with cessation of bismuth intake.

Activated carbon is used to treat oral poisonings by binding to and preventing the poison from being absorbed by the gastrointestinal tract. Charcoal biscuits were marketed in the early nineteenth century as an antidote to flatulence, and are still marketed today for diarrhea, indigestion, flatulence, and as a pet care product. Orally ingested charcoal pills are of limited effectiveness in reducing intestinal gas. This may be because the adsorptive capacity of the activated charcoal is usually fully utilized before it finally gets to the intestines where its gas adsorbing properties are needed. Fortunately, bismuth products do provide a significant advantage by binding to the sulfur compounds and eliminating them without producing offensive gas.

As with all issues of health and wellness each person needs to be assessed individually. With the advances in the human genome project it is now recognized that it is not just the genetic blueprint in the DNA that makes up the individuals uniqueness. Although humans have approximately twenty-three thousand genes these genes are also controlled by external factors in a process described as epigenetics. It is also now recognized that the human body is in essence more than just human cells. The human system includes the microbiome, the microorganisms that live on and within us. The gut-brain-microbiome-food axis demonstrates the intimate interconnectivity of these four elements. If one were to analyze the human system by the number of cells a human is comprised of we are approximately ten percent human cells and ninety percent microbial cells. If one were to analyze the system on the basis of the number of genes, humans are approximately one percent human genes and ninety-nine percent microbial jeans.

The era of personalized medicine will advance the understanding of both health and disease. The previous approach of using population based medicine will be abandoned as technology and bioinformatics allows treatments to be specifically tailored to the individual's genome, microbiome, and metabolome. The effectiveness of therapy should increase dramatically along with a significant reduction in adverse reactions to medications. This approach will also avoid the time and monetary expense of medications that did not provide a benefit, even if fortunately, they did not cause an adverse reaction. In the interval as these advances are being brought into clinical practice it remains the best approach to tailor the treatment plan to the individual. What works for one may not work for another. Until the science and technology sufficiently evolve it often takes a trial and error approach to find the best treatment approach for the individual. And it is the individual who can be the only judge if the treatment is successful or the search for a solution must continue.

Irritable Bowel Syndrome

Irritable bowel syndrome (IBS) also known as spastic colon is a functional disorder with the diagnosis based on symptoms of abdominal discomfort, bloating, and alteration of bowel habits. It may be predominated by diarrhea or constipation or alternation between the two. It is more common in women and symptoms can vary with the menstrual cycle. In the US there is an incidence of about fifteen percent of the entire population. A diagnosis of irritable bowel syndrome is made on the basis of symptoms if celiac disease, lactose intolerance, parasites, and bacterial overgrowth have been excluded and there are no signs of weight loss, gastrointestinal blood loss, infections or family history of inflammatory bowel disease.

Irritable bowel syndrome occurs more commonly after an intestinal infection, or a stressful life event. A history of sexual abuse is found in thirty percent of women with irritable bowel syndrome. A serum test for anti-vinculin antibodies, which are elevated after intestinal infections is being investigated as a possible tool to identify irritable bowel syndrome. The cause of irritable bowel syndrome is unknown and there may be several different cause and conditions all pooled together under this diagnosis until further advances are made. The most popular theory is that IBS is a disorder of the complex neuroendocrine pathway between the brain and the gastrointestinal tract. Alternative approaches to the mind-body interactions have been proposed for irritable bowel syndrome and yoga, exercise, tai chi, meditation, and other modalities may offer benefits.

Altered sensation

Altered motility

Disorders of rectal evacuation

blogs.nejm.org/now/wp Creative Commons License

Treatments have included dietary adjustments, medication and psychological interventions. FODMAP is an acronym that stands for Fermentable Oligosaccharides, Disaccharides, Monosaccharides, And Polyols. Restricting these short chain carbohydrates and related sugar alcohols, which are poorly absorbed in the small intestine. May be of benefit in irritable bowel syndrome. Many of these sugar alcohols including sorbitol, mannitol, xylitol, isomalt, and maltitol are added to commercial food products as non-nutritive bulk sweeteners. See entry on FODMAP diet for more details.

Newer prescription agents involving the neuroendocrine pathways, particularly serotonin agonist and antagonist are being studied. Other approaches using non-absorbable antibiotics such as rifaximin have provided relief for some patients, as have the use of probiotic agents to modulate the gut flora. Some believe the condition is triggered by changes in the gut flora and associated changes to the immune system. Fortunately, irritable bowel syndrome is not associated with a higher risk of cancer or other conditions that would reduce life expectancy. It has a significant impact on quality of life and the economy. In the United States irritable bowel syndrome has been estimated to cost ten billion dollars a year in direct medical costs and an additional twenty billion dollars a year in indirect costs.

CLASSIFYING IBS

The three categories

IBS with diarrhoea predominance (IBS-D) 27%

Alternating IBS and don't know (IBS-A) 39%

IBS with constipation predominance (IBS-C) 34%

* The classification of an IBS case may influence its subsequent management

media2.onsugar.com Creative Commons License

Lactase (see Lactose, Lactose Intolerance)

Lactase is an enzymes involved in the hydrolysis of the milk sugar disaccharide lactose into galactose and glucose. Lactase is located on the tips of microvilli along the lining of the small intestine. Levels of lactase decrease with weaning in a significant proportion of the human population. Other populations benefit from a mutation that is thought to have occurred over ten thousand years ago with the rise of the domestication of herd animals that allowed the continued ingestion of dairy products into adulthood. If the intake of lactose exceeds the availability of lactase to digest it, the gut flora ferments the disaccharide. This gives rise to the symptoms of lactose intolerance, gas, cramps, and possibly diarrhea.

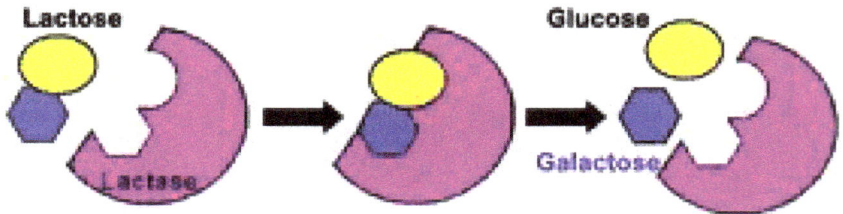

Lactose   Lactase   Glucose   Galactose

www.pharmaceutiucal-materials.com Creative Commons License

Lactose free foods are available where the lactase enzyme has already been added to the product to break down the lactose. The enzyme itself is also commercially available and should be taken with dairy products that contain lactose. Some dairy products, such as most hard cheeses, are lactose free on the basis of the production process. Acidophilus and Lactobacillus in yogurt and other foods also provides some lactase activity. Most people with lactose intolerance still have a nominal amount of the lactase enzyme and can digest lactose in very small quantities such as milk used as a creamer for coffee. Other dairy substitutes such as almond, cashew, rice, and soy 'milk' are lactose free.

Lactobacillus (see Probiotic)

Lactobacillus rhamnosus, a probiotic bacterium www.theguardian.com Creative Commons License

Lactobacillus is a Gram-positive anaerobic rod-shaped bacterium that converts the milk sugar disaccharide lactose and other sugars to lactic acid. The production of lactic acid makes its environment acidic which inhibits the growth of some harmful bacteria. In humans they are present in the vagina and the gastrointestinal tract where they make up a small portion of the gut flora. The genus Lactobacillus currently consists of over one hundred and eighty species and encompasses a wide variety of organisms. Bifidobacterium was previously called *Lactobacillus bifidus* and has a separate entry in this volume under bifidobacterium. *Lactobacillus gasseri* is a probiotic organism found in kefir, sauerkraut, kimchi, lassi, natto, miso, and tempeh that generates hydrogen peroxide and has been associated with enhanced metabolism and weight loss.

Lactose (see Lactase, Lactose Intolerance)

Lactose is the milk sugar disaccharide consisting of galactose and glucose that is found in milk, with the name derived from the Latin word lactis (milk). Milk production is a characteristic of mammals, whose name is derived from the mammary gland, commonly known as the breast. The milk secretions of the mammary gland provide key nutrition to newborn mammals, and the age of weaning off of milk varies amongst species. Humans have various cultural differences in age of weaning and it is not unusual for some mothers to delay weaning even though the child can eat a normal diet. While breast feeding can delay the return of fertility and acts as a natural birth control, it is not a reliable means of avoiding another pregnancy. The La Leche league is an organization that supports breast feeding as the proper nutrition for babies preferable to infant formula. Besides being the natural food for babies, it confers important passive immunity to the child in that it contains antibodies and immunity inducing components.

One of the important aspects is that the skin microbiome of the mother's breast becomes the source of the initial inoculation of the baby's gut microbiome. This has important lifelong benefits to the child and breast feeding should be strongly encouraged. The age of weaning is variable and is often dictated by cultural influence. As a species, humans are the only mammal that continues to ingest milk into adulthood, and the domestication of other mammals for milk production has led to the development of herding and dairy farming. Other mammals used for milk production are referred to as milch animals. These include cows, goats, camels, water buffalo, reindeer, yaks, and others. Each mammal species produces its own unique milk with varying concentrations of the key nutritional components such as fat, protein, water, lactose. Many people forget that the largest mammal is the whale, and the milk of the whale is unique in having the highest fat content as well as the lowest lactose content. Even though whale milk may be the optimal natural milk for those with lactose intolerance, the presence of a large potential market could not overcome the technical barriers of establishing a whale dairy farm.

The Compositions of Various Milks

The figures in the following table are the percent of the milk's weight accounted for by its major components.

Milk	Fat	Protein	Lactose	Minerals	Water
Human	4.0	1.1	6.8	0.2	88
Cow	3.7	3.4	4.8	0.7	87
Holstein/Friesian	3.6	3.4	4.9	0.7	87
Brown Swiss	4.0	3.6	4.7	0.7	87
Jersey	5.2	3.9	4.9	0.7	85
Zebu	4.7	3.3	4.9	0.7	86
Buffalo	6.9	3.8	5.1	0.8	83
Yak	6.5	5.8	4.6	0.8	82
Goat	4.0	3.4	4.5	0.8	88
Sheep	7.5	6.0	4.8	1.0	80
Camel	2.9	3.9	5.4	0.8	87
Reindeer	17	11	2.8	1.5	68
Horse	1.2	2.0	6.3	0.3	90
Fin whale	42	12	1.3	1.4	43

Lactose was discovered in milk in 1619 AD by Fabriccio Bartoletti. Its components and characteristics vary between mammalian species (the term derives from the distinctive characteristic of mammary glands). Lactose comprises between two to eight percent of milk by weight. It is commercially extracted from whey, several million tons of which are produced annually as a by-product of the dairy industry. Whey is the liquid remaining after milk is curdled and strained, often for the production of cheese. As a natural sugar found in milk and milk products it is found in cheese, ice cream, and processed foods, such as bread, cereal, and salad dressing. Hard cheeses typically have markedly reduced lactose content. Acidophilus milk and products that contain live Lactobacillus cultures such as in yogurts have reduced lactose content. Lactose free dairy products are also commercially available, as is the enzyme supplement lactase, which can be taken with the ingestion of lactose to help with its digestion and processing. Mammals nurse their infants on milk, which is rich in lactose. The villi of the small intestine secrete the enzyme lactase (β-D-galactosidase), which hydrolyses the lactose molecule into the simple sugars glucose, and galactose, which are easily absorbed. In most mammals the production of lactase decreases with the decreased consumption of milk associated with weaning and reaching maturity.

Humans have continued to supplement their diet with milk from other mammals, especially those cultures and populations who developed herding practices of livestock, such as cattle, sheep, goats, camels, etc. The descendants of these populations appear to have induced the genetic tendency to maintain lactase production into adulthood. Other people have lost the ability to maintain significant lactase production and when the ingestion of lactose exceeds their enzymes capacity, the symptoms of lactose intolerance become apparent. When lactose is not digested by lactase the gut flora ferments it with the production of gasses inducing bloating and flatulence. It will occasionally induce diarrhea from the osmotic properties of the sugar molecules drawing water into the digestive tract.

Any illness that damages the villi will result in a decrease of the enzymatic activity and can aggravate underlying food intolerance. A viral or bacterial gastroenteritis, commonly referred to as a 'stomach flu or bug', will damage the villi and reduce the enzymes that would normally aid in digestion. The cell lining and villi of the small intestine tend to recover rapidly and thus for the few days following an infection dairy products are best avoided until the enzyme levels have recovered. A major use of lactose is in the pharmaceutical industry where it is commonly used as inexpensive filler for pills because of its compressibility. It is also commonly used as inexpensive filler in a wide variety of food products. It is not unusual for individuals with known lactose intolerance to be unaware that they are ingesting sizable amounts of lactose in foods or pharmaceuticals. Reading the ingredient labels is important but the consumer has to be aware that lactose may be present if whey, whey protein, nonfat dry milk, milk sugar, powdered dairy product, etc. are included on the ingredient list. Unfortunately, lactose filler in pharmaceutical and nutraceutical products as well as nutritional and dietary supplements are rarely identified.

Lactose Intolerance (see Lactase, Lactose)

Lactose intolerance, also known as hypolactasia or lactase deficiency is the condition that arises when there is an insufficient quantity of the enzyme lactase, which is needed to metabolize the milk sugar disaccharide lactose commonly found in milk and dairy products. Hippocrates (460-370 BCE) was one of the first to recognize that many individuals had a difficult time digesting cow's milk. Lactase is an enzyme involved in the hydrolysis of the disaccharide lactose into galactose and glucose. Lactose intolerance is not an allergy and is not due to an immune response, it is due to the lack of a key digestive enzyme.

Lactase is located on the tips of microvilli along the lining of the small intestine. Levels of lactase decrease with weaning in a significant proportion of the human population. Other populations benefit from a mutation that is thought to have occurred over ten thousand years ago with the rise of the domestication of herd animals that allowed the continued ingestion of dairy products into adulthood. If the intake of lactose exceeds the availability of lactase to digest it the gut flora ferments the disaccharide. This gives rise to the symptoms of lactose intolerance, gas, cramps, and possibly diarrhea. Lactose is a disaccharide of galactose and glucose that is found in milk, the word being derived from the Latin word lactis (milk). Lactose was discovered in milk in 1619 AD by Fabriccio Bartoletti. Percentages of nutritional components vary between mammalian species (the term derives from the distinctive characteristic of mammary glands). Lactose comprises between two to eight percent of milk by weight. It is commercially extracted from whey, several million tons of which are produced annually as a by-product of the dairy industry. Whey is the liquid remaining after milk is curdled and strained, often for the production of cheese.

www.avonmorelactosefree.ie Creative Commons License

Mammals nurse their infants on milk, which is rich in lactose. The villi of the small intestine secrete the enzyme lactase (β-D-galactosidase), which hydrolyses the lactose molecule into the simple sugars glucose, and galactose, which are easily absorbed. In most mammals the production of lactase decreases with the decreased consumption of milk upon reaching maturity, a condition known as primary lactase deficiency. Secondary lactase deficiency arises when the intestinal villi are damaged, such as by gastroenteritis, celiac disease, parasites, etcetera. Congenital lactase deficiency is a very rare autosomal dominant inherited condition most often seen in the Finnish population. Certain populations, which developed dairy herds and persisted in milk consumption favored those who had a genetic variation now known as the lactase persistence allele. DNA evaluation of ancient skeletons revealed that this beneficial mutation developed in Europe and Russia over four thousand years ago. Seventy-five percent of African-American, Jewish, Native American, and Mexican American populations are lactose intolerant.

As a natural sugar found in milk and milk products it is found in cheese, ice cream, and processed foods, such as bread, cereal, and salad dressing. Hard cheeses typically have markedly reduced lactose content. Acidophilus milk and products that contain live Lactobacillus cultures such as in yogurts have reduced lactose content. Lactose free dairy products are also commercially available, as is the enzyme supplement lactase, which can be taken with the ingestion of lactose to help with its digestion, and processing. Humans have continued to supplement their diet with milk from other mammals, especially those who developed herding practices of livestock, such as cattle, sheep, goats, camels, etc. The descendants of these populations appear to have induced the genetic tendency to maintain lactase production into adulthood. Other people have lost the ability to maintain significant lactase production and when the ingestion of lactose exceeds their enzymes capacity, the symptoms of lactose intolerance become apparent. When lactose is not digested by lactase the gut flora ferments it with the production of bloating, flatulence and occasional diarrhea from the osmotic properties of the sugar molecules drawing water into the digestive tract.

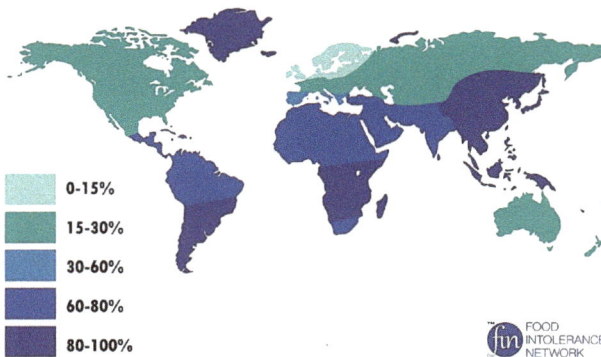

Worldwide prevalence of lactose intolerance in recent populations (schematic)

0-15%
15-30%
30-60%
60-80%
80-100%

upload.wikimedia.org/wikipedia/commons Author: NmiPortal Creative Commons License

Any illness that damages the villi will result in a decrease of enzymatic activity and can aggravate underlying food intolerance. A viral or bacterial gastroenteritis, commonly referred to as a 'stomach flu or bug', will damage the villi and reduce the enzymes that would normally aid in digestion. The cell lining and villi of the small intestine tend to recover rapidly and thus for the few days following an infection dairy products are best avoided until the enzyme levels have recovered. A major use of lactose is in the pharmaceutical industry where it is commonly used as inexpensive filler for pills because of its compressibility. It is also commonly used as inexpensive filler in a wide variety of food products. It is not unusual for individuals with known lactose intolerance to be unaware that they are ingesting sizable amounts of lactose in foods or pharmaceuticals. Reading the ingredient labels is important but the consumer has to be aware that lactose may be present if whey, whey protein, nonfat dry milk, milk sugar, powdered dairy product, etc. are included on the ingredient list. Unfortunately, lactose filler in pharmaceutical and nutraceutical products as well as nutritional and dietary supplements are rarely identified.

Lactose free foods are available where the lactase enzyme has already been added to the product to break down the lactose. The enzyme itself is also commercially available and should be taken with dairy products that contain lactose. Some dairy products, such as most hard cheeses, are lactose free on the basis of the production process. Acidophilus and Lactobacillus in yogurt and other foods also provides some lactase activity. Most people with lactose intolerance still have a nominal amount of the lactase enzyme and can digest lactose in very small quantities such as milk used as a creamer for coffee. Other dairy substitutes such as almond, cashew, rice, and soy 'milk' are lactose free. The diagnosis is based on clinical suspicion with improvement of symptoms by lactose avoidance or addition of lactase enzyme supplements, or laboratory tests such as lactose tolerance blood test, or breath hydrogen analysis breath test.

Large Intestine (Large Bowel, Colon)

The large bowel, also known as the large intestine or colon, is unlike the small intestine in that it is less involved in the digestion of foods and nutrients. It is primarily involved in the absorption of water and sodium. The colon also serves to absorb nutrients, vitamins, and metabolites produced by the gut microbiome, including Vitamin K, Vitamin B_{12}, thiamine, and riboflavin. The colon removes the excess moisture from the watery chyme, and the stool solidifies as it transits the gut. It is stored in the rectum and sigmoid colon awaiting the right opportunity to be eliminated through defecation. A process or illness that impairs the colon's absorption of water will lead to more fluid in the stool and diarrhea. If the elimination is delayed moisture continues to be absorbed by the colonic epithelium and the stools can become harder resulting in constipation.

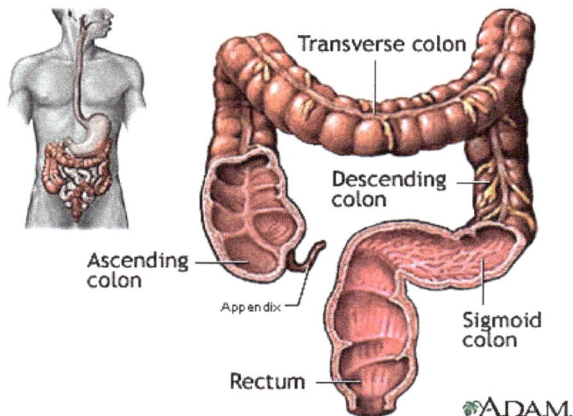

www.healthcentral.com Creative Commons License

Le Pétomane (Joseph Pujol)

Joseph Pujol (1857–1945) was a stage performer from 1887 to 1914, and first performed on the Moulin Rouge stage in Paris in 1892. He had the unusual ability to inhale air into his colon through his anus and expel it at will. With the stage name Le Pétomane, French for the fart maniac, he was also affectionately known as 'the fartiste'.

Joseph Pujol (Le Pétomane) 1857, Public Domain

With sufficient colonic inhalations and exhalations, he was able to minimize the odor and control the sounds emanating from his anus to such a degree that he could play musical tunes. To assure that there was no odor he also underwent regular colonic irrigations before performances. Appearing on stage in red cape, white cravat, and black trousers, with a pair of white gloves held in the hands, he displayed the incongruous touch of elegance that added to his charm. A program of fart impressions followed, including contrasting the hearty fart of the miller with the timid fart of the young girl.

He proceeded to demonstrate the diffidence of the fart of the bride on her wedding night (almost inaudible) compared to the fart of the bride a week later (a lusty raspberry). His musical impersonations included an imitation of a tuba player on his instrument. He stunned the audience with a majestic ten-second fart, which he likened to a couturier cutting six feet of calico cloth. He would play *Le Marseilles* on his personal human wind instrument, his colon, even though he could only produce four notes do, mi, so, and the octave do. To add to his musical repertoire, he would insert a tube offstage into his rectum and attach it to the musical instrument the ocarina. Then playing *O' Sole Mio* he would invite the audience to sing along.

Replacing the musical instrument at the end of the tube with a cigarette he used his colon to inhale. After withdrawal of the tube he would exhale the cigarette smoke out of his behind. For the grand finale he would imitate a twenty-one-gun salute, and the Great 1906 San Francisco earthquake with a thunderous roar that went on for over five continuous minutes. He would end his performance by blowing out a candle at a distance of three feet. Other than Harry Houdini, he was the highest paid stage performer in Europe and was earning a salary of twenty thousand francs per week. This was substantially more than the eight thousand francs per week salary of his contemporary Sarah Bernhardt who was considered the leading lady of the stage at that time. King Leopold II of Belgium and Edwards Prince of Wales came incognito to see Le Pétomane perform. Sigmund Freud attended a performance, and perhaps inspired, went on to describe his theory of anal fixation.

At one point he was embroiled in a disagreement with his stage manager and was going to perform in a different venue. The manager went to the courts and got a judicial injunction preventing Le Pétomane from performing elsewhere. During the court hearing Le Pétomane demonstrated his unique abilities in front of the court (the judge did not rule him out of order, or in contempt of court). Le Pétomane decided to offer his farting services and performance for free in a public display, but the manager and the court decision forbade him to fart in public.

When he died, the physicians of the day wanted to do a postmortem examination to find out how he had such remarkable anal control. The family held onto his body until enough decomposition set in that they no longer had to fear grave robbers retrieving the body for science. Joseph Pujol's memorable life lives on in the cinematic and stage arts. In Mel Brooks' 1974 movie *Blazing Saddles*, with many memorable fart scenes, there is an inside joke. It is an artistic acknowledgement to Joseph Pujol with Mel Brooks himself playing Governor William LePétomane.

Lipase

Lipase is an enzyme primarily secreted from the salivary glands and pancreas that catalyzes the hydrolysis of lipids (fats). Salivary lipase is particularly important for infants as their pancreatic lipase production is still maturing. Lipases, a category of esterases, are critical in the digestion and transport of dietary lipids such as triglycerides, fats, and oils. Lipase from the pancreas enters the duodenum to supplement the lipase from saliva where the digestion of lipids begins in humans, and gastric lipase. Lysosomal lipase is confined within its organelle to prevent auto digestion. The yeast *Candida albicans* produces a variety of lipases contributing to its effectiveness as a pathogen. Enzymes are commercially available over the counter as well as by prescription. They come in a variety of doses and potency and are usually very well tolerated.

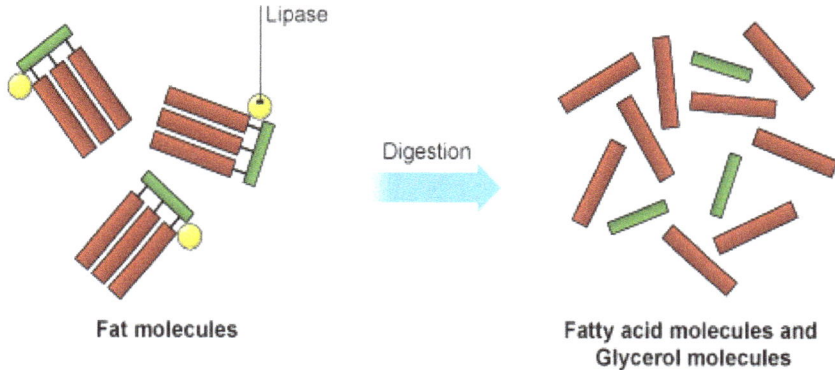

Lipase

Digestion

Fat molecules

Fatty acid molecules and Glycerol molecules

Dietary fat must be hydrolyzed in order to be absorbed by the digestive tract. Several lipases participate in the breakdown of dietary lipids. Lipases are water-soluble enzymes that hydrolyze ester bonds of water, insoluble substrates such as triglycerides, phospholipids, and cholesterol esters. Fat hydrolysis is initiated in the stomach, where triacylglycerols (TAGs) are partially digested to glycerols and free fatty acids (FFAs). Lingual lipase is secreted from the salivary glands. Most of the lipase activity that occurs in the stomach involves gastric lipase, which is responsible for ten to thirty percent of dietary fat hydrolysis.

Pancreatic lipase is synthesized by pancreatic acinar cells and is secreted into the small intestine where the enzyme completes hydrolysis of triglycerides into monoglycerides, diglycerides, free fatty acids, and glycerol. Due to the opposite polarity between the enzyme (water-soluble) and the substrate (lipophilic), bile salts act as biological detergents and emulsify dietary fats to form mixed micelles. This key step allows an easier access to the pancreatic lipase for lipid hydrolysis.

Enzymatic activity of the pancreatic lipase is inhibited by the presence of bile salts. To counteract this negative effect, the enzyme requires the presence of a cofactor, the colipase, which promotes formation of lipase-bile lipoprotein complex. The micelles formed by a mix of bile salts, fatty acids, and other breakdown products are absorbed by enterocytes at the intestinal mucosa. Fatty acids are then transported and delivered to muscles and adipose tissues as fuel or for storage. Gastrointestinal lipase inhibitors reduce nutrient digestion and systemic absorption of fat, which decrease energy intake resulting in weight loss.

Lipid

Lipids are a group of naturally occurring molecules that include fats, waxes, sterols, fat-soluble vitamins, monoglycerides, diglycerides, triglycerides, and phospholipids. The main biological functions of lipids include energy storage and as a structural component of cell membranes. Although the term lipid is sometimes used as a synonym for fats, fats are a subgroup of lipids called triglycerides. Lipids also include molecules such as fatty acids and their derivatives including triglycerides, diglycerides, monoglycerides, and phospholipids, as well as other sterol-containing metabolites such as cholesterol. Humans and other mammals use various biosynthetic pathways to both break down and synthesize most lipids. Some essential lipids such as linoleic acid (an omega-6 fatty acid) and alpha-linoleic acid (an omega-3 fatty acid) must be obtained from the diet.

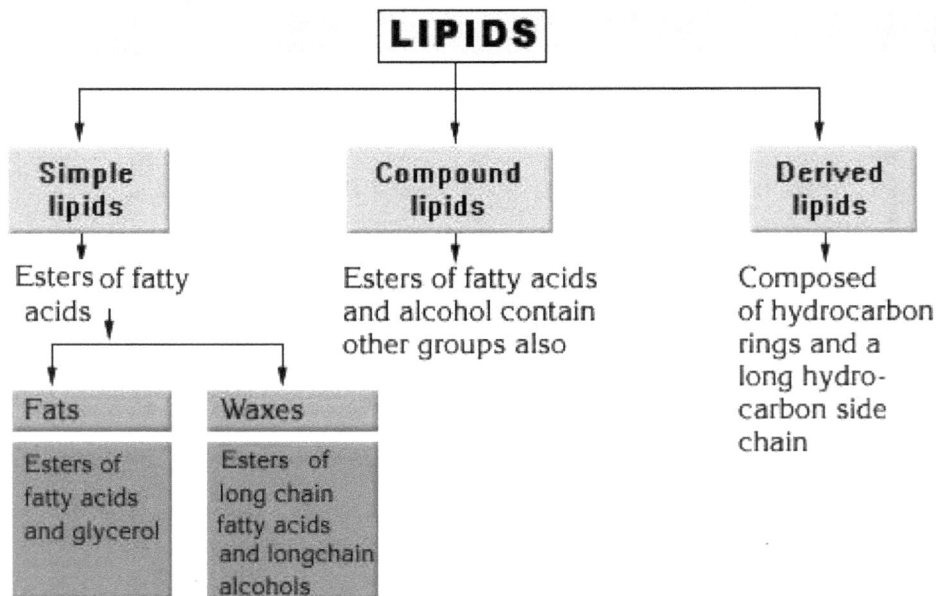

LIPIDS

Simple lipids	Compound lipids	Derived lipids
Esters of fatty acids ↓	Esters of fatty acids and alcohol contain other groups also	Composed of hydrocarbon rings and a long hydro-carbon side chain

Fats	Waxes
Esters of fatty acids and glycerol	Esters of long chain fatty acids and longchain alcohols

To lose one pound of fat you would need to burn off three thousand five hundred calories. If you think that is not too hard to do, think again. You would need to run at the high speed of just under seven miles per hour for four hours and seventeen minutes, a total distance of over twenty-five miles, to use up three thousand five hundred calories. Prefer to walk them off at a brisk three miles per hour, then prepare to walk for thirteen hours over thirty-nine miles. Prefer to bicycle at fifteen miles per hour then you have a four hour twenty-minute trip to cover sixty-five miles. If it makes you feel any better just having the extra pound of fat on your body uses up calories in its maintenance, a whopping one calorie every eight hours. By the way an equivalent weight of muscle uses three times as many calories in maintenance,

Meals that are high in fat cause the release of hormones and slows down gut motility. As the food spends more time in the digestive tract continued bacterial fermentation produces increasing quantities of gas. In addition, foods that are extremely hot or cold tend to be swallowed in smaller quantities resulting in more swallows being necessary to eat or drink the same volume at a moderate temperature. As each swallow contributes an additional quantity of air entering the esophagus and digestive tract, more swallows results in more air ingestion. Foods or snacks that require excess chewing with resultant excess swallowing of saliva, such as chewing or bubble gum, also contribute to excess air ingestion.

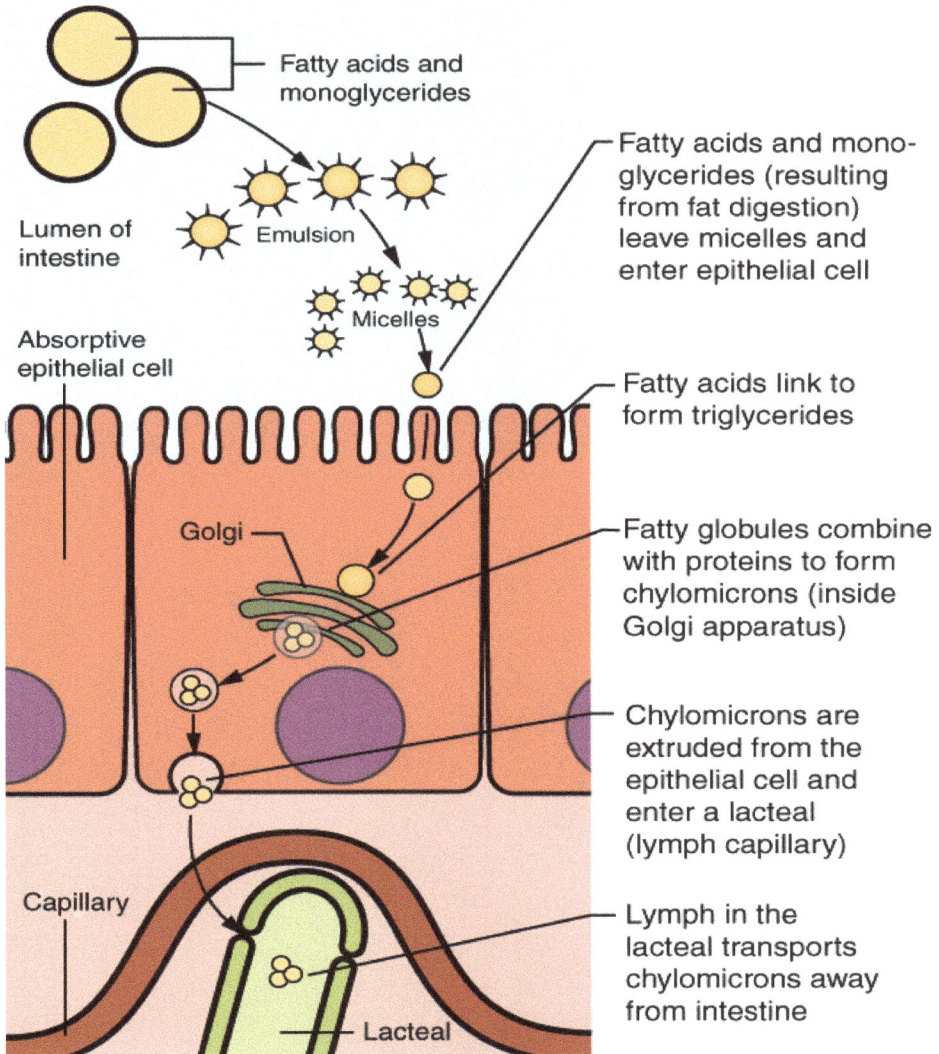

Lipid absorption of fatty acids and monoglycerides.

Fatty acids and monoglycerides enter intestinal cells via diffusion. They are combined with proteins within the cells resulting in chylomicrons, which are extruded and enter the lacteals. They are transported via the lymphatic system and lymphatic duct and subsequently enter the circulatory system. Glycerol and short chain fatty acids are absorbed into the capillary blood in villi and then transported via the hepatic portal vein.

Lower Esophageal Sphincter (see Gastroesophageal Reflux Disease)

The lower esophageal sphincter (LES) is also referred to as the cardiac sphincter and gastroesophageal sphincter. It is a ring shaped area of high muscle tone at the distal esophagus, typically just below the diaphragm that acts as a one-way valve to prevent gastroesophageal reflux, except when vomiting is necessary. The lower esophageal sphincter is under involuntary control and is usually in a closed position. It relaxes during a swallow to allow the passage of the food bolus. In cases of gastroesophageal reflux disease, it may also relax inappropriately allowing acidic gastric contents back into the esophagus causing heartburn and mucosal damage.

Lower esophageal sphincter pressure and relaxation are regulated by excitatory (e.g., acetylcholine, substance P) and inhibitory (e.g., nitric oxide, vasoactive intestinal peptide) neurotransmitters. Disorders of the lower esophageal sphincter can lead to the common disorder of gastroesophageal reflux disease (GERD), and its frequent symptom of heartburn or other atypical symptoms. It also plays a major role in other conditions such as achalasia, nutcracker esophagus, and diffuse esophageal spasm.

Esophagus

Lower esophageal sphincter

Stomach

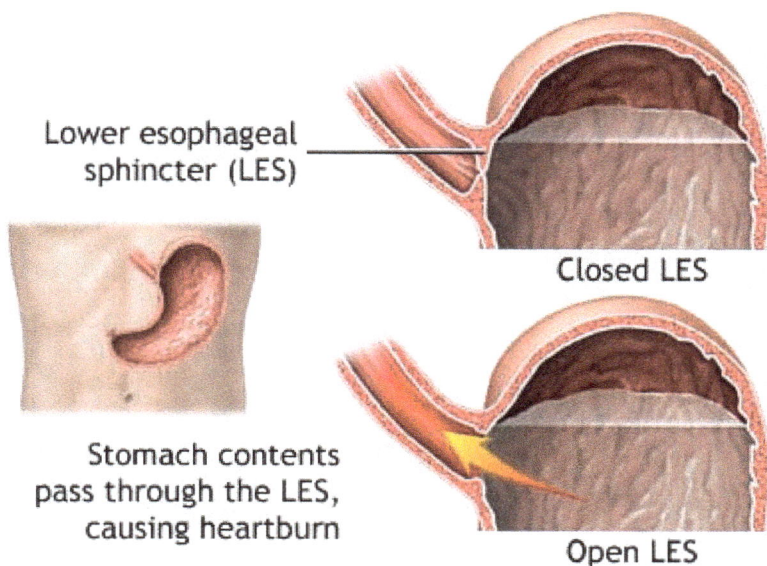

Lower esophageal sphincter (LES)

Closed LES

Stomach contents pass through the LES, causing heartburn

Open LES

Once air has been swallowed (aerophagia), or if gasses are produced in the stomach, they can only be released as an eructation (burp, belch) if the air or gas pressure can overcome the pressure generated by the upper and lower esophageal sphincters. The highest pressure is typically generated by the lower esophageal sphincter, however weakness or inappropriate relaxation of this sphincter is not uncommon. Dysfunction of the lower esophageal sphincter is very common in the conditions of hiatal hernia, and gastroesophageal reflux disease (GERD). The upper and lower esophageal sphincters are areas of high muscle tone that relax to allow the swallowing process and passage of the food bolus to take place. The upper esophageal sphincter is not as critical to esophageal health, as dysfunction of the lower esophageal sphincter alone can lead to dysphagia and gastroesophageal reflux disease.

Gastroesophageal reflux disease (GERD) is mucosal damage of the esophagus caused by the reflux of gastric acid, bile, and digestive enzymes. In Western populations GERD affects approximately ten to twenty percent of the population. The most common symptom is heartburn, formally known as pyrosis, from the Greek word πῦρ (pyro, fire). In the United States twenty percent of people have symptoms in a given week, and seven percent every day. GERD is usually caused by abnormal relaxation of the lower esophageal sphincter or hiatal hernia with contributing factors such as obesity, Zollinger-Ellison hypergastrinemia, hypercalcemia, scleroderma, and esophageal dysmotility. Carminatives, drugs, hormones, alcohol, tobacco, fried or fatty foods, and chocolate, all of which can reduce the lower esophageal sphincter pressure, can aggravate it.

Treatment is typically via lifestyle changes and medications such as proton pump inhibitors, H_2 receptor blockers, or antacids. Some antacids can be absorbed leading to an alkalosis syndrome. Antacids also generate large volumes of carbon dioxide as they neutralize the gastric hydrochloric acid. Magnesium containing antacids can cause diarrhea, aluminum containing antacids can cause constipation, and often a combination of the two is used to minimize the impact on bowel movements. Calcium based antacids can lead to a rebound of acid secretion as calcium is a potent stimulant of gastric acid production.

Surgical treatment with tightening of the lower esophageal sphincter has a similar response rate as medication therapy. If inadequately treated, GERD may progress to Barrett esophagus with intestinal metaplasia where the epithelial cells transition from the normal esophageal squamous epithelium to intestinal columnar epithelium. With the development of atypia and dysplasia this can progress to the development of adenocarcinoma of the esophagus. If Barrett esophagus has developed, screening endoscopy with biopsies to evaluate for dysplasia is suggested.

The diagnosis of GERD is usually by history with typical symptoms of heartburn and reflux. Atypical manifestations of GERD include laryngitis, unexplained chest pain, chronic cough, sinusitis, pulmonary fibrosis, earache, recurrent ear infections, asthma, and obstructive sleep apnea. Another unusual symptom is called water brash, which is a rush of salivary secretions after an episode of regurgitation to dilute and clear the acid in the esophagus. A possible cardiac cause of atypical chest should be excluded before ascribing the source to GERD. Approximately forty percent of GERD patients have a *Helicobacter pylori* infection. The eradication of *Helicobacter pylori* can lead to a worsening of the GERD symptoms since the resolving gastritis leads to an increase in gastric acid secretion.

The current gold standard for diagnosis of GERD is esophageal pH monitoring. Endoscopy is advised if any alarm symptoms are present including dysphagia, anemia, blood in the stool, wheezing, weight loss, respiratory or laryngeal symptoms. Long standing or severe symptoms would also prompt endoscopic evaluation for Barrett esophagus and dysplasia. The treatments for GERD include lifestyle modifications, medications, and possibly surgery. Initial treatment is typically with a proton-pump inhibitor or histamine two blocker that usually provides prompt and significant relief. Weight loss, avoiding large heavy meals, not lying down, bending over, or doing headstands immediately after meals, decreasing or discontinuing tobacco, alcohol, and carminative usage can be helpful. Elevation of the head of the bed, not with pillows but with wood blocks under the legs at the head of bed as long as it is not a waterbed, can be useful.

Antacids and mucosal protectants such as alginic acid or sucralfate can also be helpful, but have a more frequent dosing schedule. Prokinetic agents to enhance esophageal motility and tighten the lower esophageal sphincter (LES) can also be used. The oldest generic prokinetic metoclopramide has a high incidence of central nervous system side effects and is now rarely used. Newer prokinetics have a safer profile. The standard surgical treatment for severe GERD is the

Nissen fundoplication, where the upper part of the stomach is wrapped around the lower esophageal sphincter. This corrects the hiatal hernia by keeping the stomach and LES below the diaphragm preventing reflux. Medical therapy and surgical therapies appear to be equally effective for this often chronic condition.

Malabsorption & Maldigestion

Malabsorption is an impairment of the ability of the gastrointestinal tract to absorb one or more required nutrients. The main purpose of the gastrointestinal tract is to digest and absorb nutrients (fat, carbohydrate, protein, and fiber), micronutrients (vitamins and trace minerals), water, and electrolytes. Digestion involves both the mechanical and physiological breakdown of dietary intake. Mechanical processes include chewing, gastric churning, mixing, and transit through the small and large intestine.

Enzymatic, acidic, and microbial activity digest the dietary intake into smaller components that are amenable to absorption from the gut lumen into the enterocyte, lymphatics, blood, or intracellular spaces for transportation and metabolic utilization. Maldigestion may occur if there is a disorder of mastication (chewing), gut motility, or a quantitative or qualitative deficiency of salivary, gastric, pancreatic, small bowel, or biliary secretions. Malabsorption is the result of either maldigestion not preparing the nutrients for absorption, or a failure of the ability to transport nutrients from the gut lumen into the body proper. The differential diagnostic possibilities are exhaustive and range from mucosal damage and infiltration to enzyme deficiencies and food intolerances. Malabsorption syndromes may often be identified by symptoms of deficiencies ascribed to specific nutrients that are not being absorbed. Specific blood, stool, imaging studies, or mucosal biopsies may be diagnostic.

emedtravel.files.wordpress.com Creative Commons License

Malabsorption and maldigestion may be due to infective agents such as human immunodeficiency virus (HIV), traveler's diarrhea, a wide variety of parasites, tropical sprue, Whipple disease, intestinal tuberculosis, bacterial overgrowth with intestinal blind loop syndrome, or inflammatory bowel disease such as Crohn disease and ulcerative colitis. Infiltrative diseases such as lymphoma, amyloidosis, and eosinophilic gastroenteritis can lead to the condition, as can scleroderma and collagen vascular diseases. Surgical changes due to intestinal surgery, vagotomy, gastrectomy, and bariatric weight loss procedures such as gastric or intestinal bypass may also be causative.

Mucosal abnormality or injury from celiac disease with gluten sensitivity, cow's milk intolerance, soy milk intolerance, and fructose malabsorption are other potential causes. Enzyme deficiencies may play an important role such as lactase deficiency, sucrose intolerance, intestinal disaccharidase deficiency, and intestinal enteropeptidase deficiency. Pancreatic insufficiencies may contribute including cystic fibrosis, chronic pancreatitis, cancer of the pancreas, and Zollinger- Ellison syndrome.

Bile acid malabsorption may be due to disease of the terminal ileum such as from Crohn disease, tuberculosis, bacterial overgrowth, or primary bile acid diarrhea. The list continues with many other possibilities including systemic diseases such as hypothyroidism, hyperthyroidism, abetalipoproteinemia, carcinoid syndrome, Addison disease (adrenal insufficiency), hypoparathyroidism, diabetes mellitus, hyperparathyroidism, and gluten sensitive enteropathy also known as celiac disease, celiac sprue, and non-tropical sprue.

Meteorism (Flatulence, Intestinal Gas, Fart)

Meteorism is an old British euphemism for flatulence, and may be used when trying to be politically correct. Perhaps there is irony in the term allowing astronomy to be modified to the pun 'ass'tronomy.

*Air*Veda: Ancient & New Medical Wisdom

Methane (Natural Gas)

Methane is produced in the human intestinal tract by microbial organisms. Methanogens are microorganisms of the Kingdom Archaea, not bacteria as previously thought. They produce methane as a metabolic byproduct in anaerobic conditions when oxygen is not present. Methanogens have been found in a variety of extreme environments and thrive and reproduce in boiling water as well as in ice cores taken miles down in arctic glaciers. They are common in wetlands, where they produce marsh gas, and in the digestive tracts of animals and humans where they generate the methane content of flatulence as well as the ruminant belch. Higher methane concentrations in intestinal gas have been associated with decreased gastrointestinal tract motility and constipation.

Hydrogen and methane are combustible gasses in the presence of oxygen, and with an ignition source you have a potent flammable commodity. When methane burns it has a characteristic blue flame that you may see in a pilot light if you have a gas stove or furnace. Adolescent males and those who remain as adolescents intellectually have a fondness for demonstrating their dragon like ability to be human flamethrowers by igniting their farts. This is not a recommended activity and severe injury has resulted from successful attempts to ignite farts. Extremely rare but fatal colonic gas explosions have been reported at colonoscopy when electrical cautery to remove a polyp cause a spark that ignited the flammable gasses. Changes in bowel preparation to reduce methane and hydrogen production, as well as usage of carbon dioxide as the insufflating gas for colon distension has made the risk of explosion negligible.

Lighting a match to a pile of cow dung is not a sign of higher intelligence. The methane and hydrogen generated by the microbes active in the dung pile may accumulate to explosive levels.
youtu.be/bZI1eeV88lQ

Hydrogen and methane are the two flammable gasses that may be found in a fart making them flammable. Lighting a fart to see if one produces these gasses is actually a dangerous activity. Significant burns to the anogenital area have occurred as a result, especially when ignited without a clothing barrier. The popular television show *Mythbusters* filmed an episode confirming that many farts are indeed flammable. It appears that the network found the episode too provocative, and perhaps for liability concerns that children watching might attempt their own demonstrations decided to not 'air' the episode. On occasion dung and excrement can be more than just flammable, it can be explosive. The microorganism that produce hydrogen and methane that lead to ignitable farts continue their activity while sitting in a pile. For those foolish enough to light a match in a pile of cow dung to see what happens up close and personal the link to the video above should be convincing.

One of the more unusual injuries from a lit fart was second and third degree burns on the buttocks and a broken arm. The heavy gentlemen was sitting on the toilet defecating and farting extensively for a period of time. Being overweight his buttocks formed a firm seal around the toilet seat retaining all of the gasses in the enclosed space of the toilet bowl. He was smoking at the time and made a little space under his cheeks to innocently toss the lit cigarette into the toilet bowl. It promptly ignited blowing him off the seat, shattering the toilet bowl and causing extensive burn injuries to his buttocks. His wife called the paramedics and as he was being carried down the stairwell to the waiting ambulance he told them what caused the explosion. They laughed so hard they dropped the gurney, thus breaking his arm and adding to the injuries sustained from an exploding fart

Methane, Greenhouse Gases & Global Warming

'The primary greenhouse gases in the Earth's atmosphere are water vapor, carbon dioxide, methane, nitrous oxide, and ozone. Venus is a prime example of the planetary temperature consequences of the greenhouse effect. Nitrogen (N_2), oxygen (O_2), and argon (Ar), major components of the Earth atmosphere are not greenhouse gases because they are minimally affected by infrared radiation. Clouds, composed of water droplets or ice crystals, do contribute to the greenhouse effect since they absorb and emit infrared radiation.

Water vapor accounts for about fifty percent of the Earth's greenhouse effect, with clouds contributing twenty-five percent, carbon dioxide twenty percent, and the minor greenhouse gases and aerosols accounting for the remaining five percent. Methane has a twenty-fold greater impact on the greenhouse effect then carbon dioxide, when measured by weight. As a percentage however, methane has a much smaller effect since it is found in relatively small amounts. The most important constituents of the greenhouse gasses are water vapor, clouds, carbon dioxide, methane, and ozone. Less important contributors include sulfur hexafluoride, hydrofluorocarbons, and perfluorocarbons.

The atmospheric lifetime measures the time required to restore equilibrium in its component gas concentrations in the atmosphere. Water vapor has an atmospheric lifetime of approximately nine days, in striking contrast to carbon dioxide of thirty years, and N_2O one hundred and fourteen years. The Earth's surface temperature is partly dependent on the balance between the absorption of radiant energy from the sun, and its reflection and re-radiation of energy back to space. An earlier period of widespread glaciation (Snowball Earth) came to abrupt end about five hundred and fifty million years ago when a colossal volcanic outgassing raised the atmospheric CO_2 concentration to twelve percent, about three hundred and fifty times present day levels. The extreme greenhouse conditions resulted in the deposition of calcium carbonate as limestone at the rate of over a foot each year. This brought a close to the Precambrian eon, and was succeeded by the warner Phanerozoic times with the appearance of multicellular animal and plant life. There has not been a recurrence of such a dramatic greenhouse effect since. New volcanic carbon dioxide emissions today are less than one percent of human production.

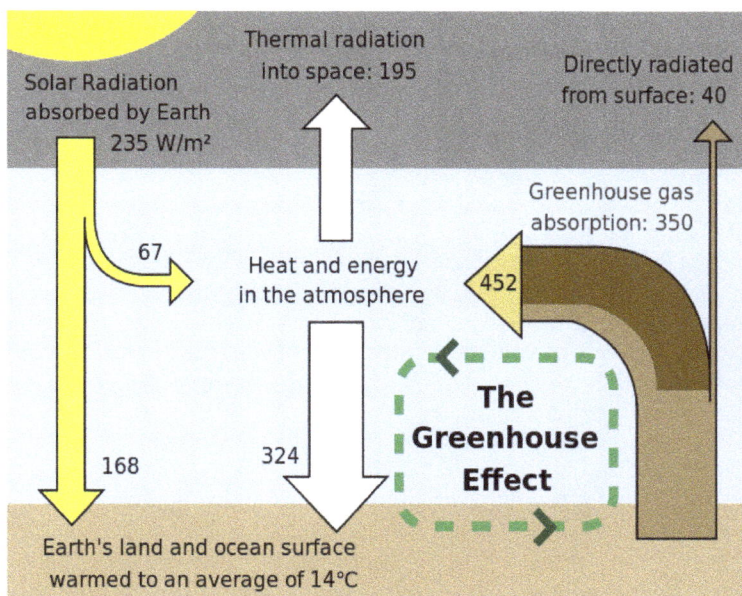

Thermal radiation into space: 195

Solar Radiation absorbed by Earth 235 W/m²

Directly radiated from surface: 40

Greenhouse gas absorption: 350

67

Heat and energy in the atmosphere

452

The Greenhouse Effect

168

324

Earth's land and ocean surface warmed to an average of 14°C

The figure shows the flows of energy between space, the atmosphere, and the Earth's surface, and how these flows trap heat near the surface and create the greenhouse effect. Energy exchanges are expressed in watts per square meter (W/m²). The sun is responsible for virtually all energy that reaches the Earth's surface. Of the surface heat captured by the atmosphere, more than seventy-five percent can be attributed to the action of greenhouse gases that absorb thermal radiation emitted by the Earth's surface. The atmosphere in turn transfers the energy it receives both into space (thirty-eight percent) and back to the Earth's surface (sixty-two percent). The process by which energy is recycled in the atmosphere to warm the Earth's surface is known as the greenhouse effect. Creative Commons License

Based on measurements from Antarctic ice cores, the concentrations of carbon dioxide in the atmosphere are now thirty percent higher than levels before the industrial revolution. The levels had not changed appreciably in over ten thousand years. Although human activity only accounts for five percent of the greenhouse gasses, the naturally occurring amount was closely balanced by the Earths capacity to utilize the carbon sink of photosynthesis. Greenhouse gas production from human activity is mainly due to deforestation, the combustion of fossil fuels, livestock enteric fermentation and manure management, and landfill emissions. In terms of biomass bacteria would be the main contributors to global warming by their methane production. Other contenders nominated have been termites, which have over two thousand species and are prolific methane producers (initial reports suggested that they produce forty percent of global methane), livestock such as cows, sheep, and pigs, and lastly dinosaurs, which are no longer around to defend their reputations.

A ruminant (Latin *ruminare* - to chew over again) is a mammal that digests plants in a multi compartment stomach through bacterial fermentation. It regurgitates the semi-digested mass, called cud, and chews it again and repeats the swallow. The process of re-chewing the cud is called "ruminating". There are about one hundred and fifty species of ruminants, which include both domestic and wild species. Ruminating mammals include cattle, goats, sheep, giraffes, yaks, deer, camels, llamas, and antelope. Ruminant fermentation is a significant contributor to global methane production, which is over twenty times as potent a greenhouse gas as carbon dioxide. Actually it is not the ruminant itself, but the protist within its microbiome that generates hydrogen from the breakdown of cellulose. Within the protist is another organism Archaea, acting as a mutualist that converts the hydrogen to methane. To incentivize efforts to reduce livestock methane production a number of countries have proposed taxes on the release of greenhouse gasses. In spite of it being labeled as a flatulence tax, the predominant source of global warming from ruminants comes from fermentation in their multi compartment stomachs. It should really be called a burping and belching tax, but that is not as newsworthy.

Carbon dioxide, methane, nitrous oxide (N_2O) and three groups of fluorinated gases, hydrofluorocarbons (HFCs), perfluorocarbons (PFCs), and sulfur hexafluoride (SF_6), are the major greenhouse gases impacted by human activity. These are regulated under the Kyoto Protocol, an international treaty that was adopted in 2005. Nitrogen dioxide (NO_2) warms the atmosphere three hundred and ten times more than carbon dioxide and methane twenty-one times more than carbon dioxide. Although CFCs are greenhouse gases, regulations were initiated because CFCs' cause ozone depletion, not because of their contribution to global warming. Ozone depletion itself has a relatively minor effect on greenhouse warming.

Methane, Natural Gas

Natural gas is a naturally occurring mixture of hydrocarbon gases that consists primarily of methane. Smaller quantities of the higher alkanes such as ethane, propane, butanes, and pentanes are also often present. Other components that are commonly removed before marketing as a fuel can include hydrogen sulfide, carbon dioxide, water vapor, nitrogen, oxygen, and helium. Natural gas is often used as an energy source for heating, cooking, and electricity generation. It is also used as fuel for vehicles and as a chemical feedstock in the manufacture of plastics and other commercially important organic chemicals. It contributes to less global warming as it produces thirty per cent less carbon dioxide than using petroleum and forty-five percent less than using coal as a fuel source.

Methane/Shutterstock/OlegDoroshin

Natural gas is found in deep underground natural rock formations or associated with other hydrocarbon reservoirs in coal beds and as methane clathrates. Petroleum is also another resource found in proximity to and with natural gas. Most natural gas was created over time by two mechanisms: biogenic and thermogenic. Biogenic gas is created by methanogen organisms in marshes, bogs, landfills, and shallow sediments. Deeper in the earth, at greater temperature and pressure, thermogenic gas is created from buried organic material.

Shale gas in the United States is rapidly increasing as a source of natural gas. Led by new applications of hydraulic fracturing technology and horizontal drilling, development of new sources of shale gas has offset declines in production from conventional gas reservoirs, and has led to major increases in reserves of US natural gas. Large quantities of methane exist in the form of hydrates on offshore continental shelves and in the permafrost of the arctic regions. Hydrates are formed in the presence of a combination of high pressure and low temperature. Technology has yet to be developed to make the extraction economically viable.

Methane, Biogas

Biogas is produced by the anaerobic breakdown of organic biomass. The breakdown may require several different organisms acting in concert. For example, the ruminant animal cannot digest cellulose without assistance from protist that reside in its gut microbiome. The protist generate hydrogen in the process of cellulose breakdown, which would be detrimental to the protist without the assistance of Archaea. The methanogenic Archaea actually reside within the protist and convert the hydrogen to methane. The sources of methane actually live in symbiotic relationships with other life, including termites, ruminants, and cultivated crops. When methane is produced with the decay of biomass it is referred to as biogas. Sources of biogas include swamps, marshes, landfills, manure, sewage sludge, and enteric fermentation.

Carbon dioxide released to the atmosphere

Methane burned for cooking or heating

Manure

Anaerobic decomposition releases methane

Biogas Generator

Carbon dioxide absorbed by plants through photosynthesis

Creative Commons License

Landfill gas has methane concentrations of approximately fifty percent. Waste treatment technologies can produce biogas of up to seventy-five percent methane. Biogas can be cleaned and upgraded to natural gas standards and is referred to as biomethane. One cow produces the manure in one day to generate three-kilowatt hours of electricity, enough to power a one-hundred-watt light bulb for twenty-four hours. If you imagine every cow having a one-hundred-watt light bulb illuminated from its digestive tract end product, you would have a new definition of a taillight.

Methane, Dinosaurs

In 1933, the Sinclair Oil Corporation had an exhibit at the World's Fair in Chicago, suggesting that the world's oil reserves were created from material from the dinosaurs of the Mesozoic Era. Sinclair Oil featured advertisements in one hundred and four newspapers and five national magazines displaying a dozen different dinosaurs, from the menacing *Tyrannosaurus rex* and three-horned triceratops to the peace loving passive yet massive forty ton vegetarian Apatosaurus (brontosaurus) with a tail thirty feet long. Sinclair used 'Dino', a big green Apatosaurus (Brontosaurus), as its official mascot and corporate symbol, trademarking the dinosaur in 1932.

P. G. Allen, developer of life-like papier-mâché animals for the motion picture industry, was working on an exhibit for the 1933 Century of Progress Exposition in Chicago, the equivalent of a World Fair. Sinclair Oil sponsored the dinosaur exhibition and to enhance the academic stature of its promotions financed the dinosaur-fossil search expeditions of Dr. Barnum Brown, curator at the American Museum of Natural History. After Doctor Brown's death in January 1963, Sinclair retained Dr. John H. Ostrom of Yale University's Peabody Museum of Natural History as consultant on the Sinclair sponsored Paleontology exhibit at New York World's Fair in 1964.

American Oil & Gas Historical Society

Sinclair's marketing was a masterstroke, but led to the common public misperception that petroleum is predominantly derived from the organic remains of the great dinosaurs. Rather than the enormous dinosaurs, it was microscopic bacteria that produced the petroleum reserves of our present time period. Single-celled bacteria evolved in the Earth's oceans about three billion years ago, and were the dominant life form on the planet until about six hundred million years ago. In fact, if dominant is qualified as largest by biomass, bacteria retain that distinction today.

As microscopic as the individual bacteria may be, the bacterial colonies known as "mats" were of enormous proportions. They had masses of millions of tons compared to the hundred tons for the largest dinosaur, the sauropods. As these massive colonies died off and decayed they subsided to the bottom of the sea and were covered by layers of accumulating sediments. Over millions of years these layers of sediment thousands of feet underground were compressed under tremendous pressure and temperature, and developed into the liquid hydrocarbons we recognize as petroleum.

The vast majority of the world's coal deposits date back to the Carboniferous period, about three hundred million years ago. The first dinosaurs would not make their grand entrance in the evolutionary timetable until seventy-five million years later. During the Carboniferous period the earth was heavily forested. With the death and decomposition of these trees and plant life buried under great pressure and temperature under heavy layers of sediment, they were transformed into solid coal rather than liquid petroleum. As the search for petroleum and coal reserves often entails drilling and excavation of deep layers of sediment, it is not uncommon for fossils of dinosaurs and other prehistoric forms of life to be uncovered. The discovery of a theropod dinosaur during fossil fuel exploration in China has been given the appropriate name Gasosaurus. It looks as though Dino's story may have come full circle.

Microbiology (see Microbiome, Pathogen)

The microbes of the gastrointestinal flora are major contributors to intestinal gas. Although unseen, an invisible world had been theorized for centuries. The ancient Greeks thought about it and wrote comprehensively about a world of atoms, molecules, and microscopic life forms far beyond the reach of the technology of their day. The glass lens makers from the thirteenth through sixteenth centuries probably developed ever improving prototypes of the microscope after first developing the telescope. It was only in late 1674 that Antoine Van Leeuwenhoek, a glass lens maker, used an improved optical microscope of his own design to identify red blood cells, spermatozoa, and microorganisms. His advance began the field of microbiology, bringing a previously invisible world into view. The field continues to bring new discoveries and understanding of life on earth and the interdependence of various life forms.

Microorganisms have been found to survive and thrive in extreme locations from many miles underground in rocks, under the ice of Antarctica, in volcanic vents under seas, and the vacuum of outer space. The world of microorganisms has expanded from knowledge of bacteria, to discovery of other microorganisms such as the virus, prion, and Archaea. The future will probably yield further discoveries as continuing research and advancing technology allow.

*Air*Veda: Ancient & New Medical Wisdom

From the time of Van Leeuwenhoek to the present, dramatic advances have taken place in the understanding of the role of microorganisms in human health and disease, as well as life in general. Louis Pasteur was a pioneering influence and identified the role of microorganisms in the fermentation process leading to enhanced production of wine, cheese, and vinegar. He developed an immunization program to protect cattle from anthrax, as well as to treat people exposed to the previously uniformly fatal rabies. He was able to disprove the prevailing theory of spontaneous generation of life, and developed the process of disabling most pathogenic organisms by boiling in a process that was named after him, pasteurization.

It took many more years for the concept of pathogenic organisms to bring hygiene to a new level of awareness. Even in medical circles there was great reluctance to embrace hand washing and the use of disinfectants. Joseph Lister was preceded by Hungarian physician and scientist Ignatz Semmelweis who fought an ignorant medical establishment that used to operate on trusting patients with their bare hands. Semmelweis was able to prove that infections were transmitted from the autopsy room to the operating room because hands were not washed. In spite of this proof he was ignored and ridiculed, which led to his mental collapse and death in a psychiatric hospital because he could not save thousands of innocent people who were condemned to death because of arrogance and ignorance.

Similar stories can be found in many areas of science and medicine where lifesaving advances were delayed for decades or centuries. The story of anesthesia is a prime example where excruciatingly painful and gruesome surgeries were performed on awake subjects who were forcibly restrained, while nitrous oxide was being used as laughing gas purely for entertainment purposes, with medical science not realizing that it could also serve as an anesthetic. The discoverer of nitrous oxide, Sir Humphrey Davies, an esteemed scientist suggested that it be studied as an anesthetic but the physicians and surgeons of his day simply ignored him. The rediscovery of it and other products as anesthetics is a remarkable story that has been the subject of several books on medical history.

Another interesting aspect of the story of microbiology is how it took hundreds of years for scientists and physicians to recognize that pathogenic organisms were responsible for many diseases. It has also taken a similar period of time for the recognition that most organisms are not pathogenic but are commensals and actually improve and preserve health. One of the pioneers in this investigation was a scientist working at the Pasteur Institute in Paris, Dr. Élie Metchnikoff (1845-1916), who received the Nobel Prize in Medicine for his work on immunity.

He investigated the extreme longevity of centenarians in Bulgaria and believed their long lives were due to the yogurt and sour milk consumed as a regular part of their diet. He identified the *Lactobacillus delbrueckii subspecies bulgaricus* organism in yogurt that is considered an ideal probiotic. His theory of aging being due to toxic bacteria, and that lactic acid producing organisms could prolong life, were very influential. His advocacy of probiotics was embraced by the Japanese scientist Minoru Shirota who developed a stronger strain of the probiotic organism *Lactobacillus casei* found in Yakult and kefir. Dr. John Harvey Kellogg, the medical director of the Battle Creek Sanitarium, also embraced Dr. Metchnikoff's theory. Dr. Kellogg administered series of colonics to cleanse the bowels, then had his patients eat half a bowl of yogurt, with the other half administered as an enema. Dr. Kellogg also advocated a high fiber high roughage diet and developed a corn flake cereal, founding the very successful Kellogg Cereal Company with his brother.

Élie Metchnikoff, Nobel Prize winning scientist at the Pasteur Institute in Paris

Unfortunately, science and medicine are replete with many instances where personality flaws, greed, arrogance, jealousy, stupidity, ignorance, and a hundred and one other human failings led to missed opportunities to prevent or cure disease, and improve human health. Even more unfortunately these failings show no sign of abating, with conflicts of interest, desire for personal financial gain, overreaching for recognition, and the securing of patents, too often leading to fraud and deception. Of course dedicated and compassionate professionals are the majority, but progress is hindered nonetheless leading to the illness and death of innocents.

Microbiome

The microbiome includes microbes, their genomes, and their environmental interactions. Gut flora consists of the microorganisms that live in the digestive tract and are the largest component of the human flora. The gut flora contains approximately one hundred trillion microorganisms in its intestines, a number much greater than the ten trillion cells of the human body. The gut flora has approximately one hundred times as many genes as the human genome.

The human genome has twenty-three thousand genes and the human microbiome genome exceeds over one million genes and still counting. Any one or a multitude of combinations of these genes, human and/or microbial, can play a very important role in health and disease. Alterations in an individual's flora may occur with changes in lifestyle, diet, illness, and age. The National Institutes of Health has embarked on the Human Microbiome Project to identify the organisms present in the human microbiome and their role in health and disease. The microbiome includes bacteria, viruses, Archaea, protist, parasites, fungi, prions, and perhaps other life forms that have yet to be discovered.

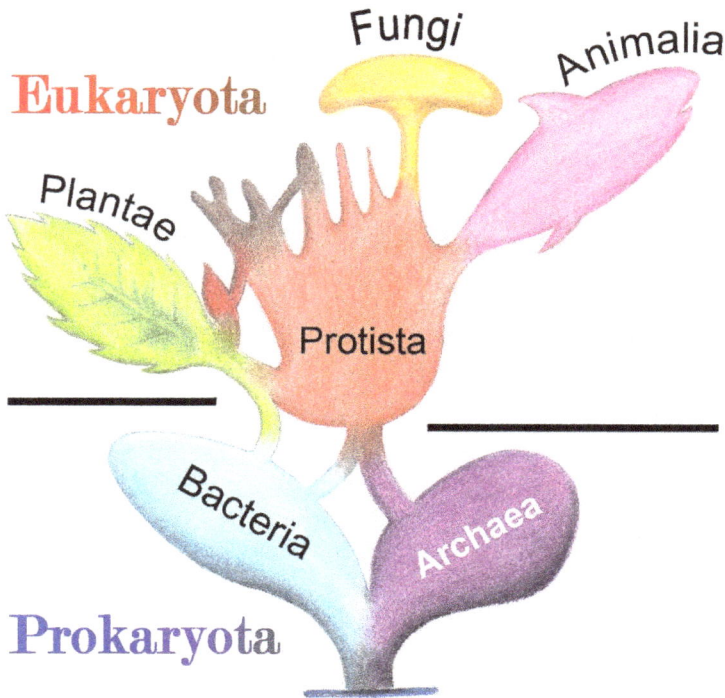

Maulucioni y Dorid Creative Commons License

Anaerobic bacteria make up most of the flora in the colon and up to sixty percent of the dry mass of feces. These bacteria perform a variety of metabolic activities that benefit the host, so much so that some scientists refer to it as the "forgotten" organ. Their metabolic activity includes extracting energy from undigested carbohydrates by fermentation and absorption of short chain fatty acids. They also synthesize vitamin B and vitamin K, as well as metabolizing bile acids and lipids. The gut flora also prevents pathogens from colonizing the intestines through competitive exclusion, also known as the "barrier effect". The bacteria stimulate the immune system lymphoid tissue to produce antibodies to pathogens, and to recognize and not develop an immune response to beneficial flora.

The human microbiome is normally established only after birth. Fetuses do accumulate a mass of sterile and odorless greenish feces like material called meconium, in their intestines. Fetuses usually pass meconium after birth but approximately twelve percent of pregnancies have yellow or green bile pigmented meconium stained amniotic fluid. The risk of meconium in the amniotic fluid increases with the length of the pregnancy. In births occurring after forty-two weeks, described as post term, the rate of meconium staining approaches fifty percent. Fetuses have amniotic fluid in their lungs until they take their first breath of air after birth. In a minority of meconium stained amniotic fluid cases potentially fatal meconium aspiration syndrome occurs. If the newborn fails to pass meconium, a congenital abnormality of the colon needs to be excluded. Hirschsprung disease may involve failure of fetal development of the ganglions of the enteric nervous system. When it involves the colon, the bowel may not relax to allow the passage of meconium or feces, and surgery may be required to remove the affected segment of bowel.

Since the digestive tract of the newborn is sterile, there are no microorganisms generating gas through cellular metabolism. All of the gas the newborn infant begins to pass is swallowed air. If an infant is bottle fed rather than breast fed, they are much more likely to swallow even more air. Baby bottles are a common cause of aerophagia in infants as they suck in and swallow air if the formula does not always cover the nipple. Burping the baby after a feeding is the means of allowing the swallowed air to escape, otherwise it will cause distension and discomfort. Some bottles are designed to use an internal plastic sleeve to prevent air from reaching the nipple, when the formula is depleted the sleeve forms a vacuum so the infant is not sucking in air.

The first exposure to microorganism that will be swallowed and begin to colonize the infant digestive tract are from the birth mother if the delivery is vaginal and breast-feeding is initiated. The microorganisms that colonize the infant become its microbiome and play a major role in its ongoing health and wellness. The initial gut flora of the infant if born via a vaginal delivery and breast-feeding is identical to the vaginal and skin microbiome of the mother. This initial flora changes over the next few months especially if formula and other milks and foods are introduced. At about three months of age the gut flora is well established, and although changes will occur it is similar to the gut flora it will have as an adult.

The gut flora helps to set the infant's immune system, and it recognizes and tolerates microorganisms that are beneficial, known as commensals. One of the theories why breast-feeding is preferable, as well as why a vaginal delivery is preferable to Caesarian section, is that the natural microbiome exposure has advantages. The immunity of infants who did not receive the natural microbiome from the mother is at a disadvantage. Some experts are advocating exposing the newborn to the mother's vaginal secretions and microbiome by swabbing after birth if the delivery was via a Caesarian section.

The gut flora is one aspect of the microbiome, with skin, ears, mouth, genitourinary, and every surface of the body exposed to the external environment developing its own unique microbiome. Infants born by Caesarean section have exposure to different organisms, which establish a microbiome that is not believed to be as beneficial as via a natural vaginal delivery. The microbiome is established rapidly upon exposure to the environment. Most people think that the digestive tract is an internal organ because it is located inside the body. They are often surprised to find out that that the digestive tract is actually considered an organ exposed to the external environment. It is a long hollow tube exposed to the external environment at both ends, and is transited by material that for the most part comes from outside of the body.

The results of cell division and multiplication are similar between cells of the body, and cells of the microbiome. Mathematically this growth pattern is described as exponential or logarithmic growth. For those more familiar with finance, it is more akin to compounding interest instead of simple arithmetic addition. If a single cell divides into two cells, those cells divide into four cells, those into eight cells, and the numbers increase rapidly. The colonization and establishment of the microbiome is extremely rapid. The limitation of cellular division and growth of human cells are controlled by genes, hormones, neurotransmitters, and a variety of other feedback control mechanisms. The microbiome is also under the influence of these mechanisms, as well as competition for habitat and nutrition.

There is an apocryphal tale told of the invention of the game of chess. Long ago in an ancient land, there lived a very wise man that happened to be the Vizier at the court of a great Sultan. Months and years passed by and the great Sultan died, and his young prince replaced him. Being young, the prince lacked experience. He started spending more than what his father used to. The wise Vizier decided to teach the brash prince a lesson! The prince set a contest and as a reward, decided to give the winner whatever he wishes, boasting of his wealth, being under the illusion that his wealth is virtually endless. The Vizier won, and asked the prince for the prize: a single grain of wheat and a chessboard!

"What?! Just a grain of wheat! Are you insulting my wealth?" yelled the prince. "No! Your majesty!" The Vizier explained. "You have to promise to double that grain of wheat until the chessboard is full, so on the first day you give me one grain of wheat on the first square of the chessboard, on the second day you double it on the second square (giving me two grains), on the third, you double that on the third square (giving me four grains), and so on, until the sixty fourth square on the chessboard." "I thought you were smart", the young prince said. "You should have asked for something more substantial. Anyway, if this is your wish I will grant you that."

And so, on the second day, the Vizier got two grains, on the third, he got four grains, and the young prince couldn't help himself making fun of the Vizier. By the sixth day, the Vizier got thirty-two grains of wheat. By the eighth day and the end of the first row, he got a mere one hundred and twenty-eight grains. By the sixteenth day and the end of the second row, he got 32,768 grains. By the end of the game the prince could not provide enough grains to give the Vizier a chessboard's worth of grains because of the power of exponential growth. The last (sixty-fourth) square alone required 9,223,372,036,854,775,808 grains. The cumulative total of all of the squares was 18,446,744,073,709,551,615 grains. Indeed, that many grains would cover the entire earth several inches deep!

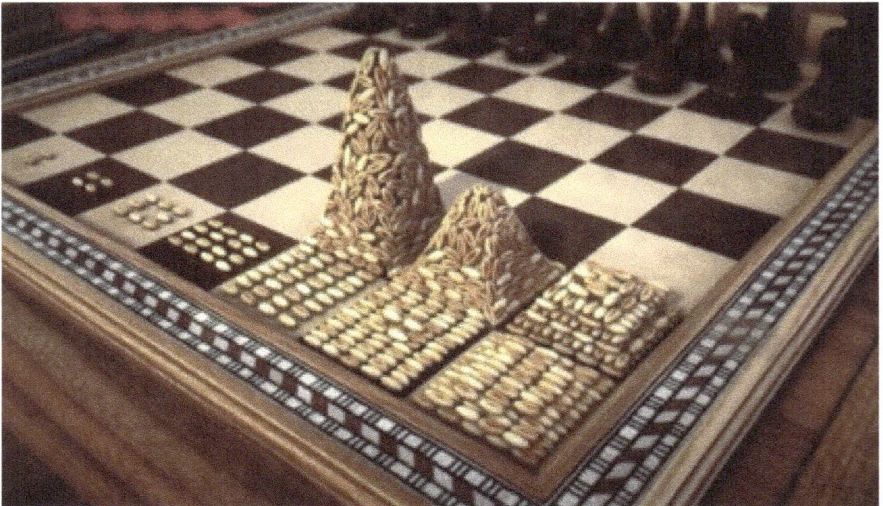

The gastrointestinal microbiome is also known as the gut microbiome and the gut flora. The gut microbiome is much more important than most people give it credit for. The microbes of the body far outnumber the number of human cells. The vast majority are commensals or are engaged with us in a symbiotic relationship from which we both benefit. The normal flora is site specific so that the microbiome of the stomach is different from the small intestine, which is different again from the colon. The appendix serves as a reservoir of the normal large intestinal bacteria flora. It represents the healthy gut microbiome from which the gut flora can be replenished after a bout of intestinal dysentery.

The effects of the microbiome include microbes, their genomes, and their environmental interactions. Gut flora consists of the microorganisms that live in the digestive tract and are the largest component of the human flora. The gut flora contains approximately one-hundred-trillion microorganisms in the intestinal tract, a number much greater than the ten trillion cells of the human body. The gut flora has approximately one hundred times as many genes as the human genome.

One of the major advances in the understanding of microbial life has come about with the recent advances in genomics technology. This technology now allows the rapid and precise identification of organisms that could not be identified because they were too fastidious and difficult to culture from stool specimens. Along with the identification of thousands of microorganisms that were not previously known to be present in the human gut microbiome is the realization that the microbial genes are in communication with the human host. Rather than genomics being a matter of just the twenty-three thousand plus human genes, is the profound implication that the millions of the additional genes found in microorganisms and food probably play an important role in human health and disease.

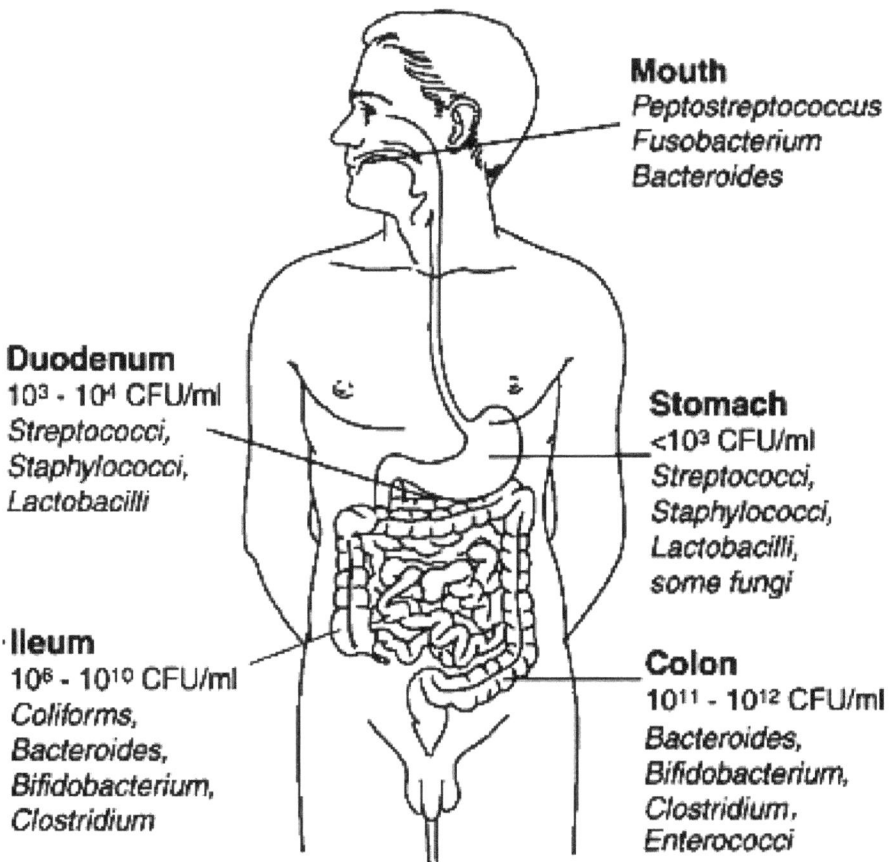

Mouth
Peptostreptococcus
Fusobacterium
Bacteroides

Duodenum
10^3 - 10^4 CFU/ml
Streptococci,
Staphylococci,
Lactobacilli

Stomach
$<10^3$ CFU/ml
Streptococci,
Staphylococci,
Lactobacilli,
some fungi

Ileum
10^6 - 10^{10} CFU/ml
Coliforms,
Bacteroides,
Bifidobacterium,
Clostridium

Colon
10^{11} - 10^{12} CFU/ml
Bacteroides,
Bifidobacterium,
Clostridium,
Enterococci

trialx.com/curetalk/wp Creative Commons License

These advances include the discovery of extremophiles, organisms that can live in extreme environments, and represent a previously undiscovered form of life called Archaea. This has prompted a reevaluation of the biological system of taxonomy, the categorizing of life forms. Most scientists now recognize six separate kingdoms: Animals (Animalia), Plants (Plantae), Fungi, Bacteria, Protozoan (Protista), and Archaea.

Significant portions of the human microbiome are not bacteria at all and are actually Archaea. In fact, the methane produced in flatus comes from the methanogenic Archaea of the gut microbiome. There will undoubtedly be major advances in the understanding of human health and diseases as the microbiome is explored and understood. The hygiene hypothesis proposes that a lack of early childhood exposure to infectious agents, parasites, and symbiotic microorganisms in the gut flora suppresses the development of the immune system. It is proposed that allergies, autoimmune disorders, and diseases seen at higher rates in the developed world may be due to excessive hygiene preventing the exposure necessary for optimal health. The hygiene hypothesis is supported by epidemiological data, yet the topic remains controversial with extensive research ongoing.

As a result of the hygiene hypothesis, helminthic infections emerged as a possible explanation of the low incidence of immunological disorders and autoimmune diseases in less developed countries. Helminthic therapy is the treatment of autoimmune diseases and immune disorders by means of deliberate infestation with a roundworm parasite. It is currently being studied as a promising treatment for several presumably non-viral autoimmune diseases including Crohn disease, multiple sclerosis, asthma, and ulcerative colitis. The anti-inflammatory effects of helminth infection are also prompting research into diseases that are not currently considered to have an immune basis. For example, heart disease and arteriosclerosis both have similar epidemiological and inflammatory profiles to the autoimmune diseases. Presently the two versions of helminthic therapy being studied are *Trichuris suis* ova and *Necator americanus* larvae.

Dysbiosis (dysbacteriosis) refers to a condition with microbial imbalances on or inside the body. Dysbiosis is most prominent in the digestive tract or on the skin, but can also occur on any surface or mucous membrane exposed to the environment such as the vagina, lungs, mouth, nose, sinuses, ears, nails, or eyes. It has been associated with different illnesses, such as inflammatory bowel disease, as imbalances in the intestinal microbiome may be associated with bowel inflammation and chronic fatigue syndrome. Microbial colonies found on or in the body are normally benign or beneficial. These beneficial and appropriately sized microbial colonies carry out a series of helpful and necessary functions, such as aiding in digestion. They also protect the body from the penetration of and infection with pathogenic microbes. These beneficial microbial colonies compete with each other for space and resources.

When this balance is disturbed by any of a variety of causes, such as antibiotic exposure, the balance of the microbial populations becomes disturbed. This can lead to an overgrowth of one or more of the organisms, which then may have a negative effect on some of the beneficial organisms. The imbalance and negative impacts can initiate a vicious cycle with further disruption from the normal flora.

Small intestinal bacterial overgrowth (SIBO) is a disorder of excessive bacterial growth in the small bowel. Risk factors include decreased motility or anatomical changes that lead to stasis, immune deficiencies, and reflux of bacteria from the colon into the small bowel such as occurs with the surgical removal of the ileocecal valve. The symptoms of bacterial overgrowth may include nausea, vomiting, bloating, flatus, chronic diarrhea, constipation, abdominal discomfort, weight loss, malnutrition, and anemia from vitamin B_{12} deficiency. Irritable bowel syndrome (IBS) may have an association with small intestinal bacterial overgrowth with some studies showing improvement after treatment. Rosacea, a dermatological condition, also appears to have an association with improvement after treatment. Small bowel bacterial overgrowth syndrome is treated with antibiotics, and if retreatment is required, various antibiotics may be given in a cyclic fashion.

Archaea

Most people have not heard of the microorganisms called Archaea, which is a kingdom of single-celled microorganisms that have no cell nucleus or membrane-bound organelles within their cells. They were first discovered in extremely hot and acidic environments in which life was not thought possible to exist. It was like a science fiction story come to life that not only were organisms found to survive in this environment but also they were actually thriving in these extreme conditions. Phylogenetics was proposed in 1965 by Linus Pauling and Emile Zuckerlan using the sequences of the genes in organisms to determine how they are related to each other.

Archaea were first classified as a separate group of prokaryotes in 1977 by Carl Woese at the University of Illinois at Urbana Champaign and George E. Fox in phylogenetic trees based on the sequences of ribosomal ribonucleic acid (rRNA) genes. Archaea were first found in extreme environments, such as volcanic hot springs. The word *archaea* comes from the Ancient Greek ἀρχαῖα, meaning 'ancient things' as the first representatives of the domain Archaea were methanogens and it was assumed that their metabolism reflected Earth's primitive atmosphere and the organism's antiquity. Archaea (singular archaeon) are prokaryote microorganisms, meaning that they have no cell nucleus or any other membrane bound organelles in their cells. Archaea cells have unique properties separating them from the other two domains of life: Bacteria and Eukaryota.

Archaea and bacteria have a similar size and shape, which may have delayed their recognition as completely separate entities. Although a few Achaea have strange and unusual shapes, such as flat and square-shaped cells, most look indistinguishable from bacteria by visual appearance. Despite a visual similarity to bacteria, Archaea possess genes and several metabolic pathways that are more closely related to those of eukaryotes. Their genetics and biochemistry are unique and there is no question but that they are an entirely different form of life.

Archaea use more energy sources than eukaryotes. These range from organic compounds, such as sugars, ammonia, metal ions, hydrogen sulfide, elemental sulfur, and hydrogen gas. They can also utilize light without photosynthesis in a process known as photophosphorylation in salt tolerant Archaea. Archaea reproduce asexually by binary fission, fragmentation, or budding; unlike bacteria and eukaryotes, no known species form spores.

Archaea were initially viewed as extremophiles living in extremely harsh environments, such as hot mineral springs, geysers, volcanic vents, salt lakes, deep ocean black smokers, oil wells, and in glaciers. Other extreme habitats included very cold arctic waters, and highly saline, acidic, or alkaline water. Even acids with the extreme limit of a pH of zero were tolerable environments. Temperatures higher than that of boiling water which was thought to sterilize and kill all bacteria was comfortable for their reproduction. In fact, they would survive in an environment as hostile as the planet Mars.

Some scientists postulate that the first Archaea may have arrived on Earth on a meteorite and are actually extraterrestrial life that came to earth from another planet or outside of our solar system. Science fiction could not be any more exciting than the actual science of studying Archaea. They have since been found in a broad range of habitats, including non-extreme environments such as soils, oceans, marshes, and the human colon and navel. Archaea are particularly plentiful in the oceans and in plankton. Archaea may play major roles in both the carbon and nitrogen cycles. They may represent up to twenty percent of the earths entire biomass. There are no known examples of Archaea acting as pathogens or parasites.

Archaea can also be commensals, benefiting from an association without helping or harming the other organism. They are often found in the role of mutualism with a symbiotic benefit for both organisms. One example of mutualism are the methanogens found in the digestive tracts where they aid digestion. In anaerobic environments within ruminants and termites, cellulose is broken down by protist with the release of hydrogen gas. The Archaea methanogens reside within the protozoan and convert the hydrogen to methane within the protozoan's organelle known as a hydrogenosome. Archaea methanogens are the primary source of the methane in the atmosphere and are major contributors to global warming. Methanogens are also used in biogas production and sewage treatment.

Extremophile Archaea are a source of enzymes that function under harsh conditions if temperature, salinity, acidity, or alkalinity. These enzymes have found many uses including research and industry. As an example amylases and galactosidases that function at over 100 °C (212 °F) may allow food processing at higher temperatures that usual. This may have commercial applications in the production of low lactose milk and whey. The enzymes from extremophile Achaea can endure high temperatures and organic solvents and have contributed to major advances in biotechnology, environmental services, and the food service industry. Archaea may also be hosts to new classes of antibiotics.

Archaea also associate with larger organisms such as corals, plant roots, and even humans. For example, the methanogen *Methanobrevibacter smithii* comprises ten percent of the prokaryotes in the human gut flora. Archaea demonstrate a high level of horizontal gene transfer between species. The mitochondria which serve as the energy power source for human cells is thought to have originated as an independent organism that entered into a symbiotic relationship. Archaea are a relatively recent discovery that has revolutionized our understanding of the microbial world and in particular the human microbiome. One of the major advances in the understanding of microbial life has come about with the recent advances in genomics technology. The discovery of extremophiles, organisms that can live in extreme environments and represent a previously undiscovered form of life called Archaea has prompted a reevaluation of the biological system of taxonomy, the categorizing of life forms. Most scientists now recognize six separate kingdoms: Animals (Animalia), Plants (Plantae), Fungi, Bacteria, Protozoan (Protista), and Archaea.

Extremophiles & Psychrophiles (Cryophiles)

Psychrophiles also called cryophiles are extremophile organisms that are can successfully grow and reproduce in the cold temperature range from −15°C to +10°C. Temperatures as low as −15°C may be found in regions of high salinity water, known as brine, that is surrounded by sea ice. Thermophiles by contrast thrive at unusually hot temperatures. Psychrophiles are very adaptive and use a wide variety of metabolic pathways to survive. These include the processes of photosynthesis, chemoautotrophy (also known as lithotrophy), and heterotrophy. This adaptive strategy allows them to survive and thrive in diverse communities throughout the colder climate zones. They are found in diverse extreme environments including soil in alpine and arctic environments, deep ocean waters at very high latitudes, polar ice fields, glaciers, and snowfields.

Grand Prismatic Mineral Hot Springs Yellowstone National Park. The striking coloration are from the extremophile Archaea that thrive in extreme environments that were previously thought to be incompatible with life. Creative Commons License

They are of particular interest to astrobiology, the science of potential extraterrestrial life, and to geomicrobiology, the scientific study of microbes active in geochemical processes. In a research study at the University of Alaska, Fairbanks a one-thousand-liter biogas digester using psychrophiles produces two hundred to three hundred liters of methane per day. Although it is only about twenty to thirty percent of the output from those in warmer climates, it is still a significant amount of biological activity in extreme cold climate zones. Most psychrophiles are either bacteria or Archaea present in widely diverse microbial lineages. Novel groups of psychrophilic fungi live in oxygen poor areas under alpine snowfields. Aristotle (384 BCE–322 BCE) wrote the first descriptive accounts of watermelon snow. It has puzzled mountain climbers, explorers, and naturalists for thousands of years.

Unusual watermelon snow pits. Author Will Beback Creative Commons License

The dramatic appearance of watermelon snow, also called snow algae, red snow, or blood snow, is *Chlamydomonas nivalis* (Latin nivalis – snow), the visible mark of the psychrophilic species of green algae. Compressing the snow by walking on it, or making snowballs, gives it a red color from a secondary red carotenoid pigment (astaxanthin), which it has in addition to chlorophyll. Psychrophiles have lipid cell membranes chemically resistant to the stiffening effect of extreme cold. They often create protein 'antifreezes' to maintain their intracellular space as liquid to protect their nuclear DNA in temperatures below the normal freezing point of water.

Methanogens

Methanogens are microorganisms of the Kingdom Archaea, not bacteria as previously thought. They produce methane as a metabolic byproduct in anaerobic conditions when oxygen is not present. Methanogens have been identified in a wide variety of extreme environments. Methanogens can thrive and reproduce in boiling water, as well as in ice cores taken miles down in arctic glaciers. They are common in wetlands, where they produce marsh gas, and in the digestive tracts of animals and humans where they generate the methane content of flatulence as well as the ruminant belch. One example of Archaea mutualism are the methanogens found in the digestive tracts where they aid digestion. In anaerobic environments within ruminants and termites, cellulose is broken down by protist with the release of hydrogen gas. The Archaea methanogens reside within the protozoan and convert the hydrogen to methane within the protozoan's organelle known as a hydrogenosome. Archaea methanogens are the primary source of the methane in the atmosphere and are major contributors to global warming. Methanogens are also used in biogas production and sewage treatment.

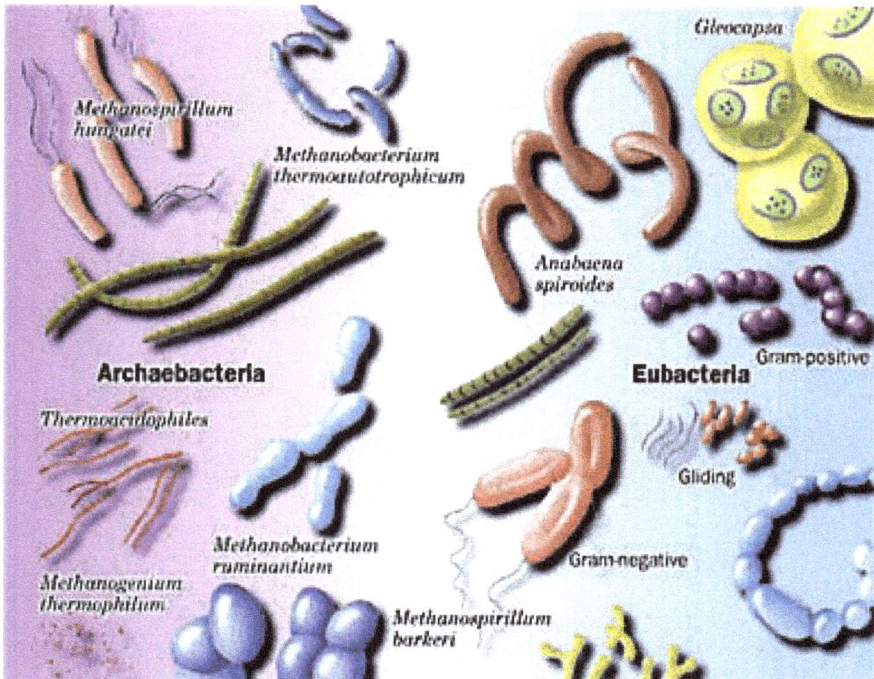

Most of the methanogenic bacteria are Archaea lawrencekok.blogspot.com Creative Commons License

Bacteria (see Pathogen)

Bacteria (Greek bakterion rod) are categorized as a large kingdom of prokaryotic microorganisms. Typically, just a few micrometers in length, bacteria have a wide variety of shapes including, rods, spirals, and spheres. Bacteria were among the earliest forms of life to appear on Earth, and are ubiquitous. They inhabit soil, water, acidic hot springs, radioactive waste, and can reside deep within rocks miles underground in portions of Earth's crust. Bacteria also live inside of plants and animals and have survived in outer space during space flights. A gram of soil typically contains forty million bacterial cells, and a single milliliter of fresh water may contain a million bacterial cells. There are approximately five nonillion, or to use a numerical version 5,000,000,000,000,000,000,000,000,000,000 (5×10 to the 30th power) bacteria on Earth. The enormous quantity of bacteria on Earth forms a total biomass that exceeds that of all plants and animals on the planet combined.

Bacteria are critical to life on Earth actively participating in many steps in the nutrient cycles that depend on these organisms, such as the fixation of nitrogen from the atmosphere. Most bacteria have yet to be identified and characterized. Advances in genomic technology and gene sequencing have markedly advanced the field of identifying new species of bacteria. The science and study of bacteria is the field known as bacteriology, and is a branch of microbiology.

There are more than ten times as many bacterial cells in the human microbiome flora as there are human cells in the body. There are more than one hundred times as many bacterial genes as human genes in the body. Very large numbers of bacteria are on the skin, and even more dramatic numbers are present as gut flora. The overwhelming majority of the bacteria in the body are commensals and do not cause disease. They are prevented from becoming pathogenic because of the protective effects of the immune system. Some bacteria are beneficial and engage in a symbiotic relationship with their human host.

Most people are not aware of the beneficial nature of the vast majority of bacteria. The recognition that several bacteria can be pathogenic and lead to disease and death has been well publicized. Several of the species of bacteria that are pathogenic and cause infectious diseases include cholera, syphilis, anthrax, leprosy, and bubonic plague. Many fatal bacterial diseases are respiratory infections, with tuberculosis alone killing about two million people a year. Antibiotics are utilized to treat bacterial infections, and are often also used in livestock farming. This has allowed antibiotic resistance to become increasingly common. In industry bacteria are important in sewage treatment, breakdown of oil spills, and the production of cheese and yogurt through fermentation. They have also been utilized in the mining industry in the recovery of gold, palladium, copper and other metals. Newer uses include biotechnology, the manufacture of antibiotics, and other proteins and chemicals.

Bacteria in the past were classified as plants in the class Schizomycetes. They are no longer considered members of the plant kingdom and at the present time bacteria are classified as prokaryotes. Prokaryotes are unlike the cells of animals and other eukaryotes. The cells of bacteria do not have a nucleus that contains the DNA based genetic information, and rarely have membrane bound organelles. The term bacteria historically included all prokaryotes. About two decades ago a major scientific breakthrough occurred with the discovery that prokaryotes actually consist of two very different groups of organisms. They are presently classified as two distinct evolutionary kingdoms, Bacteria and Archaea. The prehistoric ancestors of both bacteria and Archaea were unicellular microorganisms that first appeared on Earth about four billion years ago. For about three billion years the dominant forms of life on Earth were microscopic bacteria and Archaea. Bacteria also played a major role in the evolutionary branching of eukaryotes from Archaea.

Eukaryotes developed from ancient bacteria physically entering the cells in an internally symbiotic association. This process, which began as the engulfment of symbiotic bacteria, progressed to the development of either mitochondria or hydrogenosomes. Some eukaryotes that already contained mitochondria that had previously developed from bacteria also engulfed cyanobacteria-like organisms. This symbiotic relationship developed into the formation of specialized chloroplasts in algae and plants. Bacteria have a very wide diversity of shapes and sizes and are typically much smaller than eukaryotic cells. Most bacteria are between one half and five micrometers in length. The genus Mycoplasma has the smallest size of any bacteria, measuring only one third of a micrometer. They are so small that they are the same size as the largest viruses. Most bacterial species are either spherical cocci (Greek kókkos, grain) or rod shaped bacilli (Latin baculus stick). Elongation is commonly associated with motility. The bacteria called vibrio are rods with a slightly curved comma shape. Others bacteria called spirilla and spirochetes can be spiral shaped and tightly coiled. Several unusual species have a tetrahedral or cuboidal shape.

SHAPES OF BACTERIA

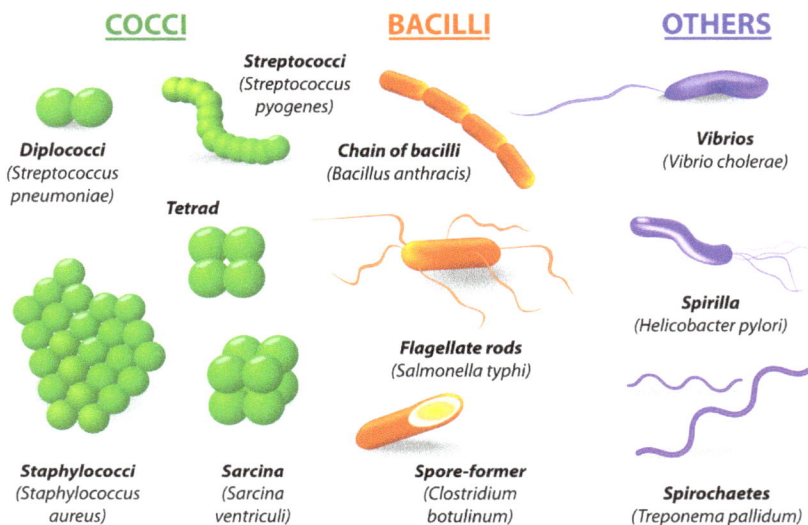

COCCI   BACILLI   OTHERS

Streptococci
(Streptococcus pyogenes)

Diplococci
(Streptococcus pneumoniae)

Tetrad

Chain of bacilli
(Bacillus anthracis)

Vibrios
(Vibrio cholerae)

Flagellate rods
(Salmonella typhi)

Spirilla
(Helicobacter pylori)

Staphylococci
(Staphylococcus aureus)

Sarcina
(Sarcina ventriculi)

Spore-former
(Clostridium botulinum)

Spirochaetes
(Treponema pallidum)

Shutterstock/designua

Recently discovered bacteria were identified deep under the Earth's crust. They grow as a branching filament with a star-shaped cross-section. These bacteria have a large surface area to volume ratio, which may be beneficial as these organisms exist in nutrient poor environments. A number of species of bacteria are found as single cells. Other species are often found in groups of multiple organisms that may associate in characteristic patterns. Neisseria organisms form pairs, Streptococcus organisms form chains, and Staphylococcus organisms group together in bunches and clusters that have the appearance of grapes. Less common species such as the genus Nocardia form complexes of branched filaments that have an appearance similar to that of fungal mycelia.

Bacteria frequently adhere to surfaces and may form a dense biofilm layer. These films may be as thin as just a few micrometers and may range up to thick bacterial mats up to half a meter (twenty inches) in depth. These film layers and mats may contain a multitude of species of bacteria, protist, and Archaea. Many bacteria living in biofilms have a complex arrangement of both cells and extracellular components. These may form complex secondary structures comprising micro colonies with networks of channels to allow the diffusion of nutrients. More recent research is suggesting that communication networks form in these large complex structures allowing the bacteria to behave in an organized manner much like a multicellular organism.

A lipid membrane known as a cell membrane or plasma membrane surrounds the bacterial cell. The cell membrane envelops and contains the contents of the cell. It acts as an environmental barrier and holds nutrients, proteins, and the other metabolically essential components of the cytoplasm within the cell. Bacteria, as prokaryotes, have few large intracellular structures and lack a true nucleus. They do not usually have membrane bound organelles in their cytoplasm such as mitochondria and chloroplasts that may be present in eukaryotic cells. Cyanobacteria may also produce gas within the cell, which forms into membrane bound vesicles. The gas vesicles may be used for locomotion by regulating their buoyancy. This allows the cell to move up or down in an aqueous environment, traveling to water layers with different light intensity and nutrient levels.

A special staining technique for the microscopic examination of bacteria was developed in 1884 by Hans Christian Gram. The Gram stain characterizes bacteria based on the structure of their cell walls. The thick layers of peptidoglycan and teichoic acids in the Gram-positive cell wall stain purple. The relatively thin Gram-negative cell wall consists of just a few layers of peptidoglycan. These layers are surrounded by a second lipid membrane containing lipoproteins and lipopolysaccharides appear pink. The endotoxin lipopolysaccharides are composed of lipid A and polysaccharides that contribute to the toxicity of Gram-negative bacteria. A bacterium in which the cell wall has been entirely removed is called a protoplast. If the cell wall is partially removed it is called a spheroplast. ß-Lactam antibiotics, such as penicillin, interfere with the formation of peptidoglycan cross links disrupting the bacterial cell wall. The enzyme lysozyme, which is found in human tears, also disrupts and digests the cell wall of bacteria. This property of the tear lysozyme is the body's main defense against eye infections.

Swimming and motile bacteria frequently move between ten and one hundred body lengths per second. On a relative scale this makes them at least as fast as fish. Flagella are whip like rigid protein structures about twenty micrometers in length and twenty nanometers in diameter that are used for motility. Fimbriae are fine filaments of protein that are found all over the surface of the cell. They appear to be involved in the bacterial cell's ability to attach to solid surfaces or to other cells. The fimbriae are essential for the virulence of some pathogens. Pili are cellular appendages that are slightly larger than fimbriae and can transfer genetic material between bacterial cells in a process called conjugation in which they are called conjugation pili or sex pili.

Certain bacteria, such as Sporohalobacter, Clostridium, Heliobacterium, Anaerobacter, can form dormant structures that are highly resistant to destruction. These structures are called endospores and have a central cytoplasm core containing the DNA and ribosomes. They are surrounded by an impermeable and rigid protective coat. Endospores appear to be in a state of suspended animation and do not exhibit any signs of metabolic activity. They can survive extreme physical and chemical stresses that would kill metabolically active organisms. They have exhibited the ability to withstand high levels of ultraviolet light, gamma radiation, heat, freezing, detergents, disinfectants, pressure, desiccation, and outer space without any reduction in their pathogenicity. Endospores in this dormant state allow these organisms to remain viable for many millions of years. Viable spores that are over forty million years old have been identified that have maintained the ability to cause disease. Examples of disease caused by dormant spores include anthrax, which can be contracted by the inhalation of *Bacillus anthracis* endospores, and tetanus, which can be contracted by contamination of deep puncture wounds with *Clostridium tetani* endospores.

In unicellular organisms growth is manifested by increases in cell size until a fixed point where asexual reproduction by binary cell division takes place. Under ideal conditions bacteria can grow and undergo cell division very rapidly. Bacterial populations can double in size as quickly as every ten minutes. This exponential growth rate allows one cell to become sixty-four cells in one hour, four thousand and ninety-six cells in two hours, 262,144 cells in three hours, 16,777,216 cells in four hours, over a billion cells in five hours, over four trillion cells in seven hours, etcetera. Certain infections can overwhelm and kill previously healthy humans and animals in a matter of just a few hours. The same power of exponential growth makes using microbes as miniature factories to produce biologic agents such as hormones, antibiotics, nutrients, etc. extremely attractive and efficient.

Bacteria are organisms that grow and multiply quickly. This feature, along with the relative ease to manipulate their DNA content, has made bacteria a model for many studies of genetics, molecular biology, and biochemistry. By creating a mutation in the DNA of bacteria a specific gene can be inactivated. By examining the effect of gene mutations, the function of genes, enzymes and metabolic pathways in bacteria can be identified. As many genes have identical functions in different organism the knowledge gained in experiments on bacteria can often be applied to more complex organisms such as humans. The scientific understanding of bacterial genes and metabolism has allowed the use of biotechnology to be commercialized. Bacteria can be bioengineered to produce a variety of therapeutic proteins, such as insulin, growth hormone, enzymes, antibodies, and other vital products.

Certain bacteria form close associations that are essential for their survival. One such mutualistic association occurs between anaerobic bacteria that metabolize a variety of organic acids. When organic acids such as butyric acid or propionic acid are metabolized hydrogen is produced as a byproduct. Increasing concentrations of hydrogen would be detrimental to the survival of these bacteria. In an association with mutual benefits methanogenic Archaea consume the hydrogen and allow the bacteria to thrive. The rhizosphere is the zone of soil that includes the root surface and soil that adheres to the root after gentle shaking. This zone contains a multitude of microorganisms that may carry out nitrogen fixation converting nitrogen gas to nitrogenous compounds. This provides an easily absorbable form of nitrogen for many plants, which cannot absorb and fix nitrogen from the atmosphere themselves.

*Air*Veda: Ancient & New Medical Wisdom

There are many bacteria that have developed a symbiotic relationship with other organisms, including humans. In the human gastrointestinal tract, the gut flora also known as the microbiome is predominantly beneficial organisms. There are over one thousand different species of bacteria in the normal human gut flora of the intestines. The organisms of the normal gut flora may contribute to gut immunity, synthesize vitamins such as vitamin K, folic acid, biotin, convert sugars to lactic acid (Lactobacillus), as well as ferment complex indigestible carbohydrates. The presence of the normal gut flora inhibits potentially pathogenic bacteria from becoming established by the process of competitive exclusion. Supplements of beneficial bacteria may be provided as probiotic dietary supplements.

Pathogenic bacteria are the cause of a number of human diseases that may lead to illness and death and cause infections such as diphtheria, tetanus, syphilis, typhoid fever, leprosy, tuberculosis, cholera, and foodborne illness. A number of known medical diseases were discovered to be caused by pathogenic bacteria many decades or centuries after the disease was first described. A recent example was the discovery that peptic ulcer disease, long thought to be caused by excess gastric acidity, was actually caused by the pathogenic organism *Helicobacter pylori*. Bacterial diseases also have a major impact on agriculture with bacteria causing fire blight, leaf spot, and wilts in plants, as well as mastitis, anthrax, Johne disease, and salmonella in farm animals.

A number of species may exist in small numbers within the normal gut flora and microbiome. They become pathogenic and cause disease with a characteristic pattern of signs and symptoms when their numbers increase substantially. Some organisms can cause a variety of signs and symptoms dependent on the location of the infection. For example, Staphylococcus or Streptococcus can cause skin infections, pneumonia, meningitis and even overwhelming sepsis. Sepsis is a systemic inflammatory response that can lead to vascular collapse and death. At the same time, in smaller numbers, these organisms are part of the normal human microbiome that is present on the skin or in the nose without causing any illness. Microorganisms have been utilized by humans for thousands of years in food production and preparation. Lactic acid is a metabolic byproduct of bacteria such as Lactobacillus and Lactococcus. These bacteria have been used for this property in combination with yeasts and molds in the preparation of fermented foods such as sauerkraut, cheese, soy sauce, pickles, wine, yogurt, and vinegar. They are commonly thought of as probiotics and may improve the gut microbiome.

Antonie van Leeuwenhoek, a Dutch lens maker, was first to observe bacteria using a microscope he designed in 1683. His scientific observations were published in a series of reports to the Royal Society of London. Scientists were fascinated by his description of animalcules in human semen and pond water. Identification and study of bacteria did not begin until over a century had passed. Christian Gottfried Ehrenberg has been credited with being the scientist who introduced the word "bacterium" in 1828. Louis Pasteur demonstrated in 1859 that the theory of spontaneous generation was incorrect. He also demonstrated that the fermentation process is caused by the growth of microorganisms, yeasts, and molds. Along with Robert Koch, Pasteur was an early advocate of the germ theory of disease. Koch was a scientific pioneer in the medical application of microbiology, and investigated the infectious causes of cholera, anthrax, tuberculosis and other life threatening conditions. Koch's research into the cause of tuberculosis proved that the germ theory was correct, for which he received Nobel Prize in 1905. Koch's postulates remain important scientific criteria to this day to prove that a specific organism is the cause of a disease. By the nineteenth century, bacteria were known to be the cause of many diseases. Unfortunately, treatments for infections with antibiotics had yet to be developed, although there were some reports that moldy foods might be helpful. In 1910 Paul Ehrlich developed the first effective antibiotic by studying and modifying dyes that selectively stained the organism *Treponema pallidum*. This is the spirochete bacteria that causes syphilis, and a dye compound Ehrlich developed selectively killed the pathogen. Ehrlich received the 1908 Nobel Prize for his work on immunology and the use of various stains to identify bacteria.

Fungi (see Pathogen)

Fungi are eukaryotes and include yeasts, mold, mushrooms. Their cell walls contain chitin, not cellulose. The science of fungi is called mycology and was once considered a subsection of botany. Over one hundred thousand species have been identified to date, and it is expected that number will rise to over five million with further exploration. A number of species can thrive in extreme environments, even the high ultraviolet light and radiation exposure of space travel. Genetic studies have revealed that fungi are actually more closely related to animals than plants. They secrete their digestive enzymes into the environment, and then absorb the dissolved nutrients. They are considered the primary decomposers in ecological systems and can have a symbiotic relationship with other plants, animals, and fungi or can act as a parasite.

Collage of fungi. Public Health England

They can produce bioactive compounds that can contaminate or spoil food sources and crops. For humans they can serve as a food, leavening agent for bread, fermentation of wine, beer, and soy sauce, or as a pathogenic source of disease. They have been used in industry in the production of antibiotics, enzymes, pesticides, and detergents. A number of species contain psychotropic compounds and have been used recreationally or in traditional spiritual ceremonies.

Parasite (see Pathogen)

Parasites (Greek παράσιτος *parasitos* 'side eating') are a common life form that depends on another living organism to serve as their host for sustenance. They do not provide any benefit to the host, and may lead to the death of the host, although that is not the parasite's primary intent. Parasites may be microbes or visible to the naked eye, and are commonly found among animals, plants, fish, fungi, and bacteria. Parasites in humans are commonly found in the intestinal tract as part of the gut microbiome. They may also infect and infest a variety of human organs and systems such as the brain, lungs, heart, skin, liver, eyes, etc.

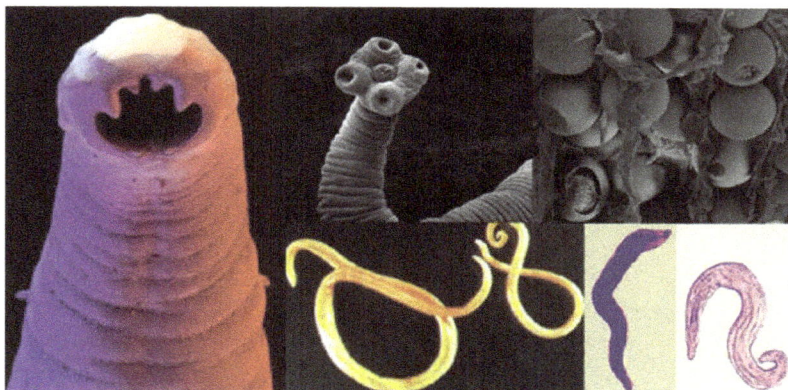
A variety of human parasites. Creative Commons License

Fortunately for humans this nasty parasite is only found in fish. It eats the tongue of the fish and stays in its mouth ready to eat anything the fish consumes. Creative Commons License

Prion (see Pathogen)

Prions are fundamentally different than a virus and contain and transmit infectious protein molecules that do not contain DNA or RNA. They can cause infections such as scrapie in sheep, bovine spongiform encephalopathy also known as mad cow disease in cattle, and chronic wasting disease in deer. In humans prion diseases include Kuru, which is acquired by cannibals eating the brain of a human infected with the virus. Other prion disease in humans includes Creutzfeldt–Jakob disease, and Gerstmann–Sträussler–Scheinker syndrome.

A prion is an infectious agent composed of protein in a misfolded form. The word prion was coined in 1982 by its discoverer 1997 Nobel laureate Stanley B. Prusiner and is derived from the words protein and infection. Prions are responsible for the transmissible spongiform encephalopathies in a variety of mammals, including bovine spongiform encephalopathy also known as "mad cow disease". In humans, prions cause Creutzfeldt-Jakob Disease (CJD), Fatal Familial Insomnia, and kuru. All known prion diseases affect the structure of the brain or other neural tissue and all are currently untreatable and universally fatal.

c0116801.cdn.cloudfiles.rackspacecloud.com Creative Commons License

Prions cause neurodegenerative disease by aggregating extracellularly within the central nervous system to form plaques known as amyloid, which disrupt the normal tissue structure. This disruption is characterized by "holes" in the tissue with resultant spongy architecture due to the vacuole formation in the neurons. Other histological changes include astrogliosis and the absence of an inflammatory reaction. While the incubation period for prion diseases is relatively long (five to twenty years), once symptoms appear the disease progresses rapidly, leading to brain damage and death. Neurodegenerative symptoms can include convulsions, dementia, ataxia (balance and coordination dysfunction), and behavioral or personality changes. All known prion diseases, collectively called transmissible spongiform encephalopathies (TSEs), are untreatable and fatal.

Current research suggests that the primary method of infection in animals is through ingestion. It is thought that prions may be deposited in the environment through the remains of dead animals and via urine, saliva, and other body fluids. They may then linger in the soil by binding to clay and other minerals. A University of California research team led by Stanley Prusiner, has provided evidence for the theory that infection can occur from prions in manure. And since manure is present in many areas surrounding water reservoirs, as well as used on many crop fields, it raises the possibility of widespread transmission. Preliminary evidence supporting the notion that prions can be transmitted through use of urine-derived human menopausal gonadotropin, administered for the treatment of infertility, was published in 2011.

Mad cow disease

Bovine spongiform encephalopathy, or mad cow disease, appears to cause a fatal human brain disease.

- **Severity** Cow begins "mad" seizures months or years after infection

- **Other livestock** Related disease called scrapie affects sheep

- **Prevention** Destroy infected farm animals; don't use animal products containing brain or central nervous system tissue as livestock feed

How it spreads

1 Person or animal eats food contaminated with brain or spinal cord tissue from infected animal

2 Disease attacks nervous system

Outer layer of brain develops tiny holes, looks spongy

SOURCES: U.S. Centers for Disease Control and Prevention, U.S. Agriculture Department, MCT Photo Service

One of the recent illnesses identified as being caused by prions is mad cow disease also known as bovine spongiform encephalopathy. It is a fatal neurodegenerative disease in cattle that causes an encephalopathy characterized by a spongy degeneration of the brain and spinal cord. Bovine spongiform encephalopathy has a long incubation period from about thirty months to eight years. It usually affects adult cattle at a peak age of onset of four to five years with all breeds being equally susceptible. In the United Kingdom, the country worst affected, more than one hundred and eighty thousand cattle have been infected and four and one-half million million slaughtered during the eradication program.

The disease may be transmitted to human beings by eating food contaminated with the brain, spinal cord, or digestive tract of infected cattle. In humans it is known as new variant Creutzfeldt–Jakob disease and by 2010 had killed more than two hundred humans. Up to five hundred thousand bovine spongiform encephalopathy infected animals had entered the human food chain before controls on high risk offal were introduced in 1989.

The epizootic condition was caused by feeding cattle the remains of other cattle in the form of meat and bone meal, which caused the infectious agent to spread. The infectious agent is remarkable for the high temperatures at which it remains viable, over six hundred degrees Celsius (about one thousand and one hundred degrees Fahrenheit). The infectious agent in bovine spongiform encephalopathy is a specific type of misfolded protein called a prion. Prions are not destroyed even if the beef or material containing them is cooked or heat-treated. Prion proteins carry the disease between individuals and cause deterioration of the brain.

Transmission can occur when healthy animals come in contact with contaminated tissues from others with the disease. In the brain, these proteins cause native cellular prion protein to deform into the infectious state, which then goes on to deform further prion protein in an exponential cascade. This results in protein aggregates, which then form dense plaque fibers, leading to the microscopic appearance of "holes" in the brain, degeneration of physical and mental abilities, and ultimately death. Cattle are naturally herbivores eating grass in pastures. Modern industrial and commercial cattle farming use various feeds, which may contain additional ingredients and supplements including antibiotics, hormones, pesticides, fertilizers, and protein additives. Meat and bone meal from the leftovers of the slaughtering process as well as from the carcasses of sick and injured cattle or sheep was often used as a protein supplement in cattle feed in Europe prior to about 1987.

In order to control potential transmission of bovine spongiform encephalopathy related variant Creutzfeldt–Jakob disease within the United States the American Red Cross has established strict restrictions on individuals' eligibility to donate blood. Because of the very long incubation period individuals who have spent a cumulative time of three months or more in the United Kingdom between 1980 and 1996, or a cumulative time of five years or more from 1980 to present in any combination of countries in Europe, are prohibited from donating blood.

Cows affected by bovine spongiform encephalopathy show progressively deteriorating behavioral and neurological signs. One notable sign is an increase in aggression with cattle reacting excessively to noise or touch. With time the cattle become ataxic and may also develop a drop in milk production, anorexia, and lethargy. At the slaughterhouse in the United Kingdom the brain, spinal cord, trigeminal ganglia, intestines, eyes, and tonsils from cattle are classified as specified risk materials and must be disposed of appropriately without entering the human food chain.

AirVeda: Ancient & New Medical Wisdom

In the US regulations prohibited the feeding of mammalian byproducts to ruminants such as cattle and goats since 1997. However, byproducts of ruminants can still be legally fed to pets or other livestock, including pigs and poultry, such as chickens. The US Department of Agriculture (USDA) has recalled beef supplies that involved the introduction of sick and dying downer cows into the food supply. Because the US standards and testing requirements are less rigorous than believed necessary to combat bovine spongiform encephalopathy many countries are hesitant to import its meat products. Sixty-five nations implemented full or partial restrictions on importing U.S. beef products. Beef consumption in the US was also affected by public concerns about food safety.

Protist (see Pathogen)

The protist are a eukaryotic microorganism that may be unicellular or multicellular and includes protozoa and amoeba. A number of these organisms may be pathogenic to humans such as chlamydia, trichomonas, and giardia. The majority are considered commensals in that they do not harm nor do they provide benefit.

http://wellcomeimages.org/indexplus/obf_images/99/db/d408763f6cfcd8e0cc232c74db20.jpg
Giardia lamblia Creative Commons License

柑橘類 • Creative Commons License Protist collage

Virus (see Pathogen)

Virus (Latin virulentus - poisonous) is a term that originally referred to poison and other noxious substances and was named by their discoverer Dmitri Ivanovsky in 1892. He mistakenly thought the illness transmitted from fluid filtered free of bacteria was a poisonous substance that the bacteria released. He did not realize that it was actually a living infectious agent much smaller than the bacteria that could not pass by the filter. Louis Pasteur was unsuccessful in his attempt to identify a bacterial cause for rabies. He speculated that the rabies pathogen may be too small to be seen using a microscope. In 1898 the Dutch microbiologist Martinus Beijerinck recognized that it was a new form of infectious agent but mistakenly thought that a virus was a liquid.

There is some controversy as to whether viruses should be considered a form of life, or nonliving organic structures that interact with living organisms. Some experts have described them as 'organisms at the edge of life' since they resemble organisms in that they possess genes, they evolve by the process of natural selection, and reproduce by creating multiple copies of their genetic code. Viruses have genes but they do not have the cellular structure that many define as the basic unit of life. Viruses do not have an independent metabolism and must invade a host cell to make new products and replicate. There are more viruses on Earth than stars in the universe. If you stacked every virus end to end they would stretch over one hundred thousand light years.

VIRUS

4. New viral particles are released, sometimes destroying the cell in the process.

3. Viral RNA uses the host cell to create new RNA and assemble more viral particles.

1. The virus enters the cell body releasing RNA.

2. Virus RNA invades the cell nucleus and takes over.

A virion is a complete virus particle. It consists of the genetic material in the form of a nucleic acid that is enveloped by a protein protective coat called a capsid. The capsid is formed from the assembly of identical protein subunits, each of which is called a capsomere. Some viruses have a protective lipid envelope that was derived from the host cell membrane. The capsid is made from proteins, the nature of which are determined by the viral genome. The shape of the virion serves as the characteristic basis for the morphological distinction and classification of viruses. The shape can range from a simple helical structure to more complex structures such as an icosahedral forms (having twenty plane faces, especially equilateral triangular ones). The average virus is only about one percent of the size of the average bacterium. Most viruses are so small that they cannot be seen directly with a standard optical microscope.

A very wide diversity of genomic structures can be seen among viral species. Viruses exhibit more genomic and structural diversity than bacteria, plants, Archaea, or animals. There are many millions of different types of viruses, yet to date only about five thousand have been described in detail. A virus may have either a DNA based or a RNA based genome, and is called a DNA virus or an RNA virus on this important distinction. The majority of viruses have RNA based genomes. Viruses are the most numerous living organisms on Earth and they outnumber all of the other life forms combined. Viruses can infect all types of cellular life including plants, animals, fungi, and bacteria. Each specific type of virus can infect only a limited range of hosts, and a number of viruses are species-specific. For example, the smallpox virus can infect only humans and it is therefore described as having a narrow host range. Other viruses that are described as having a broad range include the rabies virus, which can infect different species of mammals. The viruses that infect plants are nearly always harmless to animals. Most viruses that infect other animals are not pathogenic to humans.

Viruses may spread in a wide variety of ways including blood sucking insects and animals. When these animals or insects serve to transmit the virus, the disease bearing organisms are known as vectors. Influenza viruses are spread through the aerosolization of the virions by coughing and sneezing. Norovirus and rotavirus are two of the most common causes of viral gastroenteritis and are transmitted by the fecal oral route. They are transmitted by direct contact or by entering the body through contaminated food or water.

A bacteriophage (Greek φαγεῖν*phagein* phage devour) is a virus that infects and replicates within bacteria. Bacteriophages consist of various proteins that envelope and encapsulate a DNA or RNA genome. The bacteriophage may have a relatively simple or an elaborate structure. The bacteriophage genome may be small and encode as few as four genes, or it may be very large and contain hundreds of genes. The bacteriophage genetic material is injected into the cytoplasm and replicates within the bacteria cell. The bacteriophage infection results in the death of the bacteria.

Bacteriophages are distributed widely and found in virtually all environments that harbor bacteria, such as soil or the gastrointestinal tracts of humans and animals. Seawater has one of the highest concentrations of bacteriophages in a natural nonliving environments. Bacteriophages and other viruses have a density in seawater of up to 9×10^8 virions per milliliter. These concentrations have been found in seawater microbial mats at the ocean surface. Up to seventy percent of marine bacteria may be infected by bacteriophages. Bacteriophages have also been used for over ninety years in the treatment of bacterial infections as an alternative to antibiotics in Russia, Central Europe, and France. Bacteriophages may have a role as a possible antimicrobial therapy against strains of bacteria that have developed resistance to many antibiotics.

Drinking the waters of various rivers as an effective treatment to cure infectious diseases has been documented since ancient times. In 1896, Ernest Hanbury Hankin reported that drinking the waters of the Ganges and Yamuna rivers in India could be effective in the treatment of cholera. The antibacterial action of the river water against cholera remained even if the water was passed through a very fine porcelain filter. The antibacterial action was transmitted via the presence of microscopic viral bacteriophages in the river water. The discovery of the nature of viruses and their genetic structure and replication resulted in scientists Max Delbrück, Alfred Hershey and Salvador Luria being awarded the Nobel Prize in Physiology and Medicine in 1969. Bacteriophages are a very common and remarkably diverse group of viruses. In aquatic environments, they are the most abundant form of biological life comprising ninety percent of the biomass in the sea. In seawater they outnumber bacteria and Archaea by more than fifteen to one, reaching levels of two hundred and fifty million bacteriophages per milliliter of seawater. Most of the bacteriophages are harmless to plants and animals, yet are essential to the regulation of saltwater and freshwater ecosystems. It is estimated that viruses kill approximately twenty percent of the aquatic biomass each day.

The bacteriophage viruses infect specific bacteria by binding to surface receptor molecules on the surface of the bacteria and then entering the cell. Within a short amount of time, often measured in minutes, bacterial polymerase starts translating viral mRNA into protein. These proteins may be new virions within the cell, helper proteins that assist in the production and assembly of new virions, or proteins involved in cell lysis. Viral enzymes may aid in the breakdown of the cell membrane. In the case of the T_4 phage, overtaking the bacterial cell and producing and releasing over three hundred new virion phages could take place in less than twenty minutes from the time of infection.

Swarm of bacteriophages attacking a bacterium rafefurst.files.wordpress.com Creative Commons License

Human immunodeficiency virus (HIV) is one of several viruses that may be transmitted via several bodily fluids, including through sexual contact and by exposure to infected blood. Antibiotics are not effective in the treatment of conditions caused by a virus, but several antiviral drugs have been developed. Several examples of common human diseases caused by viruses include chickenpox, the common cold, cold sores, and influenza. Viruses cause many serious diseases such as Ebola, AIDS, avian influenza, rabies, etc. The term virulence is used to describe the relative ability of viruses to cause disease. Some viruses can lead to chronic and even lifelong infections. In chronic infections the virus is able to continue to survive and replicate in spite of the host defense mechanisms. This is seen commonly in untreated hepatitis B virus and hepatitis C virus infections. People chronically infected are known as carriers, and they can serve as an infectious reservoir for the virus to infect others. In populations where the proportion of the population that are carriers is high, the disease is said to be endemic.

Epidemiology is the area of science that deals with the study of health and disease in specific populations. Study of the transmission of viral infections in humans has demonstrated two different general categories. In the category of vertical transmission, the virus is transferred from mother to child such as via the placenta or through breast milk. In horizontal transmission the virus is transmitted from person to person. An example of the vertical transmission of a virus occurs with the hepatitis B virus and HIV. With vertical transmission occurring in utero the baby has already been infected by the virus before it is born.

The most common form of the transmission of viruses in a given population is by means of horizontal transmission. Horizontal transmission can occur with the exchange of bodily fluids during sexual activity, blood transfusion, needle sharing, saliva from the mouth, etc. Horizontal transmission may also occur via contaminated food or water, aerosolized virions being inhaled, insect vectors such as mosquitoes, etc. The incubation period is the time that elapses between the introduction of the virus to host and the first signs and symptoms of illness. Incubation periods are often of a characteristic duration for different viral diseases, and may range from a few days to weeks. The communicability period is the time when the infection can be passed from an infected individual or animal to another uninfected human or animal. It is during the communicability period that the illness is considered contagious. The knowledge of the length of time of both the incubation and communicability periods of specific viral infections is important in the control of outbreaks. An outbreak is described as an epidemic when there is an unusually high proportion of cases in a specific region, population, or community. A pandemic is the term used when the epidemic outbreaks occur on a worldwide basis.

Isolated populations that have not developed immunity to viruses can be decimated by epidemics. Among examples historically documented are the Native American populations that were devastated by contagious diseases. Smallpox was one of the infections brought to the Americas by European colonists that was particularly virulent in the native populations. The precise number of how many Native Americans were killed by infectious diseases after the arrival of Columbus in the Americas is not known, but numbered in the hundreds of thousands. It has been estimated that close to seventy percent of the indigenous population was destroyed. The decimation of the native population by diseases to which they had no natural immunity played a major role in the successful European colonization of native lands. By the way, the word decimation has an interesting history and is actually an inadequate word to describe the devastation of the native population. Decimation was a brutal form of military discipline used by senior commanders in the ancient Roman Legions to punish troops for disloyalty or desertion. Each group of ten soldiers were to draw lots to identify the one of the ten to be murdered by their fellow soldiers. Since one tenth of the soldiers involved were killed, the term decimation was derived from the Latin term meaning 'removal of a tenth.

The catastrophic 1918 influenza pandemic lasted until 1919 and was caused by an extremely virulent and deadly influenza A virus. Unlike most influenza outbreaks that target the ill and elderly, most of the victims were healthy young adults. The influenza pandemic of 1918 may have killed as many as one hundred million people, comprising five percent of the world's population at the time. The human immunodeficiency virus (HIV) is believed to have originated in primates in sub-Saharan Africa during the 20th century. HIV is a pandemic viral infection with approximately forty million people now living with the chronic disease worldwide. The United Nations and the World Health Organization (WHO) estimate that HIV has killed more than twenty-five million people since it was first recognized in 1981. It has become one of the most devastating epidemics in recorded history, but has also led to research and therapeutic breakthroughs in the management of viral diseases. Viruses are a known cause of cancer in humans and other species. Viral cancers can arise from both RNA and DNA viruses and occur in only a minority of infected persons (or animals). The risk of developing cancer is influenced by a number of factors including host immunity and genetic mutations. Viruses that are known to cause human cancers include several genotypes of the human papillomavirus, human T-lymphotropic virus, Epstein-Barr virus, hepatitis B virus, Kaposi's sarcoma-associated herpes virus, and the hepatitis C virus.

When the host immune system encounters a virus, it produces specific antibodies that bind to and inactivate the virus, making it non-infectious. This process is known as humoral immunity and is dependent on two important classes of antibodies. The first class of antibodies are known as immunoglobulin M (IgM) and are effective at neutralizing viruses. Immunoglobulin M is produced by the cells of the immune system for only the first few weeks of an infection. The second class of antibody is called immunoglobulin G (IgG) and its production can be maintained as long as necessary. The presence of IgM antibody in the blood of the host indicates a recent acute infection, whereas IgG antibody indicates the infection occurred sometime in the past.

The host immune system second line of defense is known as cell-mediated immunity and involves immune cells called T cells. The host cells of the body display self-markers consisting of short fragments of their proteins on the cell surface that identify the cells as belonging to the host. A host cell infected with a virus may also display the foreign protein from the infecting virus, which may act as an antigen to stimulate the immune response and identify the cell as being infected. The immune system T cell mediated response recognizes the foreign viral fragment on the surface of the infected host cell. As the cell has been recognized as infected it is destroyed by killer T cells. The T-cells that identify the host cells as being infected by the specific virus proliferate and intensify the immune response to the virus. Macrophages are immune cells that are specialized at antigen recognition. Interferon production is an important component of the host defense mechanism. Interferon stops viral reproduction by killing the infected cell and its close neighbors. Human immunodeficiency virus (HIV) is often able to successfully evade the immune system by frequently altering the sequence of the amino acid components of the proteins on the virion surface. With the antigenic markers on the cell surface changing regularly, the antibodies the body produced for earlier versions of the antigen are no longer effective.

Because viruses use the host cell metabolic pathways to replicate, drugs toxic to the pathway of viral replication are often toxic to all host cells as well. The most effective approach to controlling viral disease is to utilize vaccinations to provide immunity, and the use of antiviral drugs that are able to selectively interfere with viral replication. Vaccination is an inexpensive and effective way of preventing infections by viruses. Their use has resulted in the significant decline in mortality and morbidity of serious viral infections such as mumps, smallpox, rubella, measles, and polio. Vaccines are commercially available for the prevention of over one dozen major viral infections of humans, and even more vaccines are available to prevent viral infections of animals such as livestock and pets. Vaccines may consist of live but attenuated viruses, killed viruses, or antigens derived from viral proteins. Attenuated live vaccines contain forms of the virus that have been weakened to such a degree that they do not cause disease but can nonetheless confer immunity. Live vaccines have the potential of actually causing the disease they are meant to prevent, and can be particularly dangerous in causing active disease when given to people who are immuno-compromised. Antiviral drugs are often nonfunctional imitation analogues of the DNA nucleoside base building blocks. When a virus mistakenly incorporates a nonfunctioning analogue into its genome during replication, its life cycle is halted because the newly synthesized DNA is inactive.

Microfart

Microfarts are the release of intestinal gasses from very small organisms such as insects. The term is often also used to describe the nanofarts of microscopic organisms such as bacteria, fungi, archaea, and protist. Termites are major producers of methane and because of the enormous size of the termite population and biomass they are thought to be significant contributors to global warming producing over twenty-five percent of the world total methane production. Of interest, termites trapped in the sap of a tree have often been frozen in time as the sap turns to amber over the ages.

Termite farts trapped in amber have been analyzed for gas composition and indeed it is methane.

The tiny bubble of gas at the tail end of the termite entrapped in amber has been analyzed (pun intended!) and is indeed methane produced thousands of years ago from the bacterial fermentation of the wood termites ingest. The termite gut microbiome flora generates tiny bacterial nanofarts which coalesce into the termite microfarts that have been captured in amber eons ago. Even though the termites are described as the source of significant methane production that contributes to global warming, it is actually the methanogen Archaea microorganisms that resides in the guts of the termites that is the source of origin.

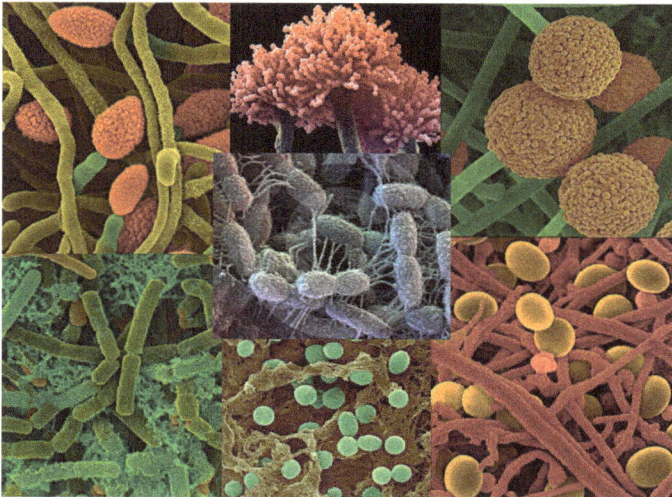

Although they do not have a digestive tract like insects, microorganisms also release gasses with fermentation and digestion of nutrients. A microorganism (Greek μικρός mikros small, ὀργανισμός organismós organism) or microbe is a microscopic single cell or multicellular organism. Microorganisms are extremely diverse and the most prolific life form on the planet. They include bacteria, Archaea, protozoa, fungi, algae, viruses, microscopic plants (green algae), and microscopic animals such as rotifers and planarians. Microorganisms live in every part of the biosphere including soil, hot springs, ocean floor, upper atmosphere, and even deep inside rocks miles underground within the Earth's crust. Those that live in otherwise inhospitable conditions are called extremophiles. Microorganisms are critical to nutrient recycling by acting as decomposers in ecosystems. Some microorganisms can fix nitrogen and are a vital part of the nitrogen cycle. Most microbes are either beneficial or compatible with human health and well-being. There are a limited number of pathogenic microbes, which are harmful and cause death and illness in plants and animals, with a significant subset that does so in humans.

Single-celled microorganisms were the first forms of life to develop on Earth approximately four billion years ago. In the Precambrian eon all organisms were microscopic. Bacteria, algae and fungi have been identified in amber that is two hundred and twenty million years old. Microorganisms have a relatively fast rate of evolution as they may reproduce rapidly with some populations doubling in size in twenty minutes. Bacteria can even freely exchange genes between widely divergent species. This horizontal gene transfer coupled with a high mutation rate and many other means of genetic variation allows microorganisms to evolve rapidly through natural selection. This rapid adaptation to new environments has allowed them to survive and thrive through the course of four billion years of the Earth's history. This rapid adaptation has also been a challenge for humans treating pathogenic microorganism as they develop resistance to therapies such as antibiotics.

The possibility that life forms exist which are invisible to the naked eye has a history of being discussed as a theoretical possibility as long as two thousand five hundred years ago. The proof that they did indeed exist occurred in the year 1675 with Dutch lens maker Antonie van Leeuwenhoek's discovery of microorganisms in pond water. Robert Hooke a contemporary of Leeuwenhoek also used the newly invented microscope to observe microbial life and coined the term cell in his 1665 book *Micrographia*. The previously widely held belief that life occurred from spontaneous generation was proven false by a series of discoveries and experiments. Lazzaro Spallanzani (1729–1799) found that boiling broth would sterilize it by killing any microorganisms it contained. He also found that new microorganisms could only contaminate the broth if it was exposed to air. Louis Pasteur (1822–1895) extended Spallanzani's findings by exposing boiled broths to the air but with filters or curved tubes. This prevented dust particles from the air carrying microbes from reaching the broth that would then rapidly spoil. The fact that nothing grew on the boiled broth proved that mold and decaying organisms did not arise from spontaneous generation but must be carried in the air as spores or on dust particles.

*Air*Veda: Ancient & New Medical Wisdom

In 1876, Robert Koch (1843–1910) established that microbes could cause disease. He found that the blood of cattle that were infected with anthrax had large numbers of the *Bacillus anthracis* bacteria. Koch found that he could transmit anthrax from one animal to another by taking a small sample of blood from the infected animal and injecting it into a healthy one. He also found that he could grow the bacteria in a nutrient broth then inject it into a healthy animal and cause illness. Based on these experiments he developed the criteria to establish a causal link between a microbe and a disease. These are known today as Koch's postulates and are still the criteria used to prove that microorganisms are responsible for specific diseases.

Prokaryotes are organisms that lack a cell nucleus and the other membrane bound organelles and are nearly always unicellular. Consisting of two domains, bacteria and Archaea, the prokaryotes are the most diverse and abundant group of organisms on Earth and inhabit practically all environments where the temperature is below one hundred and forty degrees centigrade (Celsius) (two hundred and eighty-four degrees Fahrenheit). They are found in water, soil, air, animals' gastrointestinal tracts, hot springs, and even deep beneath the Earth's crust inside rocks. Practically all surfaces that have not been specially sterilized are covered by prokaryotes. The number of prokaryotes on Earth is estimated to be around five million trillion trillion (called a nonillion in short scale for English speaking countries and quintillion in long scale for non-English speaking countries). For those who prefer numbers in numerical form it is the number five followed by thirty zeroes written as 5,000,000,000,000,000,000,000,000,000,000. They account for at least half of the biomass on planet Earth.

Prokaryote bacteria lack a nucleus and other membrane bound organelles and function and reproduce as individual cells. Their genome is a single loop of DNA while they may also have small separate pieces of DNA called plasmids. The plasmids can be transferred between cells through bacterial conjugation. Bacteria are surrounded by a cell wall, which provides structural strength and rigidity to their cells, as well as protection from the environment. Bacteria are often classified as to cell type by whether their cell walls stain Gram positive or Gram negative. They reproduce by mitosis, binary fission, or budding but do not undergo meiotic sexual reproduction with a reduction of chromosomes from diploid to haploid.

Many bacterial species can also transfer DNA between individual cells by a process referred to as natural transformation. In nature transformation usually occurs with stressful environmental conditions and appears to be a mechanism for repairing DNA damage in the recipient cells. Some species form extremely resilient spores as a survival mechanism. The spores can remain viable and able to cause deadly disease even many years later if they find their way into an opportune host. Under optimal conditions bacteria can grow extremely rapidly and can double as quickly as every twenty minutes.

Archaea are also single-celled organisms that lack a nucleus. In the past the differences between bacteria and archaea were not recognized and Archaea were classified with bacteria as part of the kingdom Monera. Archaea significantly differ from bacteria in both their genetics and biochemistry. Bacterial cell membranes are made from phosphoglycerides with ester bonds, Archaea membranes are made of ether lipids. Archaea were originally described in extreme environments, such as hot springs, but have since been found in all types of habitats. Archaea are common in the environment and are the most common form of life in the ocean. They are also common in soil and play a vital role in ammonia oxidation.

Most living things that are visible to the naked eye in their adult form are eukaryotes, including humans. A large number of eukaryotes are also microorganisms. Unlike the prokaryotes bacteria and Archaea, eukaryotes contain organelles such as the cell nucleus, the Golgi apparatus, and mitochondria in their cells. The nucleus is an organelle that houses the DNA that makes up a cell's genome arranged in complex chromosomes. When they reproduce they undergo meiosis, which reduces the diploid state of paired chromosomes to the haploid state of single chromosomes. When two haploid cells combine in reproduction they become diploid once again with newly paired chromosomes that allow for genetic diversity and evolution by natural selection. Other eukaryotic microorganisms remain and reproduce in a haploid state and some others actually have multiple nuclei.

Mitochondria are organelles vital in cellular metabolism, as they are the site of the citric acid cycle and oxidative phosphorylation. They evolved from symbiotic bacteria that over eons became incorporated into a single cell. The mitochondria retain a separate genome with DNA that is inherited in a matrilineal pattern. Plant cells have cell walls and contain organelles such as chloroplasts in addition to the organelles in other eukaryotes. Chloroplasts produce energy from light by photosynthesis, and were also originally symbiotic bacteria that became incorporated into the cell through evolution.

Unicellular eukaryotes consist of a single cell throughout their life cycle. Most multicellular eukaryotes consist of a single cell called a zygote only at the beginning of their life cycles when the two haploid germ cells unite at reproduction. Unicellular eukaryotes usually reproduce asexually by mitosis under favorable conditions. However, under stressful conditions associated with DNA damage they tend to reproduce sexually by meiosis and syngamy.

Of the eukaryotic groups, the protist are the most commonly unicellular and microscopic. They are a highly diverse group of organisms that also includes multicellular protist and slime molds that have unique life cycles that involve switching between unicellular, colonial, and multicellular forms. The full number of species of protist is unknown and new species are regularly discovered on exploration of diverse locations.

Most microscopic animals are multicellular but even so they are often too small to be seen by the naked eye. Microscopic arthropods include dust mites and spider mites. Microscopic crustaceans include copepods and the cladocera, while many worms are nematodes that are too small to be seen with the naked eye. Another particularly common group of microscopic animals are the rotifers, which are filter feeders that are usually found in fresh water. Microscopic animals reproduce both sexually and asexually and may reach new habitats as some of the eggs can survive harsh environments that would kill an adult animal. Some simple animals such as rotifers and nematodes can dry out completely and remain dormant for long periods of time, returning to active life forms with rehydration when water is present.

The fungi have several unicellular species, such as baker's yeast (*Saccharomyces cerevisiae*) and fission yeast (*Schizosaccharomyces pombe*). Some fungi such as the pathogenic yeast *Candida albicans* can undergo phenotypic switching and grow as single cells in some environments and filamentous hyphae in others. Fungi reproduce both asexually by budding or binary fission as well by producing spores. The spores are called conidia when they are produced asexually, or basidiospores when they are produced sexually.

The green algae are a large group of photosynthetic eukaryotes that include many microscopic organisms. Although some green algae are classified as protist, others are classified with embryophyte plants, which are the most familiar group of land plants. Algae can grow as single cells or in long chains of cells. The green algae include unicellular and colonial flagellates, usually with two flagella per cell. Algae can also be found in various colonial, coccoid, and filamentous forms. There are about six thousand species of green algae known to date.

Microorganisms are found in almost every habitat that exists in nature. Even in hostile environments such as the North and South Poles, deserts, geysers, inside rocks, and the deep sea. Microorganisms that have adapted to the extreme conditions and sustained colonies there are known as extremophiles. Extremophiles have been isolated from rocks as much as four and one-half miles (seven kilometers below the Earth's surface, and it has been suggested that the amount of living organisms below the Earth's surface may be comparable with the amount of life on or above the surface.

Extremophiles have been known to survive for a prolonged time in a vacuum and can be highly resistant to radiation even allowing them to survive in space. There is growing evidence to suggest that life forms very likely exist elsewhere in the universe, and that life forms may have been introduced to earth from outside of the planet's environment. Many types of microorganisms have intimate symbiotic relationships with other larger organisms; some of which are mutually beneficial (mutualism), while others can be damaging to the host organism (parasitism). If microorganisms can cause disease in a host they are known as pathogens and then they are usually referred to as microbes. With evolution symbiotic organisms may become integrated into one as evidenced by mitochondria and chloroplasts.

Extremophiles are unique microorganisms that have adapted so that they can survive and even thrive in conditions that are normally fatal to most life forms. As such they are significant beyond their extension of terrestrial life into much of the Earth's hydrosphere, crust and atmosphere. The specific evolutionary adaptation mechanisms to their extreme environment can be studied and utilized in biotechnology leading to dramatic advances in the life sciences as well as industry.

Microorganisms are vital to humans and the environment, as they participate in the Earth's element cycles such as the carbon cycle and nitrogen cycle, as well as fulfilling other vital roles in virtually all ecosystems, such as recycling other organisms' dead remains and waste products through decomposition. Microorganisms are used in brewing, winemaking, baking, pickling and other food-making processes. They are also used to control the fermentation process in the production of cultured dairy products such as yogurt and cheese.

Many life forms on Earth are also dependent on the nitrogen cycle in soils, which requires the fixation of atmospheric nitrogen. One way this can occur is in the nodules in the roots of legumes that contain symbiotic bacteria of the genera Rhizobium, Mesorhizobium, Sinorhizobium, Bradyrhizobium, and Azorhizobium. Symbiotic microbes such as fungi and algae form an association in lichen. Certain fungi form mycorrhizal symbioses with trees that increase the supply of nutrients to the tree. Microorganisms can form an endosymbiotic relationship with other larger organisms. For example, the bacteria and Archaea that live within the human digestive system contribute to gut immunity, synthesize vitamins such as folic acid and biotin, and ferment complex indigestible carbohydrates. Some forms of bacteria that live in animals' stomachs help in their digestion. For example, cows have a variety of different microbes in their multi-chambered ruminant stomachs that aid them in their digestion of grass and hay.

As important as the human genome is in understanding human health and disease, it has become apparent that the microbiome and its genomics may well play a critical role as well. We are continually learning more about how humans are impacted by the approximately twenty-three thousand genes in the human genome. We are just at the dawn of understanding how we are impacted by the over one million genes of the human microbiome, the microorganisms and macroorganisms that share our bodies as welcome or unwelcome guests.

Mountain Climbing (see Atmospheric Pressure, Ideal Gas Law)

Those who travel to higher altitudes, whether by climbing a mountain, driving up a mountain road, or traveling by air, experience an increase in flatulence. The underlying principle is the same, according to the gas laws of physics a reduction in atmospheric pressure results in an increase in the volume of intestinal gas. For those climbing hills and mountains with fellow travelers the incline usually means the person behind has their nose at about the same level as the butt of the person in front. The practical take home message is that it is to your olfactory advantage to always be in the lead.

Shutterstock/MyGoodImages

Another important consideration for those engaged in high altitude activities is the recognition that the oxygen content of air decreases with an increase in altitude. For those with underlying circulatory or lung conditions the additional stress of low oxygen content of the air can be potentially life threatening. Altitude sickness can also develop rapidly and is a life-threatening condition requiring an immediate descent in altitude.

Many air travelers are under the false impression that pressurization of the aircraft means the oxygen content of the air is the same as that on the ground at sea level. The aircraft is typically pressurized to maintain a cabin pressure equivalent to an altitude of approximately eight thousand feet. This leads to a reduction in the oxygen content of the air on the aircraft. Some normal individuals find this reduction in oxygen uncomfortable and develop headaches and other symptoms. Others are more sensitive, or recognize that their underlying medical condition requires that they have access to supplemental oxygen for their safe travel.

Nitrogen (see Nitrogenation)

Nitrogen is a chemical element with symbol N and atomic number seven is a colorless, odorless, tasteless, gas constituting seventy-eight percent by volume of Earth's atmosphere. The element nitrogen was discovered by Scottish physician Daniel Rutherford, in 1772. Nitrogen is the largest volume component of atmospheric air, and as would be expected, represents an identically high proportion of the gasses swallowed through aerophagia. Once in the body the carbon dioxide of the air is absorbed and eliminated. The nitrogen however is a very poorly absorbed gas, and in essence will either come back up as a burp, or will sooner or later, comes out the other end as a fart.

The oxygen in the air, representing nearly twenty-one percent of the air gasses swallowed during aerophagia, is absorbed slowly, as the gut is not nearly as efficient as the lungs for respiration. As the carbon dioxide and oxygen are absorbed the percent of the gastrointestinal tract air that is nitrogen increases. As soon as the digestive process begins, hydrochloric acid of the stomach is neutralized by sodium bicarbonate of the duodenum and pancreas. Large volumes of carbon dioxide gas are generated, as are smaller quantities of hydrogen, methane and other aromatic gasses. The carbon dioxide generated is absorbed, enters into solution in the blood, travels to the lungs, and is exhaled through the alveoli into the atmosphere.

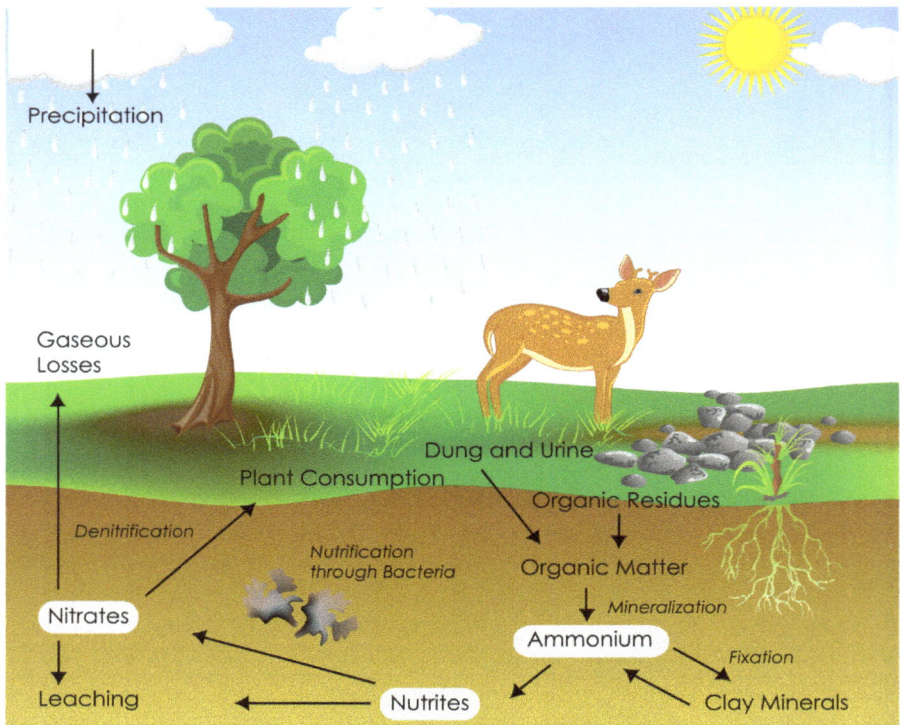

Nitrogen Cycle/Shutterstock/snapgalleria

The nitrogen cycle is one of the most important nutrient cycles found in ecosystems. Living organisms use nitrogen in the production of complex organic molecules like amino acids, proteins, and nucleic acids. The mass of nitrogen found in the atmosphere as a gas is about one million times larger than the nitrogen contained in living organisms. Nitrogen is often the most limiting nutrient for plant growth because most plants can only take up nitrogen in two solid forms: ammonium ion (NH_4^+) and the ion nitrate (NO_3^-). Animals receive the required nitrogen they need for metabolism, growth, and reproduction by the consumption of living or dead organic matter that contains material partially composed of nitrogen. The characteristic odor of animal flesh decay is caused by putrescence and cadaverine, which are breakdown products of the amino acids ornithine and lysine, respectively.

Nitrogen occurs in all organisms, primarily in amino acids, proteins, and in the nucleic acids DNA and RNA. The human body contains about three percent by weight of nitrogen, the fourth most abundant element in the body after oxygen, carbon, and hydrogen. It is a large component of animal waste (for example, guano) in the form of urea, uric acid, and ammonium compounds, which are valuable fertilizers. Nitrogen compounds were well known by the Middle Ages. Alchemists knew the mixture of nitric and hydrochloric acids, called aqua regia (royal water) could dissolve gold (the king of metals). Nitrogen compounds were used in saltpeter for gunpowder, and later as fertilizer. Nitrogen gas is used in beer due to the smaller bubbles it produces, which makes the beer smoother and headier.

When inhaled at pressures higher than four atmospheres nitrogen can act as an anesthetic agent causing nitrogen narcosis, a temporary semi-anesthetized state of mental impairment similar to that caused by nitrous oxide. Nitrogen also dissolves in the bloodstream and body fats. Rapid decompression in the case of divers ascending too quickly, or astronauts decompressing too quickly can lead to life threatening decompression sickness, formerly known as caisson sickness or the bends, when nitrogen bubbles form in the bloodstream, nerves, joints.

Nitrogenation (Nitrogenized)

During fermentation yeast in the brewing vat metabolizes sugars from the liquid (called wort or sweet barley tea) resulting in the production of alcohol and carbon dioxide. Before the beer is transferred from the fermentation vessels to a settling vessel called a bite tank it is force carbonated or nitrogenated, often to a ratio of thirty percent carbon dioxide and seventy percent nitrogen for canning or bottling. Carbon dioxide has traditionally been used as the infusion gas because of its high solubility in liquids, low expense, ready availability, and ease of use with relatively modest temperature and pressure requirements. Carbon dioxide in solution leads to the formation of carbonic acid which enhances an acidic taste.

The alternative of nitrogen-infused beverages originated in Ireland and historically included beer, ale, stout, and lager. The nitrogenation (nitrogenized) trend has increased in popularity, and advanced from large breweries to craft beers and coffee shops. Nitrogenated beer is beer that has been infused with a mixture of twenty-five to thirty percent carbon dioxide and seventy to seventy-five percent carbon dioxide. In the beer trade, they may be referred to as

'Nitrobrews'. Nitrogenated beer can be sold in kegs to pubs and bars, or in cans and bottles.

Carbonation with carbon dioxide results in larger bubbles and increased acidity with the formation of carbonic acid. Nitrogenization provides smaller longer lasting bubbles with enhanced mouthfeel, with a sweeter less acidic taste. Photo courtesy Deschutes Brewery, used with permission.

Nitrogenation does not have the carbonic acid generating properties of carbon dioxide and thus gives the beverage a sweeter taste. The poor solubility requires that it be placed under much greater atmospheric pressure requiring lower temperature and specialized equipment for infusion. The size of nitrogen bubbles is much smaller than carbon dioxide bubbles, and gives the beverage a much smoother, sweeter, and silkier texture, and a much longer lasting lush rich tasting froth head. The description of the beverage character called mouthfeel is considerably thicker and velvety with nitrogen than with carbon dioxide. The nitrogen infusion replacing the oxygen in the beverage also enhances stability with longer shelf life. It does so by preventing oxidation and thus slowing the degradation of organic compounds with bitter and sour tastes.

Nitrogenation has now become popular at coffee bars, giving coffee beverages a creamier and richer texture than regular cold brew coffee. Carbon dioxide was problematic with coffee because the carbonic acid production curdled any milk content and added to the acidic taste. Nitrogen bubbles are more stable than carbon dioxide bubbles, because the atmosphere is already about seventy-eight percent nitrogen reducing gas diffusion out of the bubbles. Carbon dioxide bubbles are short lived because the high concentration gradient of carbon dioxide inside the bubbles rapidly diffuse into the exposed air, which is less than one percent carbon dioxide. In order to serve nitrogenated beverages a more expensive mixed gas system and special faucet are required for high pressure of around thirty pounds per square inch. Nitrogenation in bottles and cans requires the presence of a small device called a widget that causes the nitrogen to form tens of thousands of fine bubbles upon opening and release of the high pressurization.

As predicted by the gas laws of physics the pressure and temperature of the beer will dictate the extent of the bubbling and head. The warmer the beverage temperature and the lower the atmospheric pressure the greater the bubbling. If you travel in an airplane the cabin pressure is usually reduced to the atmosphere pressure equivalent of eight thousand feet above sea level, and the excessive bubbling of carbonated soft drinks is very noticeable. The identical pressurized beverage will have a visibly greater effervescence and head if enjoyed in Denver, Colorado at an altitude one-mile-high, than at a sea level beach. A notable example of the reverse effect was a champagne celebration in a high atmospheric pressure deep sea diving chamber where everyone was disappointed that the champagne was flat without bubbles. They did not discover that the bubbles were suppressed by the high pressure of the chamber until they started their return to the surface and the bubbles reappeared with a vengeance inside their stomachs!

Olestra

Olestra is a fat, cholesterol, and calorie free fat substitute that offers the mouth feel of fat without its nutritional consequences. It has been used in the preparation of otherwise high-fat content snack foods such as potato chips since it gained Food and Drug Administration (FDA) approval for use as a replacement for fats and oils in 1996. A popular olestra containing snack named Wow became the source of reports of gastrointestinal complaints including oily anal leakage and pungent intestinal gas. Subsequent studies suggested the gastrointestinal side effects might have been due to excessive intake of the product. Consumer concerns contributed to prohibition of the use or sale of olestra products in the European Union and Canada.

Triglycerides consist of three fatty acids bonded to glycerol, which acts as its backbone. Olestra uses the sugar sucrose as its backbone and bonds between six to eight fatty acids in a radial arrangement. This makes the molecule too irregular and too sizable to be absorbed by the intestinal lining, and it passes through the gut undigested. As it is not absorbed, it has no nutritive or caloric value. Because it contains fatty acids it can absorb and carry fat-soluble vitamins such as Vitamins A, D, E, and K with it as it transits the gut. Most products containing olestra are fortified with lipid soluble vitamins because of this effect, which could otherwise lead to malabsorption of these necessary nutrients.

Orlistat

Orlistat is a pharmaceutical designed to treat obesity. In the United States it is marketed as a prescription drug under the trade name Xenical, and is sold over-the-counter as Alli. Orlistat is a local inhibitor of gastric and pancreatic lipases and prevents the hydrolysis of triglycerides into absorbable free fatty acids. The triglycerides are excreted undigested in the feces along with the orlistat, which is not absorbed systemically. Taken three times daily before meals it prevents approximately twenty-five percent of dietary fat from being absorbed, resulting in modest weight loss in conjunction with a reduced calorie diet.

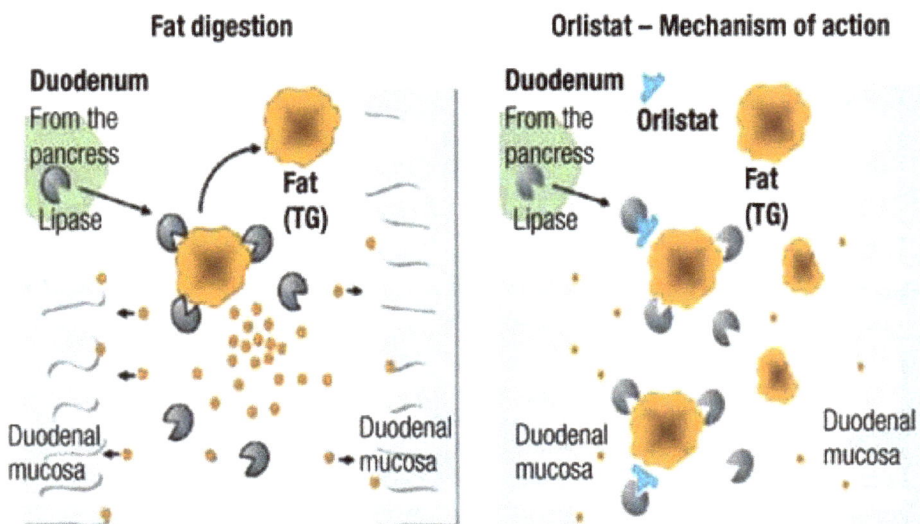

Creative Commons License

As expected with inhibition of fat absorption, Orlistat is notable for steatorrhea, oily, loose, and foul smelling stools. These decrease with time, especially with the learned aversion of fatty foods, one of the behavioral modifications that lead to the desired weight loss. Absorption of fat-soluble vitamins and other fat-soluble nutrients are inhibited by the use of orlistat. A multivitamin tablet containing vitamins A, D, E, K, and beta-carotene should be taken once a day as a supplement when using orlistat.

Oxygen

Oxygen is a chemical element with symbol O and atomic number eight that forms dioxygen a colorless odorless, and tasteless gas. It was mistakenly named Oxygen (the Greek ὀξύς (oxys) "acid", and γόνος (gonos) "producer"), by Antoine Lavoisier who thought that all acids required oxygen (they require hydrogen). It was discovered by Carl Scheele Sweden in 1773 but his publisher delayed publication for two years. This inadvertently allowed British clergyman Joseph Priestley, who independently discovered it a year later, to be given priority as its discoverer because his work was published first. Oxygen is a highly reactive element that forms compounds with most elements except the noble gases. Oxygen is a strong oxidizing agent and only fluorine has greater electronegativity. Oxygen is the third-most abundant element in the universe, after hydrogen and helium. On Earth's surface it is the most abundant element making up half of the earth's crust, and makes up nearly twenty-one percent of the air.

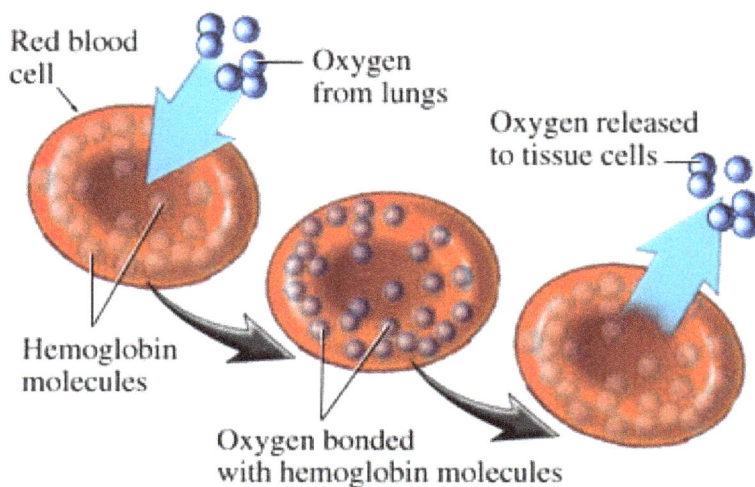

Red blood cell

Oxygen from lungs

Oxygen released to tissue cells

Hemoglobin molecules

Oxygen bonded with hemoglobin molecules

Oneminutecure.com Creative Commons License

For free dioxygen to remain in Earth's atmosphere it needs to be replenished by the photosynthetic action of cyanobacteria, algae and plants. Free elemental oxygen only began to accumulate in the atmosphere about two and one-half billion years ago with the Great Oxygenation Event. Towards the end of the Carboniferous period three hundred million years ago oxygen levels reached their highest levels of thirty-five percent and allowed insects to grow to a size with over a two-foot wingspan. One would suspect that a mosquito that size would cause a human to pass out from blood loss if there were any humans to bite back then.

Cold water holds more dissolved oxygen, which is the reason the polar waters support a much higher density of life then tropical waters. The marine Cyanobacteria and green algae generate up to seventy percent of the free oxygen produced on Earth. In humans and vertebrates, the O_2 changes the oxygen carrying hemoglobin to a bright red color. In mollusks and some arthropods like crabs, hemocyanin gives a deep blue color when oxygenated. Hemocyanin uses copper, which has only one quarter of the oxygen carrying capacity as the iron in hemoglobin. If an iron nail is allowed to rust it will gain weight as it demonstrates its oxygen binding.

Pancreas

The pancreas has several vital functions in the body, including the endocrine control of blood sugar (glucose) levels by its release of the hormones insulin and glucagon. It also releases a multitude of key enymes and their precursors called zymogens, that are utilized in the digestion of carbohydrates, proteins, and lipids. If the pancreas is diseased or injured the lack of glucose control can lead to diabetes mellitus, and the lack of digestive enzymes can lead to maldigestion and malabsorption. The lack of the lipid digesting enzymes such as lipase can lead to steatorrhea, a form of diarrhea caused by unabsorbed fats. It can also cause symptoms of excessive intestinal gas, with a pronounced foul odor due to the malabsorption of aromatic fatty acids.

Another important function of the pancreas, is the production of large volumes of a sodium bicaronate solution which neutralizes gastic (stomach) hydrochloric acid. The neutralization results in the production of water and large volumes of carbon dioxide gas. The gas production may contribute to the bloating and fullness common after a large meal. Since the carbon dioxide gas is readily absorbed by the small intestine it enters into solution in the bloodstream and is exhaled in the breath when it reachs the alveoli of the lungs. The pancreas was first identified by Herophilus (335–280 BC), a Greek anatomist and surgeon and named by Rufus of Ephesus, another Greek anatomist. Its name is derived from the Greek πᾶν ("all", "whole"), and κρέας ("flesh") because of its fleshy consistency. The pancreas, having two separate functions has distinct tissues for each. The exocrine function for producing digestive juices make up ninety-eight percent of the pancreas, but the two percent of tissue that is endocrine for hormone production is critical.

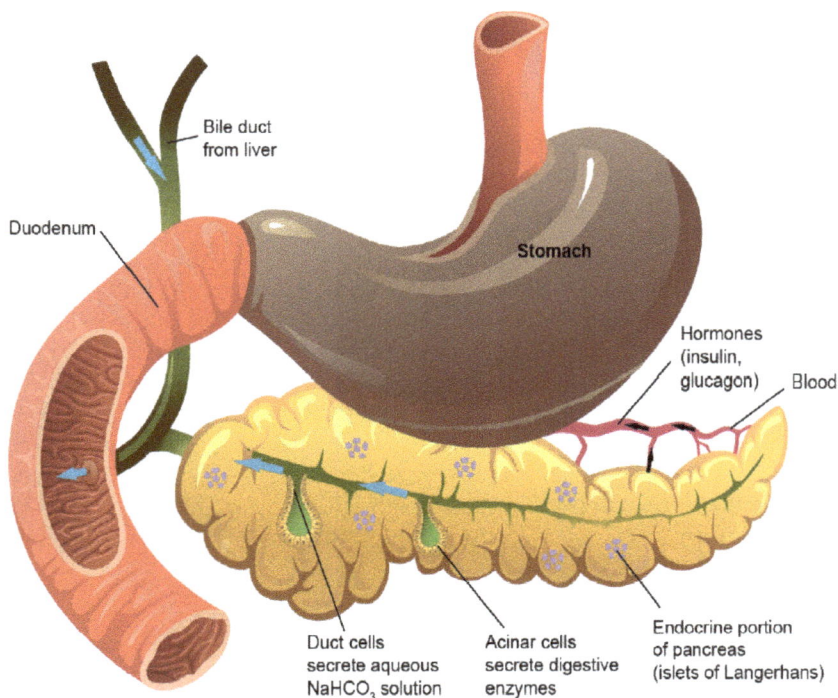

The endocrine tissue has approximately three million cell clusters called the islets of Langerhans, which are scattered throughout the pancreas, and on occasion in ectopic locations elsewhere in the body. They secrete the hormones insulin, glucagon, somatostatin, and pancreatic polypeptide directly into the bloodstream.

The exocrine pancreas secretes its digestive enzymes and juices into the gut via a system of ducts. The bile ducts and pancreatic ducts usually share a common duct with the sphincter of Oddi controlling the entry point into the duodenum. There are several important illnesses associated with the pancreas. Diabetes mellitus type 1 (Juvenile Diabetes) is a chronic autoimmune disorder in which the insulin secreting beta cells in the Islets of Langerhans are damaged and destroyed. Diabetes mellitus type 2 is common among overweight adults, reaching epidemic proportions because of the obesity prevalent in Western society. This development of insulin resistance in body tissues is best controlled with weight reduction, but oral medications are available if it has not progressed to a need for insulin itself.

Pancreatitis, inflammation of the pancreas is a dangerous condition in which activated pancreatic enzymes begin to auto-digest the organ. Gallstones and alcohol, particularly in excess, are the two most common causes. Pancreatic cancers unfortunately have a very high mortality rate and are predominately of the exocrine tissue. Pancreatic endocrine tumors are rare, usually benign, and can present with excess secretion of various hormones, which usually leads to their early detection and surgical cure. Cystic fibrosis is a genetic disorder which often demonstrates deficiency of pancreatic enzymes among its clinical manifestations. Commercial preparation of pancreatic enzyme replacement is available.

Pancreas, Insufficiency

Pancreatic enzyme replacement along with nutritional and vitamin supplements are commercially available over the counter as well as by prescription. Pancrease and lipase come in a variety of doses and potency and are usually very well tolerated. Exocrine pancreatic insufficiency is the lack of digestive enzymes normally produced by the pancreas leading to the inability to properly digest food. Cystic fibrosis and Shwachman-Diamond Syndrome with chronic pancreatitis are the most common causes in humans, and result from a progressive loss of the pancreatic acinar cells that produce digestive enzymes. This disease is also found frequently in dogs, especially the German Shepard breed, as an inherited disorder, and is caused by pancreatic acinar atrophy.

The deficiency of digestive enzymes leads to maldigestion and malabsorption of nutrients. The most sensitive and specific test is the measurement of fecal elastase, which can be done with a single stool sample. The condition is treated with commercially available pancreatic enzyme replacement products such as pancrealipase. They include pancreatic lipases to break down and digest lipids (fats), proteases to digest proteins, and amylases and carboxylases to digest carbohydrates into their smaller subunits which can then be absorbed by the gastrointestinal tract.

In dogs the cause of pancreatic insufficiency appears to be an inherited immune mediated pancreatitis. Symptoms begin to appear after eighty-five to ninety percent of the pancreas is unable to secrete its enzymes. The loss of digestive enzymes leads to maldigestion and malabsorption of lipids, proteins, carbohydrates, and vitamins. steatorrhea, and anemia. With the inability to digest lipids the fat rapidly transits the bowel leading to particularly foul smelling oily yellow-gray diarrhea called steatorrhea. In dogs poor hair coat is also noted. the best treatment is to supplement its food with dried pancreatic extracts. Symptoms usually improve within a few days but lifelong treatment is usually required.

Pancreas, Secretions

Pancreatic juice is a water solution of enzymes and electrolytes, primarily sodium bicarbonate. It neutralizes the acidic chyme to provide the optimal environment for activation of the pancreatic enzymes. The pancreatic enzymes are released in inactive form to prevent autodigestion and are activated in the lumen of the duodenum. Trypsinogen is activated to trypsin and procarboxypeptidase is activated to carboxypeptidase. Additional active pancreatic enzymes secreted include amylase, lipases, and nucleases. These enzymes require ions or bile for optimal activity.

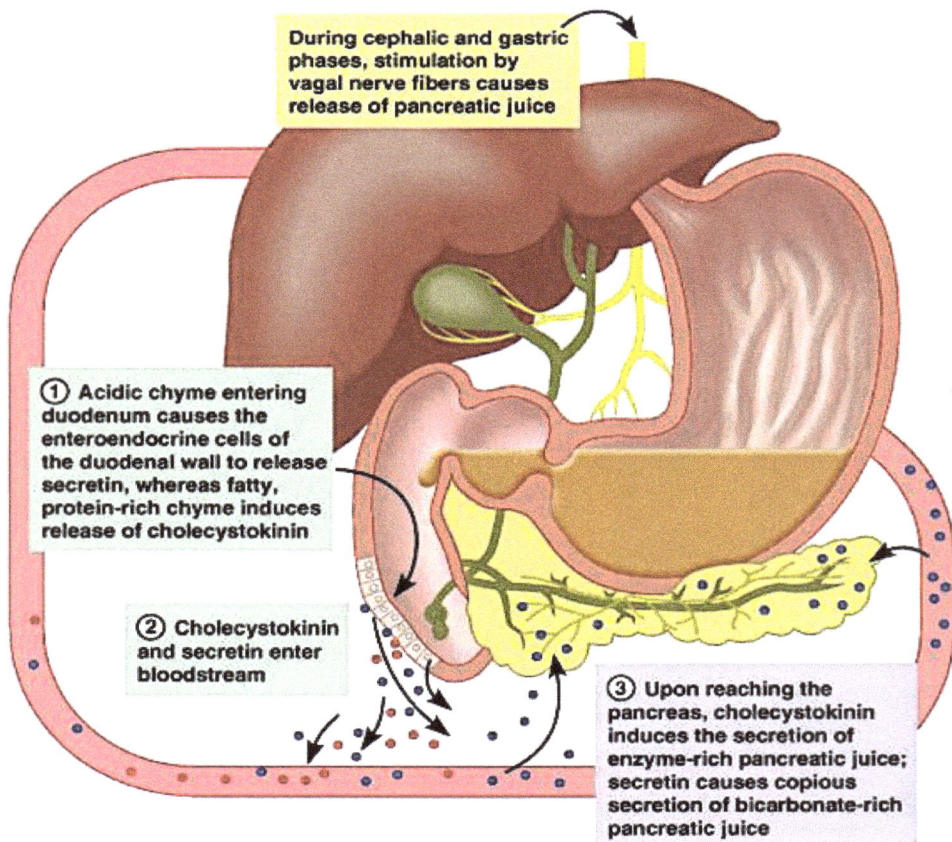

During cephalic and gastric phases, stimulation by vagal nerve fibers causes release of pancreatic juice

① Acidic chyme entering duodenum causes the enteroendocrine cells of the duodenal wall to release secretin, whereas fatty, protein-rich chyme induces release of cholecystokinin

② Cholecystokinin and secretin enter bloodstream

③ Upon reaching the pancreas, cholecystokinin induces the secretion of enzyme-rich pancreatic juice; secretin causes copious secretion of bicarbonate-rich pancreatic juice

Pancreatic juice secretion is regulated by the gastrointestinal hormones secretin and cholecystokinin (CCK), which are released when fatty, or acidic chyme enters the duodenum. CCK and secretin enter the bloodstream and upon reaching the pancreas, CCK induces the secretion of enzyme rich pancreatic juice. Secretin causes secretion of sodium bicarbonate rich pancreatic juice. Vagal nerve stimulation also causes the release of pancreatic juice. The pancreas synthesizes and secretes insulin, glucagon, pancreatic polypeptide, and somatostatin. It synthesizes and secretes about one and one-half liters of pancreatic juice per day. The alkaline juice neutralizes the gastric acid present in the duodenal chyme and contains enzymes for digesting proteins, fats and carbohydrates.

The pancreas is innervated by the parasympathetic vagus nerve that stimulate cholinergic neurons within the pancreas. Sympathetic nerve impulses inhibit and parasympathetic nerve impulses stimulate pancreatic juice secretion.
Acid in the duodenum below a pH of three triggers the hormone secretin to stimulate the release of large volumes of pancreatic juice, which is rich in sodium bicarbonate but low in pancreatic enzymes. Cells in the duodenum and proximal jejunum, in response to digestive products of fatty acids of between eight and ten carbon lengths and peptides rich in the amino acids phenylalanine and tryptophan, release CCK. It stimulates the acinar cells of the pancreas to secrete their zymogens, which are then converted to the active enzymes.

The cephalic phase of gastric acid secretion is stimulated by the visual, olfactory, gustatory, auditory, and tactile senses as well as cognition of food. Cholinergic fibers of the vagus nerve and enteric plexus mediate this phase through the secretion of acetylcholine. A decrease in the degree of stimulation of parasympathetic activity by vagotomy will block the cephalic phase response. The cephalic phase stimulates the pancreas to secrete sodium bicarbonate and pancreatic enzymes. The cephalic phase is about fifty percent of the pancreas maximal response when tested with the administration of intravenous CCK and secretin.

Parasite (see Microbiome, Pathogen)

Pathogen (see Microbiology, Microbiome)

In biology, a pathogen (Greek: πάθος pathos "suffering, passion" and -γενής -genēs "producer of") is a living agent that can produce disease. Typically, the term is used to describe an infectious agent such as a virus, bacterium, prion, fungus, protist, or parasite that causes disease in its host. The host may be a human, an animal, a plant, a fungus, or even another micro-organism. Although the vast majority of the millions of species of microbes are harmless or beneficial, a relatively small number can cause significant disease morbidity and mortality. Not to be underestimated, the relatively small number of pathogens infects billions of humans each year and leads to millions of deaths. Children, the elderly, and the immunocompromised are at highest risk. Transmission of pathogens occurs through many different routes, including airborne, direct or indirect contact, sexual contact, through blood, breast milk, or other body fluids, and through the fecal-oral route.

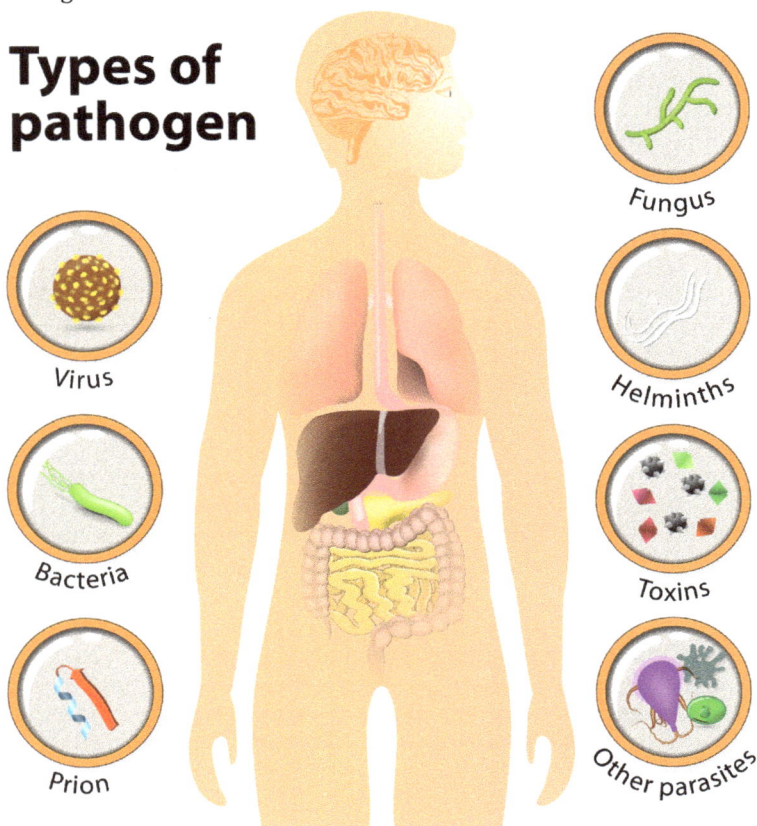

Shutterstock/designua

Bacteria

Bacteria are much smaller than the average human cell, and typically range between one and five micrometers in length. To put this size in perspective there are twenty-five thousand four hundred micrometers in one inch. In spite of this small size bacteria cause a high disease burden. Tuberculosis, caused by the bacterium *Mycobacterium tuberculosis* infects over two and one-half billion humans, one third of the human population. It kills about two million people a year, mostly in sub-Saharan Africa. Other pathogenic bacteria contribute to other globally important diseases, such as pneumonia, which can be caused by bacteria such as Streptococcus and Pseudomonas, and foodborne illnesses, which can be caused by bacteria such as *Shigella dysenteriae, flexneri, boydii, sonnei* (gastroenteritis), *Campylobacter jejuni, coli* (gastroenteritis), and *Salmonella enterica, bongori* (gastroenteritis). Pathogenic bacteria also cause infections such as *Clostridia tetani* (tetanus), *Salmonella typhi* (typhoid fever), *Corynebacterium diphtheriae* (diphtheria, *Treponema pallidum* (syphilis), and *Mycobacterium leprae* (leprosy).

Virus

Some of the diseases that are caused by virus pathogens include smallpox, influenza, mumps, measles, chickenpox, ebola, and rubella. Pathogenic viruses are diseases mainly those of the families of: Adenoviridae, Picornaviridae, Herpesviridae, Hepadnaviridae, Flaviviridae, Retroviridae, Orthomyxoviridae, Paramyxoviridae, Papovaviridae, Poliovirus, Rhabdoviridae, Togaviridae. Viruses are much smaller than bacteria and typically range between 20-300 nanometers in length. They are too small to be seen with a standard microscope that can visualize bacteria, and require scanning electron microscopes to be seen.

Fungus

Fungi comprise a eukaryotic kingdom of microbes that are usually saprophytes (consume dead organisms) but can cause diseases in humans, animals and plants. Fungi are the most common cause of diseases in crops and other plants. The typical fungal spore size is 1-40 micrometers in length.

Prion

Prions are infectious pathogens that do not contain nucleic acids. These abnormally folded proteins are found characteristically in some diseases such as scrapie, kuru, bovine spongiform encephalopathy (Mad Cow disease, and Creutzfeldt–Jakob disease.

Parasites

Billions of humans are infested and infected with parasites, frequently with multiple species. The highest incidence is in areas of limited access to clean water and food supplies and higher levels of poverty. Although parasites can be a major cause of disease morbidity and mortality, there is growing evidence that low grade parasite loads can offer humans survival advantages and disease prevention by manipulating the human immune response. The 'good hygiene hypothesis' suggests that the enhanced hygiene of western societies has reduced the exposure to parasites, with a resultant increase in allergies and immune modulated disorders associated with inflammation such as arthritis, heart disease, atherosclerosis, cancer, inflammatory bowel disease, and others.

The most common human parasites are classified as protist or helminth. Intestinal parasites are among the most common found in the human population and can arise with ingestion, skin exposure to contaminated soil, inhalation of aerosolized pathogens, transmission by insect vectors such as mosquitos, fleas, ticks, etc., sexual contact, and other avenues. Protist are single cell microscopic organisms and although the vast majority are not human parasites the species associated with human infection and disease include *Plamodium falciparum, vivax, ovale, malariae, knowlesi* (malaria), *Entamoeba histolytica* (amoebiasis, amoebic dysentery), *Giardia lamblia* (Giardiasis), *Trypanosoma brucei* (Trypanosomiasis African sleeping sickness), *Trypanosoma cruzi* (Chagas Disease), *Toxoplasma gondii* (Toxoplasmosis), *Leishmania donovani* (Leishmaniasis), *Babesia microti* (Babesiosis), *Cryptosporidium fragile, hominis, muris, parvum* (Cryptosporidiosis), *Cyclospora cayetanensis* (Cyclosporiasis), N*aegleria fowleri* (amoebic meningoencephalitis)

The term helminth is a generic term describing wormlike organisms. It is not considered a correct term in taxonomy, as it is not based on genetic or evolutionary characterization. It includes over one million widely divergent species. Common helminth parasites include *Ascaris lumbricoides* (Ascariasis), *Enterobius vermicularis* (enterobiasis, pinworm), *Strongyloides stercoralis* (Strongyloidiasis), *Toxocara canis, cati, leonina* (Toxocariasis), *Dracunculus medinensis* (Guinea Worm, Dracunculiasis), *Ancylostoma duodenale & Necator americanus* (Hookworm), *Taenia solium* (pork tapeworm), *Taenia saginata* (beef tapeworm), *Diphyllobothrium latum* (fish tapeworm), *Echinococcus multilocularis, granulosus, shiquicus* (echinococcosis, hydatid cyst disease), *Trichuris trichiura* (Whipworm), *Schistosoma mansoni, japanocum, haematobium, indicum* (Schistosomiasis), *Gnathostoma spinigerum, hispidum* (Gnathostomiasis), *Paragonimus westermani* (Paragonimiasis), *Fasciola hepatica* (Fascioliasis).

Pepsin, Pepsinogen

Pepsin (Greek - peptein: to digest) is a protease enzyme discovered in 1836 by Theodor Schwann, the first enzyme to be discovered. Pepsin is stored as the inactive zymogen pepsinogen in the chief cells so it does not digest the cell's own proteins. The hormone gastrin and the vagus nerve trigger the release of both pepsinogen and gastric hydrochloric acid when food is ingested. The pepsinogen released from the gastric chief cells is activated to pepsin by the hydrochloric acid released from the gastric parietal cells. Pepsin, chymotrypsin, and trypsin are the proteolytic enzymes that break protein down into the peptides and amino acids readily absorbed by the small intestine. Pepsin is inhibited by high pH and by feedback inhibitor compounds that are products of protein digestion. Commercial pepsin is extracted from pig stomachs and is a component of rennet used to curdle milk during the manufacture of cheese. Pepsi-Cola was originally formulated with pepsin and cola nuts.

Peristalsis

Peristalsis (Greek peri-, "around" and stallein, "to place") is the propulsive wave of muscular contraction and relaxation, which advances digestive material through the intestinal tract. Earthworms use a similar mechanism in their movement. The process of peristalsis is controlled by the medulla oblongata of the brainstem. Segmental contractions are used to mix the chime with digestive juices and enzymes, and to bring additional nutrient material in contact with the villi and microvilli of the small bowel mucosa. Digestive material is called chime, but the portion being advanced by peristalsis is often called a bolus. The peristaltic wave in the esophagus advances the bolus in a wave lasting less than ten seconds. In the small intestine peristaltic waves lasts for a few seconds and the bolus is advanced a few centimeters. It serves to mix the chyme as well as provide access to the villi and microvilli of the intestinal lining as digestion and absorption of nutrients occurs during the transit through the small intestine.

Migrating motor complexes (MMC) are waves of gastric emptying followed by peristaltic activity that sweep through the stomach and small intestines in between meals. They each last for a moment or two and occur in a cyclic pattern several times an hour, advancing any remaining food residue or chyme through the small intestine into the colon. The maintenance of regular peristaltic activity during meals, and intermittently during fasting, is also thought to prevent the migration of colonic bacteria into the terminal Ileum. The hormone motilin triggers the migrating motor complexes, as can motilin like agonists such as the antibiotic erythromycin. The at times audible borborygmi from the migrating motor complexes are also referred to as stomach rumbles or growls, and are also commonly thought of as hunger pains since the cramps occur during a fasting state.

Muscular contractions of digestive tract (peristalsis)

www.healthcentral.com Creative Commons License

Gastrointestinal motility is under the control of local enteric neurons that coordinate intestinal motility. Cholinergic neurons cause asynchronous contraction and shortening of the circular muscle layer, shortening of longitudinal muscle, and distension of the intestine. As chyme enters the duodenum, carbohydrates and proteins are only partially digested, and limited fat digestion has taken place with the salivary and gastric lipases. Digestion continues in the small intestine where hypertonic chyme has a low acidic pH before being neutralized by sodium bicarbonate, and mixing is required for the enzymes and substrates to interact.

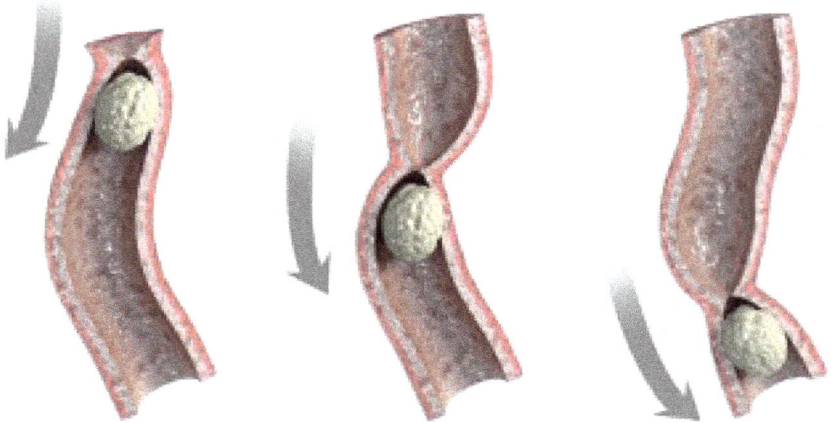

The most common motion of the small intestine is the motility action called segmentation. It is initiated by intrinsic pacemaker cells (Cajal cells) with the segmentation mixing the contents while peristaltic activity moves the bolus distally towards the ileocecal valve.

After the bulk of the nutrients have been absorbed the gastroileal reflex and the hormone gastrin relax the ileocecal sphincter and allow chyme to pass into the large intestine. The colon absorbs the water and electrolytes from the still liquid chyme that is increasingly solidified by water absorption as it transits the large intestine. The colon also serves to absorb nutrients, vitamins, and metabolites produced by the gut microbiome. The vitamins absorbed include Vitamin K, Vitamin B_{12}, thiamine, and riboflavin. Haustral contractions are slow segmenting movements that move the contents of the colon by peristaltic activity towards the rectum. The haustra sequentially contract as they are stimulated by distension. The defecation reflex is triggered by distention of rectal walls by feces. When stimulated the defecation reflex contracts the rectal walls and relaxes the internal anal sphincter. Voluntary signals stimulate relaxation of the external anal sphincter and defecation occurs.

The transit time is the general period of time it takes, from the swallow of ingestion to the elimination at defecation, for food to pass through the gastrointestinal track. Normal ranges are from half a day to two days but individuals vary. Certain conditions especially those with diarrhea may have a more rapid transit time, while those with neurologic conditions or diabetes mellitus may have a slow transit time. Diabetics are particularly prone to a condition called gastroparesis diabeticorum, where the delay is primarily in gastric emptying. Although it is not uncommon to see certain undigested foods passed, like kernels of corn, more undigested foods may be seen with a rapid gut transit time.

Personalized Medicine

As with all issues of health and wellness each person needs to be assessed individually. With the advances in the human genome project it is now recognized that it is not just the genetic blueprint in the DNA that makes up the individuals uniqueness. Although humans have approximately twenty-three thousand genes, these genes are also controlled by external factors in a process described as epigenetics. It is also now recognized that the human body is in essence more than just human cells. The human system includes the microbiome, the microorganisms that live on and within us. The gut-brain-microbiome-food axis demonstrates the intimate interconnectivity of these four elements. If one were to analyze the human system by the number of cells, a human is comprised of approximately ten percent human cells and ninety percent microbial cells. If one were to analyze the system on the basis of the number of genes, humans are approximately one percent human genes and ninety-nine percent microbial jeans.

The era of personalized medicine will advance the understanding of both health and disease. The previous approach of using population based medicine will be abandoned as technology and bioinformatics allows treatments to be specifically tailored to the individual's genome, microbiome, and metabolome. The effectiveness of therapy should increase dramatically along with a significant reduction in adverse reactions to medications. This approach will also avoid the time and monetary expense of medications that did not provide a benefit, even if fortunately they did not cause an adverse reaction. In the interval, as these advances are being brought into clinical practice it remains the best approach to tailor the treatment plan to the individual. What works for one may not work for another. Until the science and technology sufficiently evolve it often takes a trial and error approach to find the best treatment approach for the individual. And it is the individual who can be the only judge if the treatment is successful, or if the search for a solution must continue.

Physics

The laws and principles of physics apply to living as well as inanimate systems. An understanding of these principles explains many natural phenomena that are otherwise a source of mystery and confusion. When it comes to intestinal gas in particular, understanding the gas laws goes a long way in helping to manage this very common concern. Using Boyle's law, you can calculate into how much the volume the gas will compress as you go deeper underground or underwater. You can likewise calculate how much a gas will expand, as you go higher in altitude and the atmospheric pressure decreases. Using Charles Law, you can calculate what happens to the gas in a cold drink when it is swallowed and then expands as it is raised to body temperature.

Boyle's Law

Creative Commons License

Charles's Law

-10 ℃   250 ℃

Creative Commons License

Pneumaturia

The release of air bubbles from the urethra, most often in the urinary stream, is an unusual occurrence but may occur with development of a fistula, an abnormal passageway, between the bladder and vagina, colon, or rectum. Potential causes include inflammatory bowel disease, diverticular disease, trauma, inflammation, cancer, or infection. If the air passage is from the bowel it may have the characteristic feculent odor of flatus.

Prebiotic

Prebiotics are foods or products that support and encourage a healthy gut flora and microbiome. They typically have a high content of non-digestible material such as fiber. They are often utilized along with probiotics, which are the live organisms themselves, which are being introduced into the gut to establish themselves as part of the gut flora. Prebiotics are non-digestible food ingredients that stimulate the growth and/or activity of bacteria in the digestive system in ways claimed to be beneficial to health. They were first identified and named by Marcel Roberfroid in 1995. A prebiotic is a non-digestible selectively fermented food ingredient that promotes the populations and activity of bifidobacteria, lactic acid bacteria, and other beneficial species in the gut microbiome.

Top 10 Foods Containing Prebiotics	
Food	**Prebiotic Fiber Content by Weight**
Raw Chicory Root	64.6%
Raw Jerusalem Artichoke	31.5%
Raw Dandelion Greens	24.3%
Raw Garlic	17.5%
Raw Leek	11.7%
Raw Onion	8.6%
Cooked Onion	5%
Raw Asparagus	5%
Raw Wheat bran	5%
Whole Wheat flour, Cooked	4.8%
Raw Banana	1%

Food	Amount of food to achieve 6 g serving of prebiotics
Raw Chicory Root	9.3 g (0.33 oz)
Raw Jerusalem Artichoke	19 g (0.67 oz)
Raw Dandelion Greens	24.7 g (0.87 oz)
Raw Garlic	34.3 g (1.21 oz)
Raw Leek	51.3 g (1.81 oz)
Raw Onion	69.8 g (2.46 oz)
Cooked Onion	120 g (4.2 oz)
Raw Asparagus	120 g (4.2 oz)
Raw Wheat Bran	120 g (4.2 oz)
Whole Wheat Flour, Cooked	125 g (4.4 oz)
Raw Banana	600 g (1.3 lb)

Dietary sources include soybeans, Jerusalem artichoke, jicama, chicory root, raw oats, unrefined wheat, unrefined barley, onion, asparagus, banana, raw wheat bran, leek, garlic, dandelion greens, and yacon. Examples of prebiotics include inulin, galactooligosaccharide, fructooligosaccharide, xylooligosaccharides, polydextrose, lactulose, and tagatose. The sudden addition of substantial quantities of any product to the diet, including prebiotics, may result in an increase in gas, bloating, or change in bowel movements.

"Short-chain" prebiotics like oligofructose contain fewer links per saccharide molecule. They are fermented more quickly during transit through the gastrointestinal tract and have most of their activity in the ascending colon. Longer-chain prebiotics like inulin, contain more links per saccharide molecule and are fermented more slowly with their activity predominantly in the descending colon. Oligofructose-Enriched Inulin, the prebiotic on which most research is based, is designed to provide a full spectrum of chain lengths providing activity throughout the colon.

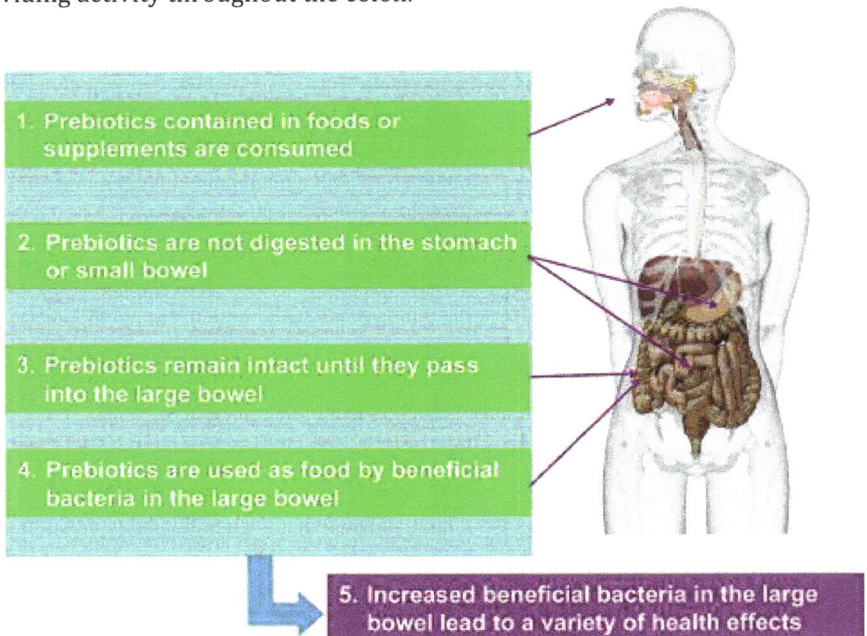

1. Prebiotics contained in foods or supplements are consumed

2. Prebiotics are not digested in the stomach or small bowel

3. Prebiotics remain intact until they pass into the large bowel

4. Prebiotics are used as food by beneficial bacteria in the large bowel

5. Increased beneficial bacteria in the large bowel lead to a variety of health effects

e-brainpages.com/types Creative Commons License

Lactulose is a synthetic prebiotic non-digestible disaccharide of fructose and galactose that remains undigested until it reaches the large intestine. In the colon beneficial bacteria like Bifidobacteria and Lactobacilli ferment and metabolize lactulose to produce short-chain fatty acids. It is an osmotic laxative that increases stool volume and gas, and shortens transit time. Lactulose is sold over the counter in most countries in the world. In the United States and Austria, it requires a prescription. Common side effects are abdominal cramping, borborygmus, gas, and diarrhea.

Inulins are prebiotic oligosaccharides from plants that have nutritional value as carbohydrates. They are polymers of the plant sugar fructose known as fructans. Chicory roots and Jerusalem artichokes have high concentrations of inulin and frequently are used as its commercial source. With its natural sweetness and its value as a mixable and smooth flowing prebiotic fermentable fiber, it is often used to replace sugar, fat, and flour in powdered nutritional supplements. Inulin contains only a fraction of the calories of another carbohydrate or fat. It is fermented and metabolized by the gut microbiome into short-chain fatty acids, which have anti-inflammatory properties as well as the ability to increase absorption of calcium, magnesium, and iron, metabolizes it. Inulin provides additional benefits by promoting Lactobacillus and Bifidobacterium populations in the gut flora.

Prion (see Microbiome, Pathogen)

Probiotics

Probiotics (Latin pro "for" and Greek βίος bios, "life") are live microorganisms that colonize the gastrointestinal tract and may provide a health benefit. Lactic acid bacteria (LAB) and bifidobacteria are the most common types of microbes used as probiotics. In 1935 certain strains of *Lactobacillus acidophilus* were found to be very active when implanted in the human digestive tract. Werner Kollath first introduced the term probiotics in 1953. Popular commercially available fermented dairy products and fortified foods may contain live probiotic cultures. Freeze dried cultures are available in capsules and powders.

Milk fermented lactic acid bacteria are known to inhibit the growth of proteolytic bacteria because of the acidic environment they create. Russian scientist and Nobel laureate Élie Metchnikoff advocated a sour milk and yogurt diet early in the twentieth century because of his observations that populations who regularly consumed fermented dairy products had unusual longevity. As a professor at the Pasteur Institute in Paris he proposed that the gut flora be replaced with lactobacillus to prevent proteolytic 'intestinal auto-intoxication' that he believed led to aging and a shorter life span.

Certain probiotic strains digest lactose providing a benefit to the lactose intolerant. Other probiotic strains can also synthesize Vitamin K, folic acid, and Vitamin B_{12}, which can be beneficial. The other health claims are heavily marketed and have led to dramatic probiotic sales growth even though the claims have not passed the regulatory scrutiny of the U. S. Food and Drug Administration or European Food Safety Authority. Global sales of probiotics have exceeded twenty billion dollars a year with the marketplace growing twenty percent a year as well. Over three thousand species of beneficial bacteria have been identified in the gut flora. The use of probiotics concomitantly with antibiotics when they are required has reduced the incidence of antibiotic associated diarrhea by over forty percent. Research into the potential health effects of probiotics has accelerated and science based knowledge will hopefully soon replace unsupported marketing claims.

Shutterstock/niloo

Yogurt is a popular probiotic product. The label live and active cultures is placed on yogurt by the National Yogurt Association to certify that you are eating real, fresh yogurt with at least ten million organisms per gram at the time of manufacture. Some yogurts are pasteurized which destroys all of the microorganisms including the beneficial ones, but extends the product's shelf life. The most common organisms are *Lactobacillus bulgaricus*, *Lactobacillus gasseri*, *Streptococcus thermophilus*, and *Bifidobacterium bifidus*. These are lactic acid producing bacteria that can ease lactose intolerance, enhance immunity, reduce cholesterol, and may serve as anti-carcinogens. Besides yogurt other popular foods that have probiotic benefits include soft fermented cheeses like Gouda, fermented soybean paste soups like Miso, unpasteurized pickled foods like sauerkraut and Kimchi, sourdough breads, buttermilk, acidophilus milk, Kefir, tempeh, and others.

To put probiotics in perspective, it is important to have a clear understanding of the human microbiome. The microbiome is the world of microorganisms, too small to be seen with the naked eye, that exist in our environment, as well as on, in, and within our body tissue. The fact that we are surrounded by and immersed in a world of microbes has been known for a long time. What is new and surprising is the revelation that we are much more interdependent with the microbiome than science and medicine ever knew or believed.

The most remarkable finding is that the human body and its microbiome are in nearly constant communication with each other. It would not be an overstatement to describe these discoveries as revolutionary, and our understanding of health and disease is being dramatically altered. In fact, even how we consider what it means to be human, and the nature of our body, is being revised and redefined. But before we explore our relationship with the microbiome in detail, let's get some more background information, and start by taking a closer look at where microbes are within the remarkable evolutionary diversity of life on our planet Earth. The forms of life on the planet range from the simplest organisms of a single cell or less, to multicellular organisms of increasing complexity and size. There are also a variety of major life forms that were previously classified as Kingdoms, ranging from the commonly known plants, animals, fungi, bacteria, viruses, and protozoans. Over the last few decades' scientific advances have also identified new life forms including the controversial prions that are the cause of exotic diseases such as mad-cow disease (Bovine Spongiform Encephalopathy) and kuru. Even more surprising has been the discovery of a new life form called Archaea (Latin for 'ancient one'). The reason this was such an unexpected discovery is that they are in fact commonplace, and thrive in places where life was not even thought possible.

One of the reasons they were not recognized, even though found in abundance, was that their external appearance is similar to bacteria. It was only with the advent of genomic sequencing that it was recognized that Archaea were not just a little bit different than bacteria, but so totally different that it appears as if they came from an alien planet. As strange as that thought might sound, there is a field of science called astrobiology that theorizes that that is exactly what happened. Archaea live and thrive within fuming volcanic vents, boiling hot springs, even deep inside of rocks mined miles underground. They have been transported to outer space and lived and thrived when left exposed to the unearthly vacuum outside of the International Space Station. Because they survive and thrive in extreme environments, they have been designated as extremophiles (Latin - loving extremes).

As you may recall from the theory of evolution, developed by Charles Darwin and others, life began on the planet Earth from the simplest of organisms, to single and then multicellular organisms of increasing complexity. From submicroscopic viruses and prions that can only be visualized with extraordinarily powerful electron microscopes to enormous individual plants and fungi that literally stretch for miles, the abundance of life diversity on the planet is astounding. It is a testament to the miracle of life, and the power of evolution and genetics, that all living things on the planet are distant relatives, all arising as the progeny of the very first single organism. Over the millions of years of evolution, you should not be surprised that you do not recognize your one-billionth cousin, one million times removed.

Probiotic Benefits

ACIDOPHILUS AND OTHER PROBIOTIC BACTERIA SECRETE: ANTIVIRAL ANTIBACTERIAL AND ANTIFUNGAL CHEMICALS.

PROBIOTICS FORM A PHYSICAL BARRIER TO HINDER INVASION OF BACTERIA AND YEASTS

PROBIOTICS LIKE ACIDOPHILUS CREATE AN ACIDIC MICROENVIRONMENT WHICH PROMOTES IRON AND OTHER MINERAL ABSORBTION.

C.H. Hassell www.drhassell.com Used with permission

Even if you restrict your consideration to life forms that are visible to us, the diversity of appearance and activities is staggering. Humans as a species are very sensitive to physical appearance, both as a social as well as a biological consideration. Numerous studies show that our preferences for mate selection are highly driven by physical appearance. This is partly based on appearance correlating to physical and mental health, and the ability to provide support and protection. Although we have great variability in skin, hair, eye, nose, ears, height, weight, etcetera, we are virtually the same genetically. Even one of our closest evolutionary relatives, the chimpanzee, has ninety-nine percent genetic similarity to humans.

Humans are one of the largest animals in physical size. Of course we are relatively small compared to blue whales and elephants, but compared to a mouse or ants we are gigantic. There's an even more heavily populated much smaller world, invisible to the naked eye, which contains microbes. Seen by humans only with the assistance of a microscope, their invisible individual presence has a profound effect on our health and wellness. Its ability to overwhelm an organism many times its size is partly due to its rapid rate of reproduction.

The population pattern displayed by microbes, as well as other cells, is known as exponential or logarithmic growth. One cell divides and become two cells, the two cells divide and become four, the four become eight, and so forth. The power of exponential growth is often underestimated. A side story of the development of the game of chess will serve as an excellent demonstration. When the inventor of the game presented it to his King as a gift hundreds of years ago, the king was so grateful for the gift that he asked the inventor what he would like in return. The inventor asked the king for one grain of rice to be awarded him for the first square of the chessboard, two grains of rice for the second square, and each subsequent square to be given twice the amount of rice awarded for the square before. There are sixty-four squares on the chessboard and the sequence of doubling would begin with the series of numbers 1, 2, 4, 8, 16, 32, 64, 128, 256, 512, etcetera.

After the first ten squares had been added up that was less than one thousand grains of rice, and the King said he would grant him what he requested, and he was surprised that the inventor was not so smart after all and asked for such a small reward. What the King did not recognize about the power of exponential growth bankrupted his kingdom. By the time the numbers had finished doubling on the sixty-fourth square the king owed the inventor eighteen quintillion grains of rice, a number with eighteen zeros, 18,000,000,000,000,000,000! The rice would have covered the entire continents of Asia and Europe, and there was not that much rice in the entire world.

Although the microbes are diminutive in size, they are metabolically active and their impact is magnified because of their enormous populations. The entire human population of the Earth is under eight billion. If you pick up a handful of soil you pick up an entire world with more microbes than the earthly human population. You have also given those microbes an experience of an earthquake of astronomical proportions! Now put them down gently, and savor an instance of power that few mortals have ever experienced and appreciated.

It should not surprise you that your skin has microbes on it; after all it is exposed to the external environment. What might surprise you are the variety and population numbers of microbes that consider your skin home. When the microbes on or in the body have established themselves as residents they are considered the microbiome, the microbial populations in that environment. If you have not heard of the term microbiome before, please add it to your vocabulary now; you will be hearing a lot more about it over the years to come.

The skin microbiome is just one of the many microbiomes of the body, and one of the most accessible. When you bathe, shower, or wash your hands you remove many of these microbes, but a sizable population remain and have made you their permanent home. Don't be upset with them however, as they are actually providing you with a valuable service in exchange for your hospitality. The vast majorities of microbes are actually beneficial to humans, and live with us in a relationship described in biological terms as symbiotic when they provide a benefit, and commensal when they do not provide a benefit but at the same time do no harm. When microbes go badly in their guest relationship with humans we describe them as pathogens. Just like plants, where the majority of plants are beneficial or do no harm, and there are just a few harmful ones like poison ivy, the microbial pathogens are very few in number.

Kimchi, a probiotic food/Shutterstock/Foodio

The skin has different features and characteristics dependent on body location, and the microbiome is unique to each area as well. Various skin products including soaps with anti-microbial activity, lotions, massage oils, as well as swimming, bathing, clothing, and other environmental factors can influence the skin microbiome. Various oils and botanicals applied in massage and skin therapy undoubtedly affect the skin microbiome, as well as being absorbed systemically. The skin is considered one of the largest organs of the body, and its large surface area serves as both protection as well as access to the environment. Skin exposure to toxins and pollutants can lead to illness, and likewise the skin can be the mode of application of remedies and beneficial products.

Although the skin was originally thought to have the larger surface area, it is actually the digestive tract surface area that is by far and away the largest. If you were to flatten out the villi, the finger like projections of the gut lining, and the microvilli, the microscopic finger like projections that cover each villus, the surface area of the gut exceeds that of championship tennis court. As Mark Twain once famously described Switzerland, it would be a large country if they ever flattened out their mountains.

What many people find surprising is that the intestinal tract, normally considered an internal organ, is actually an external organ just like the skin as far as the body is concerned. The reason for this 'inside out' logic is that the external environment continues all the way through the gut, from mouth to anus. The material within the digestive tract is considered outside of the body until it is absorbed through the intestinal lining. Because this is a potential source of infection and allergies, the body has a powerful and vigilant immune system that is extremely active in the gut. As you can imagine, a lot of microbes live in the mouth, between the teeth, under the gums, in the nasal passages, etcetera. A large number of microbes entered your mouth on the surface or within the food you ate, joining with the microbes who have already established this part of your body as their permanent home. These microbes are feasting on small particles of food and debris left over from the chewing process, even when you brush and floss well.

The microbes in the mouth and within the food are regularly swallowed and travel down the digestive tract on an amazing voyage that would make any theme park ride pale in comparison. For many of the bacteria this is a nightmare journey at the ends of their lives, and for others it is the equivalent of being transported to heaven. The microbes making this journey contribute to the gut microbiome, which is the largest microbiome of the body, numbering over one hundred trillion organisms. This astronomical number is greater than the number of stars in the universe, and collectively weighs in at about three pounds.

Measured by cell populations the average human is ten percent human cells and ninety percent microbial cells. If you look at a more important factor, gene activity, the human genome has about twenty-five thousand genes, and the microbiome well in excess of a million, making us only one percent human by gene count. The gut microbiome is much more than just fermenting or metabolizing food products our own intestinal tract cannot digest. Amazingly, the gut microbiome engages in an active two-way communication with the human brain, and through epigenetics with every aspect of the human experience.

Communication is one of the hallmarks of higher animals, and language has traditionally been thought to be a uniquely human trait. Science is exploring the communication of other animals and it appears that they also use language of a limited vocabulary that is primarily used to warn of danger. More research is ongoing into the modes of communication of other animals, from the vocalization of whales that communicate over distances of many miles at sea, to the recently discovered elephant communication at extremely low frequency below the range of human hearing.

Humans and other species frequently communicate, as we do routinely with pets. This is especially clear when cats command their human servants to feed them. From dog whisperers and trainers, to the simple dog facial expressions of joy and remorse, nonverbal communication is a regular occurrence. Even plants communicate with each other, often through the air by releasing volatile chemical messengers warning of pathogens and danger. In the case of the microbiome, the communication takes place in the common language of most living organisms, chemical neurotransmitters, hormones, and metabolites. This is a language the microbes, body, and brain instantly recognize and understand. The gut microbiome weighs in at about three pounds, roughly the same weight as the human brain, and interestingly enough, is part of what is now commonly known as the 'second brain' comprised of the gut-microbiome-brain axis. This 'second brain' is adding a scientific understanding to what has commonly been described as gut feelings or gut instincts.

TOP 10 PROBIOTIC FOODS TO ADD TO YOUR DIET

 1 YOGURT

 2 MISO SOUP

 3 MICOALGAE

 4 KEFIR

 5 KOMBUCHA

 6 PICKLES

 7 SAUERKRAUT

 8 POI

 9 KIMCHI

 10 TEMPEH

Shutterstock/Kninwong

The digestive tract can be thought of as the opposite of an assembly line, as the food is broken down into its basic parts for ease of absorption and metabolism. As efficient as the digestive tract is, a large portion of the energy stored in food is not processed and metabolized by the human system. Undigested food travels through the intestinal tract and is often fermented and metabolized by our allies in the gut microbiome. These microbes have the ability to digest and metabolize the food content we cannot, and release absorbable nutrients for our benefit as well as waste products for elimination. A number of these metabolites, such as Vitamin K, cannot be produced by humans yet are critical for our survival. It is not an understatement to say that the gut microbiome is as much a benefit to us, as we are to it by providing it with a home and nourishment.

The nerve cells and fibers within the digestive tract are known as the enteric nervous system. It is directly connected to the brain and spinal cord of the central nervous system. The vagus nerve, autonomic, sympathetic, and parasympathetic nervous systems are all intimately interconnected. What many people find surprising is the degree of gut involvement with the two major neurotransmitters of the human body. It is impressive that fifty percent of the dopamine in the body is found in the brain, and the other fifty percent in the gut. What is particularly striking is that only five percent of the serotonin of the body is found in the brain, and the other ninety-five percent is found in the gut. There are over thirty active neurotransmitters found throughout the enteric nervous system. With further exploration of the remarkable enteric nervous system, perhaps we will need to reconsider what is considered the second brain and what is the first brain.

The populations and varieties of organisms in the gut microbiome is staggering. The advances in the field of genomics now allows for the identification of organisms that were previously hidden from view or simply unknown. Before this technology, the number of species of microbes in the human intestine was thought to number a few dozens. To date over five thousand different species have been identified, and some scientists expect the number may reach a million or more before the counting is complete. The populations and diversity vary by location within the gut, as well as age, diet, and a multitude of other factors. Much like a fingerprint, it appears that the gut microbiome may be unique for each individual. It is also clear that the gut microbiome can be disrupted by illness, change in diet, and in particular following the ingestion of antibiotics.

Besides the important role in digestion and fermentation of food content, the microbiome plays a critical role in metabolism. The microbes generate metabolites that can serve as neurotransmitters, hormones, and other products that have bioactive properties. When the microbes in the intestinal tract create them, the absorptive process brings them from the external environment of being inside the lumen of the tube of the digestive tract, into the cells and circulation of the body. When a blood specimen is analyzed using genomic sequencing scientists were surprised to find that twenty percent of the metabolites in the circulation were of microbial origin. The interplay within the gut, microbiome, and brain is striking, but one of the most surprising findings is the direction of communication. Although we like to think our brains are in charge, the vast majority of communication was not from the brain to the gut, but in the other direction!

The influence of the diet on the microbiome is profound, and is perfectly logical. Much like us, the microbes rely on the human diet for all of their nutritional needs. A good portion of the diet we ingest is actually not digestible by humans, such as the fiber often found in plant based foods. Although they are not digestible by us, they are digestible by microbes and are critical for their health and survival. As we are just as dependent on a healthy gut microbiome, the nutrients needed by the microbes, known as prebiotics, are critical for our welfare as well. One of the more interesting findings of microbiome research was that the microbes might actually be influencing our dietary behavior, much like sending our brains a shopping list of what they would like to be on the menu. Some peculiar dietary habits such as a craving to eat non-edible products such as dirt, starch, paper, etcetera are described as a pica, and may be influenced by the microbiome. It is somewhat similar to cravings during a pregnancy, where a strong stimulus creates a dietary diversion for pickles. One curious aside is that traditional pickles, sauerkraut, and the Korean fermented cabbage kimchi are very rich in healthful probiotics.

Prebiotics are not typically considered nutritive for humans, but are definitely so for the microbes. Even though they may carry labels saying they are calorie free, that may no longer be true once the microbes are finished with them. For example, if you were to eat hay or grass the cellulose of the plant would not be digestible because humans do not have the necessary enzyme called cellulase to break it down into absorbable sugars. Horses, cows, and sheep have this enzyme as well as a ruminant digestive tract that can process that form of diet into absorbable simple sugars by microbial fermentation. When we eat prebiotic fiber (do pass on the hay) the microbes ferment and digest it into simpler sugars that we can absorb as calories. So even though on paper we cannot digest it, thus allowing it to be labeled as zero calories, the microbes may not have read the label and provide us with calories we may not have counted on.

The field of genomics and the microbiome is expanding very rapidly. We are just beginning to identify and understand which organisms may be associated with various conditions of good or ill health. The concept of systems biology describes complex organisms with a multitude of variables, such as humans. There are so many variables it is unlikely for the remaining unexplained diseases to be caused by a single microbe pathogen, like past discoveries salmonella, shigella, or cholera. It is much more likely to be a combination of various factors such as genetics, environment, diet, activity, hormones and a host of other factors. When it comes to the input from the microbiome it will most likely be from a variety of microbes interacting with each other in the proper proportions to have a recipe or formula for optimal health, or when out of balance for illness and disease. The use of genomics and systems biology will hopefully allow the implementation of personalized precision medicine where diet, microbiome, and prescription medicine can be individualized for optimal outcome.

As we are still discovering previously unidentified microbial species in the gut microbiome, the balances of species mix and proportions for optimal health are not known. We also realize that the proper balance will be different for each individual based on his or her genomics, epigenetics, immunity, previous illnesses, activity, medications, etcetera. As much as one would like to know what the optimal probiotic to take as a supplement is, the science has not yet provided an answer. When science does not provide a clear answer, health concerns and products meet in the marketplace with confusion, misinformation, and big business to promote a new industry. The probiotic industry has arrived, for better or for worse, but mostly for the better.

There is a long history of experience with a number of the probiotics that are most popular today. The long track record, documented scientific research identifying benefits, apparent lack of adverse reactions, and millions of consumers self-reporting benefits who continue to use these products is more than sufficient evidence for an individual to consider a trial to see the response. An important point to remember is that each individual is unique. There are tremendous variations in our genetic makeup, environmental exposures, existing microbiomes, medical history, and dozens of other variables that may confound our response to individual probiotics. While there may be some general categories of probiotics that have benefits, the identification of the ideal microbiome for each individual is still some time off in the future. The research into identification of the organisms of the microbiome is still in its infancy. Their association with health and disease, as individual organisms and in combinations with others, will be assessed over the years to come as many such studies are just beginning.

The selection of the right probiotic, or mix of probiotics, for a general population is as challenging as being asked to select a perfume or cologne that is right for a large community of individuals. The answer is that most of the population will do well with certain base fragrances such as jasmine or musk, but the concentration of the essence, and the final aroma is dependent on the other ingredients and the chemistry of the individual. With that general disclaimer, there are a number of probiotics that contain microbes generally thought to be beneficial to human health.

The pioneer in the effort to identify the optimal organism of the gut microbiome was Ukrainian scientist Élie Metchnikoff) (1845-1916) who received the Nobel Prize in Medicine or Physiology in 1908 for his earlier pioneering work in immunology. He discovered than immune cells were able to surround and devour microbes, described as phagocytosis, as a protective mechanism against pathogens. In this age of discovery of microbes and their role in infections and disease, his discovery of phagocytosis was as striking as if science fiction became reality. Indeed, many leading scientist of the day, including Louis Pasteur the namesake of pasteurization, took years to be convinced that he was right.

Appointed to a prestigious position at the Pasteur Institute in Paris, and with his international stature already assured, he began to study a previously unexplored area of medicine, aging and longevity. He is credited by some sources with coining the term gerontology to describe this field of research. His interest in longevity is somewhat curious in that he tried to shorten his life, not lengthen it, by attempting suicide on two occasions. Fortunately for science and posterity, his many talents did not include success at these endeavors. He traveled to Bulgaria to study the large population of centenarians, individuals who lived for a century and beyond. He noted that a common component of their diet was called sour milk, what we describe today as yogurt, and he suspected that this might hold an important clue. He took samples of the sour milk back to his laboratory and was able to culture a new subspecies of microbe, never identified before, which he named *Lactobacillus delbrueckii bulgaricus*.

Metchnikov developed his popular theory that toxic bacteria in the gut cause aging, and that lactic acid generated by microbes could prolong life as evidenced in the Bulgarian centenarians. He drank sour milk every day and wrote a landmark paper *The Prolongation of Life: Optimistic Studies*, in which he promoted the potential life-lengthening properties of lactic acid bacteria. His work inspired Japanese microbiologist Minoru Shirota (1899-1982) to develop a stronger strain of lactic acid bacteria, named *Lactobacillus casei shirota*. He believed the lactic acid production could destroy the harmful bacteria living in the intestines and improve health and longevity. Shirota developed Yakult, kefir and other fermented milk products as the first probiotics brought to market in 1935, which developed a worldwide interest and popularity.

Another pioneer of prebiotic and probiotics was John Harvey Kellogg (1852-1943). A graduate of New York University Medical School, he was the medical director of a Seventh Day Adventist medical facility in Battle Creek, Michigan with a particular focus on nutrition, exercise, and intestinal health. Kellogg was an advocate of vegetarianism and following the research of Élie Metchnikoff advocated yogurt for its beneficial probiotic benefits. The Battle Creek Sanitarium became an internationally renowned center for health and wellness. Part of the regimen at the sanitarium was colonic cleansing, with several large volume enemas a day to clear the intestine. Kellogg's unique application of yogurt by mouth as well as by enema was meant to assure that the gut microbiome was saturated with beneficial organisms.

He recognized the value of probiotics, as well as the need for prebiotics to provide sustenance to the microbes. His best-known invention was a process for flaking cereal, inventing corn flakes with his brother William Keith Kellogg. Kellogg promoted whole grain cereals and fiber for intestinal health, and with his brother founded the Kellogg Cereal Company, which grew into one of the world's most successful enterprises. (For those interested in biography the life and times of the Kellogg brothers is an amazing and colorful story with surprising twists and cameo appearances of many noted figures).

The most popular probiotics today belong to two large groups Lactobacillus and Bifidobacterium. There are thousands of species and subspecies of these and other probiotics, and the ones with optimal benefit are dependent on the many variables of each individual. The uniqueness of the individual is the basic premise of the valuable concept of personalized precision medicine. Unfortunately, at present there is no way other than an individual identifying what works best for themselves by the trial and error approach. The marketplace for probiotics is expanding rapidly with hundreds of products coming to market. Many companies are identifying and patenting subspecies and strains to deter competition and to market their products as unique. There is minimal regulatory oversight, and the marketing typically over promises and under delivers.

In general, the mantra in medicine is 'above all do no harm'. I would suggest trying the probiotics with the longest tract record of safety, Lactobacillus and Bifidobacterium. First one at lower doses, increase as tolerated. If the response is not satisfactory try the other. Combing both is reasonable if one alone did not provide sufficient benefit. Branching out to other probiotics is reasonable, but obviously back off if the results are not satisfactory. The good news is that the gut microbiome can be changed rapidly with probiotics and can also be changed again if the results are less than desired. In the coming years there will be clear identification of specific diets and probiotics which will bring us 'back to the future', fulfilling the ancient adage of Hippocrates, the father of modern medicine: "Let food be thy medicine!"

Proctology

Shutterstock/LisaF.Young

Proctology (Greek πρωκτός Proktos anus, λόγος Logos science), also known as colorectal surgery, is a field in medicine dealing with disorders of the rectum, anus, and colon. Physicians specializing in this field of medicine are called colorectal surgeons or proctologists. In the United States to become a board certified colorectal surgeon a physician has to complete a five-year general surgery residency as well as a subsequent multiyear colorectal surgery fellowship and certification examinations.

Protist (see Microbiome, Pathogen)

Rectum

The rectum (Latin rectus straight) is the pelvic part of the large intestine of the alimentary tract and is continuous proximally with the sigmoid colon and distally with the anal canal. The rectosigmoid junction lies anterior to the third sacral vertebra. At this point, the teniae of the sigmoid colon spread out to form a continuous outer longitudinal layer of smooth muscle, and the fatty omental appendices are discontinued.

The rectum follows the curve of the sacrum and coccyx, forming the sacral flexure of the rectum. The roughly eighty-degree anorectal flexure is an important mechanism for fecal continence, being maintained during the resting state by the tonal contraction of the puborectalis muscle. This muscle is also actively contracted during peristaltic intestinal activity to prevent defecation. In spite of the Latin meaning of the word rectum meaning straight, it is anything but linear. With the flexures of the rectosigmoid junction superiorly, and the anorectal junction inferiorly, the rectum has an S shape when viewed laterally.

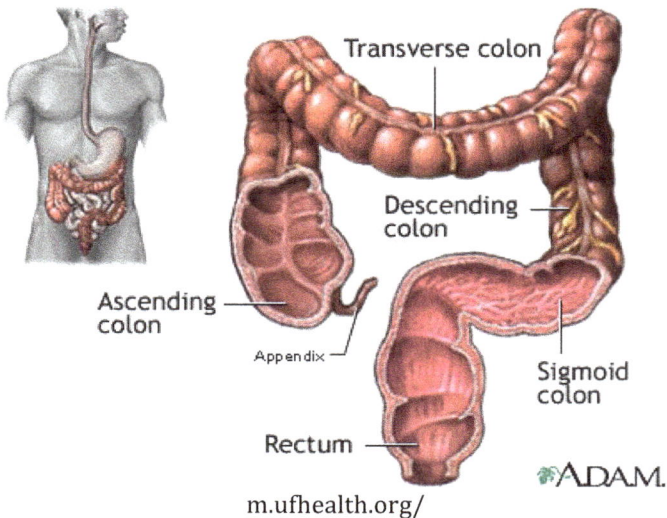

m.ufhealth.org/

Rumination Syndrome

Rumination syndrome is an unusual condition and can lead to excessive air swallowing. Because the initiation of the rumination process itself requires the relaxation of the lower esophageal sphincter, burps and belches are common findings. Rumination is typically seen in herbivorous livestock, which have compartmented stomachs to aid in the fermentation and digestion process. These animals regurgitate what is called the cud or partially digested food from the foregut stomach compartment to be chewed and swallowed again for further processing.

Humans can develop voluntary control of the esophageal musculature to retrieve stomach contents and swallow them again as if they were ruminant animals. The ability to train the esophageal muscles is most noted in yogi masters and circus performers, but it is a learnable skill. Postprandial regurgitation is a symptom of rumination syndrome. For the others who subconsciously develop the rumination habit, excessive air swallowing is simply the unavoidable result of the excessive swallowing that is part and parcel of the rumination syndrome. There are considerable psychological and psychiatric aspects of rumination disorders.

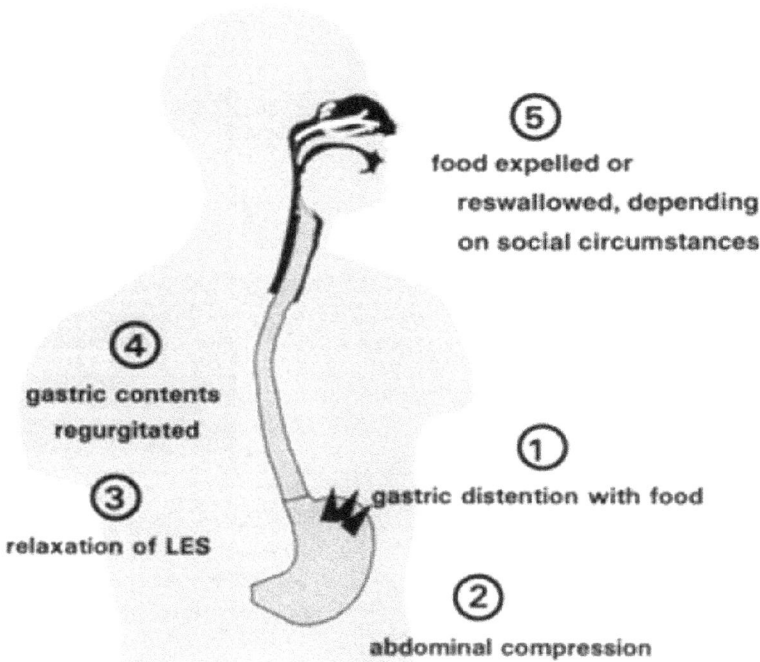

⑤ food expelled or reswallowed, depending on social circumstances

④ gastric contents regurgitated

① gastric distention with food

③ relaxation of LES

② abdominal compression

Rumination syndrome. Creative Commons License

Saliva

The production and swallowing of saliva contributes to intestinal gas with approximately three to five milliliters (one teaspoon) of air ingested with every swallow. The stimuli of food smell and appearance, and the sounds of food preparation can prepare the digestive tract by initiating salivation even before any food or drink is consumed. Saliva is a mixture of both serous fluid and mucus that in addition to providing the lubrication for chewing (mastication) and swallowing (deglutition) contains the digestive enzyme amylase. Smell, taste, or the sight of food is a well-recognized trigger of salivation. As demonstrated by Ivan Pavlov with his experiment ringing a bell every time he fed dogs, just the cephalic brain stimulus of the bell ring by itself could stimulate salivation.

Human saliva is 99.5% water, while the other 0.5% consists of electrolytes, mucus, glycoproteins, enzymes such as amylase and lipase, and antibacterial compounds such as secretory IgA, lactoferrin, lysozyme, and peroxidase. Saliva also protects the teeth from bacterial decay and serves a lubrication function. The salivary glands secrete one to two liters of saliva per day (pH 6 to 7) at a rate of 0.1 milliliter/min at rest to 4 milliliters/min during a period of active stimulation during a meal. The saliva produced at rest is more viscous than the watery saliva produced during meal stimulation. The tongue is very sensitive to changes in pH so the ingestion of anything acidic will stimulate the release of saliva to return the pH back to its normal baseline.

Salivary glands are exocrine glands that produce and release saliva into the mouth and during the chewing (mastication) and swallowing (deglutition) process. In addition to lubrication and oral hygiene, the salivary glands secrete the enzymes amylase for carbohydrates and lipase for lipids. The three main pairs of salivary glands are the parotid glands around the mandible, the submandibular glands beneath the lower jaws, and the sublingual glands under the tongue.

Shutterstock/reddogs

Saliva is a mixture of both serous fluid and mucus. Even though the parotid glands are larger it produces twenty-five percent of saliva, compared to seventy percent by the submandibular glands, and five percent by the sublingual glands. The parasympathetic and sympathetic arms of the autonomic nervous system innervate salivary glands. The mouth of animals harbors many bacteria, some pathogenic. Human bites are considered more dangerous than other animal bites, and because of the number and types of bacteria present are treated with antibiotics. The salivary secretions of cobras, vipers, and poisonous snakes are venomous and injected by fangs or by spitting. Some snakes can spit accurately, aiming for the victim's eyes, up to a distance of eight feet. The large lizard the Komodo Dragon kills by biting, but the fatality often comes about as a result of overwhelming sepsis from the virulent microbes in its saliva. Some spiders and caterpillars create thread from their salivary glands.

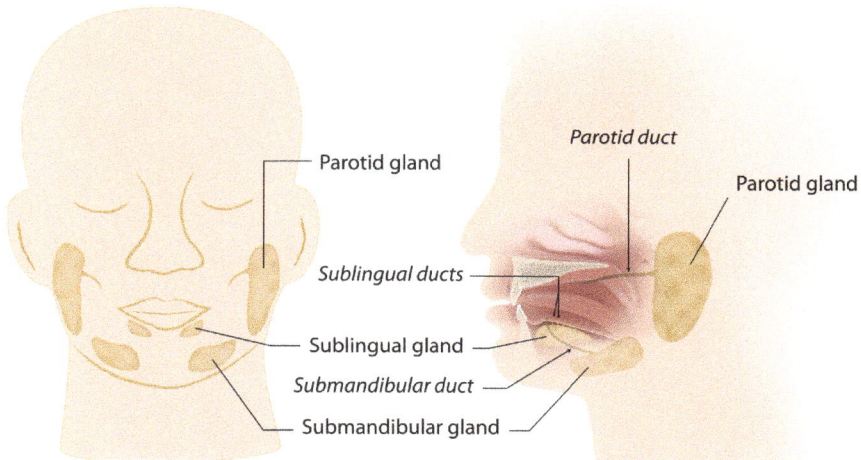

Salivary Glands - Shutterstock/Alila Medical Media Group

Their saliva is the basic material from which the swallow and swiftlet birds build their nests. Traditional Chinese cuisine has made bird nest soup a delicacy, which has been ascribed health benefits including aiding digestion, enhancing libido, and strengthening the immune system. When dissolved in water, the birds' nests have a gelatinous texture from the high mucus content of the bird's salivary laminae cement. In addition, the nests have high levels of calcium, iron, potassium, and magnesium. Hong Kong and the United States are the largest importers of these nests, which are amongst the most expensive of food delicacies. Formerly harvested from enormous limestone caves on the island of Borneo, the commercial development of habitat for swallows to build nests have become a major industry in other parts of Indonesia.

Scatology (Coprology)

Scatology or coprology Greek σκώρ 'feces' is the study of feces that can be used to determine diet, parasites, and migratory patterns. In psychology the term is used to describe the study of obsessions with excretion or excrement. In literature, "scatological" is a term to describe works that make particular reference to excretion or excrement, as well as to toilet humor. The name of the chemical which gives feces (excrement, shit, poop, and hundreds of other euphemisms.) its characteristic odor is called skatole similarly derived from the Greek το σχατος - feces.

For those who have an interest in learning more about the end result of the digestive process ***The Scoop on Poop! Flush With Knowledge*** provides a fascinating and entertaining wealth of information. For those who would enjoy a more provocative and cheeky title, especially if offered as a unique gift to others, the identical content is also published as ***You Don't Know Sh*t! Until You Read This Book***.

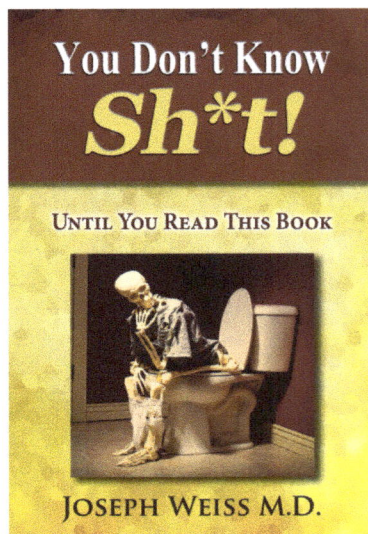

Scuba Diving (see Atmospheric Pressure, Ideal Gas Laws)

Scuba diving can be a very enjoyable activity, but it does require an understanding of the behavior of gasses and the laws of physics for safety. The atmospheric pressure changes associated with diving activity are pronounced and require close attention. Unfortunately, errors in judgment in scuba diving can be very unforgiving, and lead to fatal consequences if safety precautions are overlooked.

Boyle's Law was named after Robert Boyle, a chemist and physicist who published his discovery in 1662. The law describes that the pressure and volume of a gas are inversely proportional, if the temperature is kept constant. As the pressure on a gas increases its volume decreases, and vice versa, if you increase the volume of the gas, the pressure decreases.At the surface of sea level (zero feet) the pressure is one atmosphere (ATM). At a depth of thirty-three feet underwater the pressure is two atmospheres, the sum total of one ATM of air pressure and one ATM of water pressure. If a balloon with gas at the surface is submerged it will be one-half of the original volume at thirty-three feet depth, and one-third the volume at sixty-six feet depth. On ascent the balloon volume will be one and one-half times greater on going from sixty-six feet depth to thirty-three feet depth. It will have a volume three times greater at the surface than it did at sixty-six feet depth.

O ft ~ 1 atm — Volume x1 — Volume x 3

33 ft ~ 2 atm — Volume x 1/2 — Volume x 1.5

66 ft ~ 3 atm — Volume x 1/3 — Volume x 1

Creative Commons License

The diver experiences the effect of these pressure changes firsthand. As one descends the air in the facemask is compressed giving rise to the phenomenon known as mask squeeze. The pressure changes in the air spaces of the ear canal can be very significant if they are not purposefully equalized during descent and ascent. Severe ear injury including perforated or ruptured eardrum can result from unequaled air pressure. The air pressure on both sides of the eardrum known as the tympanic membrane, can be equalized by performing the Valsalva maneuver of attempting to exhale against a closed glottis. This is the same procedure many people use when straining to have a bowel movement. Head cold, allergies, sinus congestion, and other conditions that reduce the patency of the Eustachian tubes can prevent equalization of air pressure and should preclude diving activity.

The air volume in buoyancy control devices requires adjustment to maintain neutrality. The gas laws also explain why divers are advised to exhale while ascending as the gasses in the lung can over expand if the breath is held and result in severe internal injury. Dive bubbles increase in size as the gasses expand because of the reduced atmospheric pressure as they ascend. The gasses in the bubble are following the gas laws that dictate their behavior with changes in pressure, temperature, and volume.

William Henry was an English physician and chemist who proposed what is now called Henry's law in 1803. The law states that at a constant temperature, the amount of a given gas dissolved in a liquid is directly proportional to the pressure of that gas. As the gas pressure increases, the solubility of the gas in the liquid increases. As the temperature increases, the solubility of gas in liquid decreases. The greater the pressure, the greater the quantity of a gas that can be absorbed by a liquid. The cooler the liquid, the greater the amount of gas that it can absorb. As the temperature of liquid increases, the solubility of the gas decreases forming bubbles that allow it to escape. Henry's Law explains why carbon dioxide in a pressurized container, such as in a can or bottle of a carbonated beverage remains in solution until it is opened. As soon as the container is opened the pressure is reduced causing the carbon dioxide gas to lose its solubility and escape in the form of bubbles or fizz. It also explains why so much gas is released when you drink a cold carbonated beverage and it is warmed to body temperature in the stomach.

Creative Commons License

In a similar manner as a diver descends nitrogen inhaled is under increasing pressure and becomes soluble in the bloodstream, muscles and tissues. This is not a problem until the diver begins an ascent and the pressure is reduced allowing the nitrogen in the body to form bubbles. If the diver ascends too quickly this can lead to Decompression Sickness also known as Caisson Disease or the bends. This is the reason why divers are advised to ascend gradually, to allow the nitrogen to be exhaled out of the lungs rather than to form bubbles in the bloodstream or tissue. Henry's Law also explains why after a dive the diver should not be exposed to higher temperatures such as a sauna, hot bath or shower or engages in strenuous activities or exercise. The increase in body temperature may cause the nitrogen to become less soluble and increase the risk of Decompression Sickness. Likewise diving in colder water enhances the absorption of nitrogen into the body, which should be adjusted for by shorter dive times or shallower dives.

Charles' Law states that at a constant volume, the pressure of gas varies directly with the temperature. While a French philosopher named Joseph Louis Gay-

Lussac published this law, Lussac attributed the law to an unpublished work by Jacques Charles. Jacques Alexander Charles was a French scientist, mathematician, inventor, and balloonist who studied the effects of temperature on the volumes of a gas. He formulated and published what became known as Charles' Law in 1787. Charles wrote about the law after observing the effects of temperature on balloons. When a balloon is filled with gas and exposed to heat, the molecules of the gas cause the balloon to expand. When the balloon is exposed to colder temperatures, the molecules of the gas cause the balloon to deflate. The law states that at a constant pressure, the volume of a gas increases or decreases by the same factor as its temperature increases or decreases. Charles' law helps to explain the hazard of leaving scuba tanks out in the sun, or in the trunk of a car. The gas already under high pressure will have a further increase in pressure if subjected to heat, which can cause the tank to explode. The law also explains why scuba tanks increase in temperature when being filled with compressed air.

An extreme example of the laws of physics on the volume of a fart occurs in the case of the giant blue whale. The whale is an enormous mammal and as can be expected of such a large animal, its farts are also quite large. The Blue Whale is the largest animal on Earth, up to one hundred feet (thirty meters) long and three hundred and forty thousand pounds (154,545 kilograms or one hundred and seventy tons). The blue whale is a mammal that ingests and digests up to sixteen thousand pounds (7,272 kilograms or eight tons) of plankton per day. The whale digestive tract generates large quantities of gas and when the blue whale releases a fart the bubble expands as it rises to the surface. The blue whale will fart deep underwater in the ocean where the high atmospheric pressure compresses the fart. As the fart bubble rises from the depths of the ocean, the atmospheric pressure decreases and the fart expands, as predicted by Boyle's Law. Fisherman who have been exposed to the results of a whale fart breaking the surface of the ocean describe the bubble as huge enough to engulf and asphyxiate a large horse. The smell is just as powerful as its giant size would predict. Now that is a true whale of a story for even a fisherman to tell.

Shart

The word shart is a portmanteau, a word created by the combination of parts of two separate words. In the case of shart it is more than just the literal combination of the two words shit and fart. It is also the combination of the two verbs, when one farts the anal sphincter may relax too much and unintended defecation occurs. This occurs more commonly with diarrhea, with the passage of liquid or semi-solid feces. It can also occur with the passage of solid well-formed stool.

Simethicone (see Bubbles, Surface Tension)

Simethicone is an oral over the counter product that is used as a treatment to reduce bloating, discomfort, or pain caused by intestinal gas. Simethicone is a mixture of polydimethylsiloxane and hydrated silica gel, and is an anti-foaming agent that decreases the surface tension of gas bubbles. Surface tension is the property seen in water and other fluids that causes the formation of form semi-spherical droplets and bubbles. The reduction in surface tension does not eliminate the bubbles, nor does it cause them to become smaller.

Creative Commons License

Counterintuitively, it actually causes them to combine into larger bubbles, and the presumptive relief is most often from being able to burp or belch up the larger bubble from the stomach more easily. There have been studies suggesting that simethicone increases the transit time so that intestinal gas may be more readily eliminated as flatus. Simethicone is not absorbed by the body and does not enter into the bloodstream. It is often used for infants with colicky symptoms thought to be due to swallowed air causing intestinal gas.

Creative Commons License

Although simethicone has been promoted and marketed as a treatment for colic in babies, the actual cause of colic has yet to be clearly identified. Simethicone solutions of differing concentration also have industrial applications for reducing foaming in certain chemical processes, in detergents, as well as in medical imaging studies of the gastrointestinal tract.

Singultus (Hiccup)

Singultus, a hiccup, is an involuntary contraction of the diaphragm that may occur singly or in bouts. It is caused by a strong contraction, known as a myoclonic jerk, of the diaphragm. The diaphragm contraction increases the negative pressure in the chest cavity that causes it to act as a vacuum inflating the lungs when inhaling a deep breath. Within milliseconds the epiglottis and vocal cords abruptly close creating a hic sound and cutting off the flow of air. A hiccup is an onomatopoeia; a word that was created to imitate the sound it is describing.

Hiccups are believed to be an evolutionary trait inherited from fish and tadpoles. The phrenic nerve which controls the diaphragm extends from the base of the skull and travels through the chest cavity. This design appears to have been derived from fish ancestors with gills closer to the neck. Interestingly enough as the human embryo develops the vestigial gills can be easily identified. The hiccup itself may have arisen from our evolution through the amphibian phase. The characteristic pattern of muscle and nerve activity of hiccups occurs in tadpoles that use both lungs and gills to breathe. When tadpoles use their gills they shut the glottis to close off the breathing tube while sharply inspiring. In essence tadpoles breathe with their gills using an extended form of a hiccup.

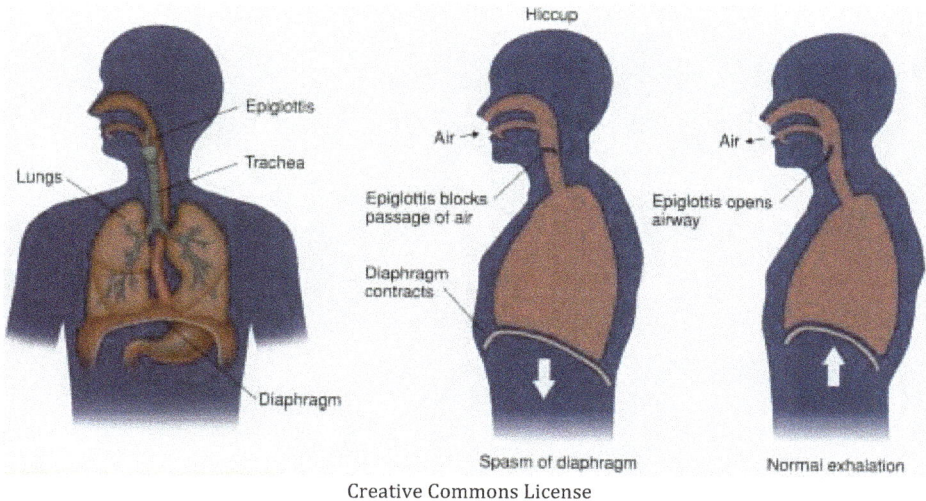

Creative Commons License

Hiccups resolve spontaneously in the vast majority of cases, yet dozens of home and medical remedies exist that are not particularly effective. A recent theory proposes that hiccups developed as a reflex to allow the escape of swallowed air from the stomach during the suckling and feeding of infants. Pope Pius XII was seriously ill with a hiatal hernia and virtually uncontrollable hiccups in 1954.

Common home remedies include: holding one's breath and exhaling slowly, holding the nose, breathing into a paper bag, sucking on ice cubes or hard candy, drinking water from the far side of a glass, gargling, pulling on the tongue, biting on a lemon, swallowing granulated sugar, swallowing hard bread crust, sneezing, peeling onions, bending over so that the head is lower than the chest, frightening the person with hiccups, and slapping the person with hiccups on the back.

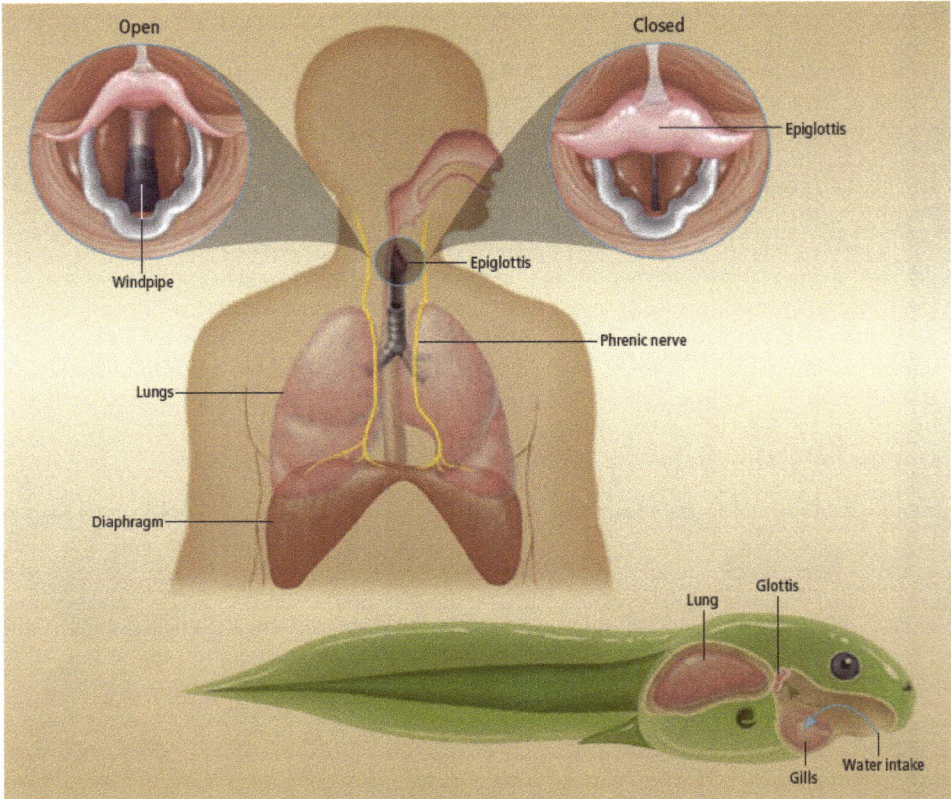

Creative Commons License

Skatole

Skatole (from the Greek το σχατος = feces), or methylindole, is a mildly toxic organic compound belonging to the indole family. It is the primary source of the odor of feces and is produced from the breakdown of the important amino acid tryptophan, the precursor of the neurotransmitter serotonin. Surprisingly, in low concentrations skatole has a very pleasant flowery smell and is found in orange blossoms, jasmine, and other flowers and essential oils. It is used as a fragrance in many perfumes.

Skatole is attractive to males of various species of bees, who gather the chemical to synthesize pheromones. It is also an attractant to gravid (pregnant) mosquitos. The U. S. military has used skatole as a non-lethal malodorant weapon. The German physician Ludwig Brieger, who also identified cadaverine and

420

putrescence, discovered skatole in 1877. His neighbors were probably not pleased with the smell coming from his laboratory as the names he gave his discoveries were derived from their source material.

Skatole also plays a major role in the aroma of pork obtained from mature male pigs (boars). After puberty, under the influence of the male hormone androstenone, the gut microbiome of the male pig generates skatole. This odorant is deposited in the fat and muscle giving it an offensive smell and taste known as taint. Because it cannot be sold at market, male pigs are typically castrated at a young age or slaughtered before puberty. The male of the human species, under similar hormonal influence is also a larger producer of skatole contributing to the enhanced offensive potency of male farts after puberty.

Of particular interest to some scientists is that androstenone, and its effect on skatole, appear to have a pheromone like effect on the human female. Much like color-blindness, there appear to be some odors that cannot be smelled by all people. Initial studies suggested that about thirty percent of human females could not sense androstenone. Further studies revealed that the majority of the non-scenters could be trained to identify it, yet there remained a small proportion of less than five percent who could not perceive the scent. The ability to sense androstenone was found to be genetic and the gene responsible was identified.

The sense of smell in the human female is intimately tied to the menstrual cycle. The height of olfactory sensitivity peaks at the time of ovulation. The androstenone and skatole scents are perceived to be less offensive or more attractive at the time of ovulation. The androstenone skatole connection also explains why the feces and flatus of males are considered more powerful or offensive than that of females. Diet also plays a role in that the ingestion of more meat and fat also leads to more skatole production than a diet with higher fiber content. This is partly due to the diet containing more tryptophan, the amino acid precursor of skatole, as well as the diet induced change in the microbiome. Androstenone also occurs naturally in some plants, including celery, parsnip, and truffle. The celery has long had a reputation as an aphrodisiac dating from Greek and Roman times.

Small Intestine (Small Bowel)

The small intestine, also known as the small bowel, is the section of the gastrointestinal tract between the stomach and the large intestine. The small intestine is divided into three anatomical segments, the short first portion immediately following the stomach is called the duodenum The term duodenum comes from the middle Latin duodenum digitorium 'space of twelve digits', a translation of the Greek dodekadaktylon, literally 'twelve fingers long', as described by the Greek physician Herophilus (c. 353-280).

It has the critical function of receiving the highly acidic gastric contents and mixing in the pancreatic and biliary secretions of digestive enzymes, bile, and large volumes of sodium bicarbonate to neutralize the potent stomach acid. The jejunum, the middle portion of the small intestine between the duodenum and the ileum, was given its name after the Latin word jējūnus, which meant empty or poor, so called because it was always thought to be empty after death.

The ileum, from the Latin ilium meaning flank or groin, is the final segment of the small intestine and enters the cecum of the colon close to the appendix at the ileocecal valve. The small intestine is described as small because the lumen is narrower than the lumen of the large intestine. The average length of the small intestine is twenty-three feet (seven meters) and is approximately one inch (two and one-half centimeters) in diameter. It is substantially longer than the approximately five-foot length of the large intestine, also called the colon.

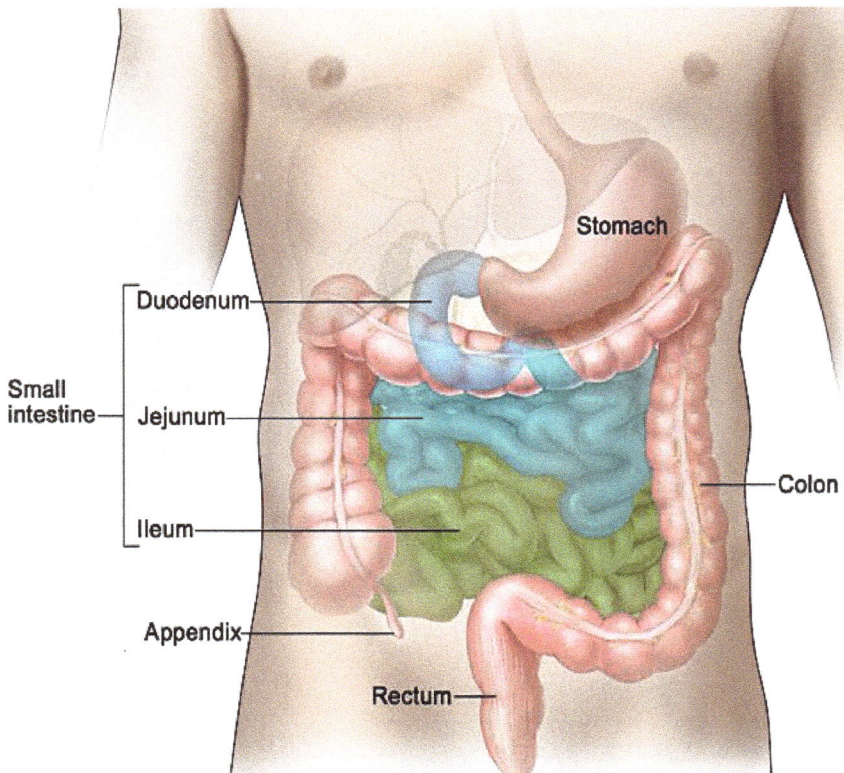

m.cancer.gov Public Domain

In spite of the relatively long length of the small intestine its absorptive capacity would not be sufficient to maintain nutrition for an organism the size of a human without modifications to increase its surface area. The deep circular folds of the mucosa and submucosa are known as plica circulares or plica. The fingerlike extensions of the mucosa called villi, in conjunction with the microscopic projections of the mucosal cell plasma membranes called microvilli, dramatically increase the surface area. The surface area thus available for digestive processes, enzymatic activity, and absorption of the human small intestine exceeds that of a championship tennis court.

The small intestine receives chyme from the stomach and is the primary location where digestion and absorption of nutrients takes place. Gastric content leaves the stomach via the pyloric sphincter and enters the duodenum, which also receives gallbladder bile and pancreatic juice via the sphincter of Oddi. The pancreatic juice contains sodium bicarbonate to neutralize the stomach acid as well as digestive enzymes. The small intestinal mucosal epithelial cells consist of absorptive cells, mucus secreting goblet cells, enteroendocrine cells that secrete gastrointestinal hormones, and interspersed intraepithelial lymphocytes and T cells important in the immune response. The immune response of the gastrointestinal tract is critical for human health as the gut is exposed to the vast majority of foreign pathogens introduced into the body.

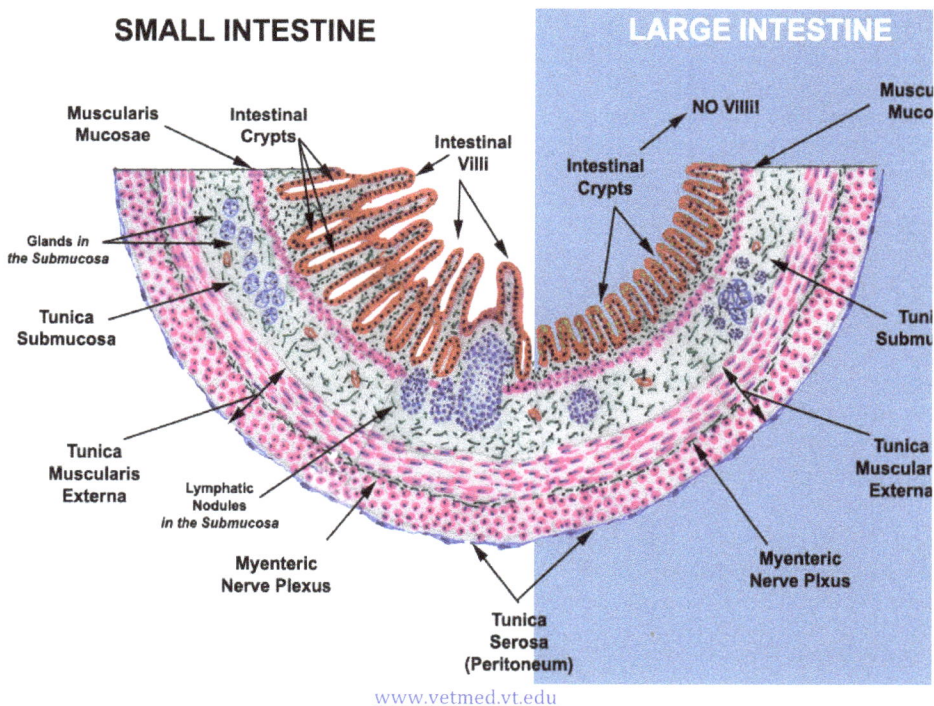

www.vetmed.vt.edu

The cells of the intestinal crypts secrete intestinal juice in response to distension or irritation of the mucosa. This solution is slightly alkaline and isotonic with blood plasma. It is largely water, contains mucus, and very little in the way of enzymatic activity. A number of intestinal infections or inflammatory processes may stimulate the release of intestinal juice with diarrhea resulting. The liquid chyme with over ninety percent of its nutritional value digested and absorbed, leaves the ileum of the small intestine via the ileocecal valve into the cecum of the colon. Non-absorbed carbohydrates and non-digested material are fermented by the gut flora to short-chain fatty acids (mainly acetic, propionic, and n-butyric acids), carbon dioxide, hydrogen and methane. The colon will absorb nearly all of the short-chain fatty acids with the butyric acid being utilized as the main source of energy for colonic epithelial cells.

Brunner glands (duodenal glands) are compound tubular submucosal glands found in the proximal duodenum. The main function of these glands is to produce a mucus rich alkaline secretion containing sodium bicarbonate that protects the intestinal mucosa by neutralizing the acidic content of chyme leaving the stomach. Brunner glands also secrete the hormone polypeptide urogastrone, which inhibit the parietal and chief cells of the stomach from secreting hydrochloric acid and their digestive enzymes. The hormone can be identified and isolated from the urine as a fluorescent pigment and is derived from epidermal growth factor. Peyer patches are organized lymphoid nodules in the ileum of the small intestine. There are approximately thirty Payer's patches, each a few centimeters long, distributed in the laminae propria layer of the mucosa and extending into the submucosa. They contain B and T lymphocytes and are involved in the gastrointestinal tract immune surveillance, response, and defense mechanism. They are found only in the ileum and are not present in the duodenum or jejunum.

Because the lumen of the gastrointestinal tract is contiguous with and exposed to the external environment it is an avenue for potentially pathogenic microorganisms. Peyer patches are covered by specialized epithelial cells called microfold cells (M cells). These cells allow the sampling of antigens, which may stimulate a response from the Peyer patches T cell, B cell lymphocytes, and memory cells. Activated lymphocytes stimulate and magnify the immune response and pass into the mesenteric lymph nodes and travel via the lymphatic thoracic duct into the blood stream. From here they circulate throughout the body and gastrointestinal tract as a defense. Pathogenic microorganisms and other antigens entering the intestinal tract also encounter macrophages, dendritic cells, B-lymphocytes, and T-lymphocytes from Peyer patches, and other Mucosa Associated Lymphoid Tissue (MALT) all of which provide immunological defenses.

Spelunking

Spelunking, the exploration of caves, has become an increasingly popular activity and can take place above or below sea level altitudes. Some of the deepest explored caves have vertical drops in excess of one thousand feet. Although changes in atmospheric pressure are noticeable, this effect is one of the least dangerous aspects of the sport activity. The exploration of underwater caves known as cave diving, combines spelunking with scuba diving, and is a particularly demanding and challenging activity. In this activity understanding the potential effects of atmospheric pressure changes becomes critically important.

Creative Commons License

41.media.tumblr.com Creative Commons License

Stomach

Stomach (Greek stomachos (στόμαχος), from stoma (στόμα), "mouth"). The words gastro- and gastric (meaning related to the stomach) are from the Greek word gaster (γαστήρ). The stomach is a strong muscular organ that can be distended up to many times its resting size when food or fluids are ingested. It is unique in that it has three separate layers of smooth muscle while the rest of the digestive tract has only two. The stomach is located in the abdomen, just below the lower esophageal sphincter at the level of the diaphragm. If a hiatal hernia is present a portion of the stomach and lower esophageal sphincter may be in the chest, and thus subjected to negative intra-thoracic pressure acting as a vacuum.

Parts of the Stomach

The gastric chief cells secrete the zymogen pepsinogen, which is activated to the active protease pepsin by the hydrochloric acid released from the gastric parietal cells. The zymogen Prorennin is also activated to rennin, which digests the milk protein caesinogen (soluble) into casein (insoluble), curdling the milk. The stomach produces multiple hormones, and intrinsic factor necessary for the absorption of vitamin B_{12}. Depending on the quantity and character of the meal the stomach will release the partially digested chyme through the pyloric channel into the duodenum within minutes to hours.

The stomach is under the influence of multiple stimulant and inhibiting pathways including the autonomic and parasympathetic nervous system via the vagus nerve, multiple hormones, and feedback loops of digestive products and distention. Ruminants have an even more complex stomach with multiple chambers where microbial fermentation of ingested food may take place. Gasses generated are released by eructation such as burps and belch or as flatus. Some species, especially birds, have a powerful muscular gizzard, often containing stones purposefully swallowed to help grind up food.

Sucrase

Invertases and sucrases are closely related enzymes that catalyze the hydrolysis of sucrose (table sugar) to fructose and glucose. Hydrolyzed table sugar is referred to as inverted sugar. Invertases are commonly found in plants, and for commercial uses are typically derived from yeast, and hydrolyze the fructose bond. Bees use invertase to make honey from nectar. Sucrases found in humans and higher animals hydrolyze the glucose bond.

Sucrose

Sucrose (saccharose) (Latin sucrum = "sugar"), also known as table sugar, is a disaccharide composed of the monosaccharides glucose and fructose. Sucrose forms caramel upon melting. The enzymes sucrase, invertase, and isomaltase glycoside hydrolases, as well as gastric acidity, converts sucrose to glucose and fructose during digestion. Sucrose is digested rapidly but it has a low glycemic index because its fructose has a minimal effect on blood glucose. Fructose has approximately twice the sweetness of glucose, making sucrose distinctively sweet.

Around 500 BC in India sugar cane was processed into easier to store and transport raw sugar crystals. In the Indian language these crystals were called khanda (खण्ड), which is the origin of the word candy. Sugarcane plantations were an integral part of the history of the slave trade and colonization. Sugar beet production became increasingly important with the industrial revolution and mechanized sugar production.

Venezuelan sugar cane (Saccharum) harvested for processing. Author: Rufino Uribe Creative Commons

Sucrose Intolerance, Sucrase Deficiency

Sucrose intolerance, also called Sucrase-isomaltase deficiency, is the condition in which the enzyme required for proper metabolism of sucrose is not produced in the small intestine. It is more common among the native Inupiat people in Alaska. Sucrase deficiency is usually an autosomal recessive genetic disorder. Sucrose is a disaccharide composed of glucose and fructose, which are bonded together. The common table sugar made from beets and cane is sucrose. When sucrase deficiency leads to sucrose intolerance, symptoms may include abdominal cramps, bloating, diarrhea, and excess gas production. Other symptoms may include constipation, vomiting, hypoglycemia, headaches, poor weight gain, and delayed growth. Dietary modifications and enzyme replacement therapy are often suggested.

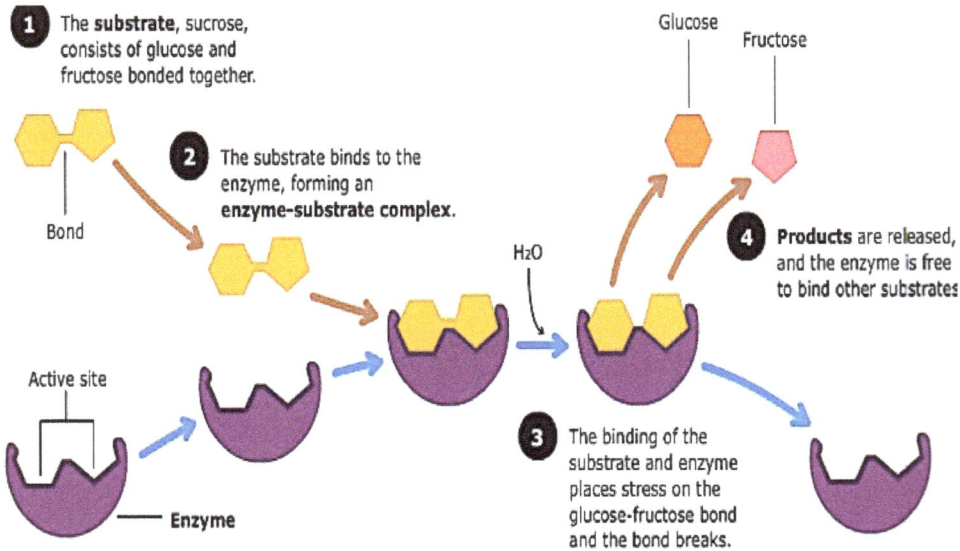

1 The **substrate**, sucrose, consists of glucose and fructose bonded together.

2 The substrate binds to the enzyme, forming an **enzyme-substrate complex.**

Glucose

Fructose

Bond

H_2O

Active site

4 **Products** are released, and the enzyme is free to bind other substrates

Enzyme

3 The binding of the substrate and enzyme places stress on the glucose-fructose bond and the bond breaks.

Surface Tension

Surface tension is a physical property exhibited when certain liquids are in contact with a gas. It is particularly pronounced when liquid water is in contact with the gasses of the air. Each water molecule contains two hydrogen atoms and one oxygen atom, giving rise to its familiar chemical shorthand of H_2O. Because of their atomic structure the negative charge of the electrons of the hydrogen atoms are attracted to the positive charge of the oxygen atom, creating was is known as a hydrogen bond. The electric charges also create an attractive force between water molecules, causing them to want to remain close together. These forces are balanced out when a water molecule is surrounded by other water molecules.

Surface tension allowing to go over brim of glass without spilling. Andre Roberto Doreto Santos www.flickr.com Creative Commons License

Booyabazooka Unbalanced charges on water molecules at the surface of a liquid gas interface.
Creative Commons License

When the water molecules on the surface are exposed to the gasses of the air above them they are no longer exposed to balanced charges. The water molecule on the surface exposed to the air is only subject to the electric charge pulling it down, keeping it in the liquid. This resistance to leaving its fellow water molecules behind gives it the property known as surface tension, a tension that prevents it from being separated from the remaining liquid. This surface tension is visible when you see water assume the shape of a droplet, or when you fill a glass to the brim and the fluid builds up above the lip of the glass before it begins to overflow. It is also the principle that allows insects such as the water glider to walk on water, because the surface tension acts as a walkable surface and the insect's weight is not enough to overcome the surface tension. Surface tension also is the force that allows the creation of bubbles. Surfactants are products that have the property of reducing surface tension and are used in detergents, as well as in anti-bubble and anti-gas products such as simethicone.

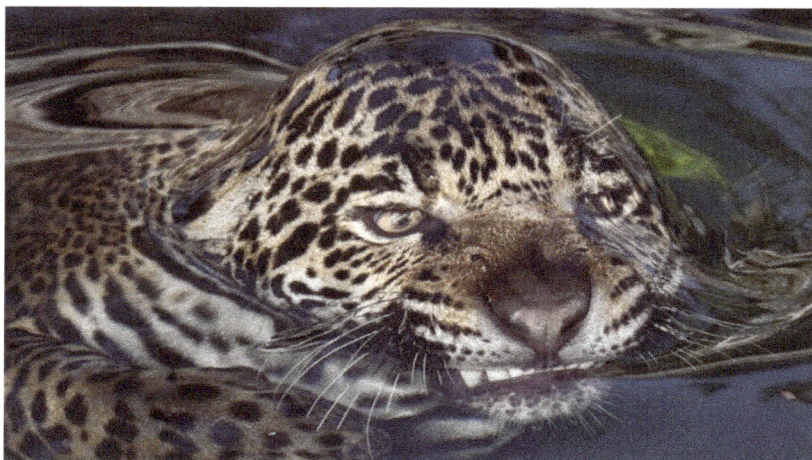

Photograph of surface tension effect. i.imgur.com Creative Commons License

Thiol, Sulfhydryl, Mercaptan

The sulfur hydrogen functional group may also be referred to as a thiol group or a sulfhydryl group. Thiols are also referred to as mercaptans. The term mercaptan (Latin mercurium captans 'capturing mercury') is used because the thiolate group bonds so strongly with mercury compounds. Hydrogen sulfide is known for its characteristic odor of smelling like rotten eggs. Surprisingly women tend to produce more hydrogen sulfide then men. Diet certainly plays a role as cruciferous vegetables such as broccoli, cabbage, cauliflower, and Brussels sprouts are common offenders. Dried fruits such as apricots are often treated with sulfur products that create odiferous gasses. Red meat, beer, garlic, and aromatic spices are other significant contributors. The offensive smell of sulfur products led to religions ascribing an association between the devil and sulfur.

Hydrogen sulfide is a toxic substance in high concentrations yet very valuable and beneficial on a cellular level when present in minute quantities. The human nose is exceptionally sensitive to this toxin and can identify it in minute concentrations, such as in a fart. When present in very high concentrations the olfactory cells are overwhelmed and can no longer sense it. This has led to a sever hazard for farmers and workers in animal waste manure pits and sewage treatment facilities. A worker collapses on exposure to the high concentration of hydrogen sulfide and fellow workers coming to their aid are likewise stricken because there was no olfactory warning. With a toxic potency equivalent to cyanide workers in such hazardous occupations are urged to use self-contained breathing apparatus to avoid exposure.

Volatile thiols have distinctive and strong garlic like odor. The spray of skunks consists mainly of thiols and derivatives. These compounds are detected by the human nose at concentrations as low as ten parts per billion. Human sweat contains methyl-sulfanylhexan (MSH), found in higher concentrations in females, and has a fruity onion-like odor. Not all thiols have unpleasant odors. The aroma of roasted coffee is due to thiols as is the characteristic scent of grapefruit. Dimethyl sulfide has an aroma that is often described as sweet. Natural gas distributors were required by law to add odorants such as thiols to odorless natural gas after a tragic school explosion in New London, Texas, in 1937 occurred without warning from a leaking gas line.

Most natural odorant additives used today contain mixtures of mercaptans and sulfides. T-butyl mercaptan is often utilized as the main odorant constituent. The characteristic and pungently offensive odor of animal flesh decay is caused by putrescence and cadaverine. Putrescence and cadaverine are the breakdown products of the amino acids ornithine and lysine, respectively. Cadaverine and putrescence were also used as odorant additives for natural gas before improved odorants became commercially available.

Methanethiol (methyl mercaptan) is a flammable, colorless gas with a powerful smell like rotten cabbage or decomposing vegetables. It is a natural substance found in certain foods such as some nuts and cheese, and is released from decaying organic matter. Methanethiol is also a byproduct produced by the metabolism of asparagus. The change in the odor of urine may be apparent within thirty minutes of eating asparagus. It is one of the main chemicals responsible for bad breath and the smell of feces and flatus.

Natural gas and propane are colorless and odorless, and an undetected leak can lead to tragic consequences. To serve as an odorous marker that a leak is occurring small amount of methyl mercaptan or ethyl mercaptan may be added as an odorant. The addition of an odorant is often required by law to prevent the danger of natural leaks going undetected.

Toilet (see Anal Hygiene)

Toilet is derived from the French word toilette meaning the act of washing, dressing, and preparing oneself. In Western society human feces waste management is usually a matter of a toilet with indoor plumbing, and a sewer or septic system. Anal cleansing after defecation was historically accomplished with sticks, leaves, stones, clay, corncobs, water, or literally whatever was available at hand. Contrary to popular belief Thomas Crapper did not invent the indoor flush toilet. It had been developed hundreds of years before he established his manufacturing company in Victoria England. The advance his product offered was an improvement in the siphon flush function. The average person goes to the toilet 2,500 times per year, and spends a total of three years of their lifetime sitting on the toilet. For those musically inclined most toilets flush in the key of E flat. Other trivia of note, one third of Americans flush the toilet while still sitting on it, and there are 40,000 injuries a year while sitting on the toilet seat. The toilet faucet handle has four-hundred times more bacteria per square inch than the toilet seat.

Anal cleansing after defecation was historically accomplished with sticks, leaves, stones, clay, corn cobs, water, or literally whatever was available at hand. The ancient Greeks used clay and stone. Romans used a water soaked sponge on a stick. Toilet paper may be used for the cleaning of the anus and urethra after elimination. The first recorded use of toilet paper was in China in the sixth century. The bidet is commonplace in many countries including Spain (thirty percent), Portugal (seventy percent), Greece (eighty percent), Italy (ninety five percent), and Japan (fifty percent). In Japan automated and high technology toilets incorporate water washing as well as air blow drying and other features. The water bidet is also very popular in the Middle East, and growing in popularity in the United States. On the Indian subcontinent, in spite of lack of bidets, over ninety-five percent of the population uses water for anal cleansing. Many also use soap with the water for cleansing after defecating. Use of paper is rare in this region and hand washing after cleansing is critically important to prevent illness.

Ancient Roman toilets at Ephesus Turkey shutterstock/AbelFeyman

Stories of snakes navigating domestic plumbing are quite common. Rats and other rodents often populate sewers and the snakes go into the sewer system to prey on the rodents. The only barrier between a toilet and the rest of the sewer system is the bend in the pipe known as the 'S' or 'U' bend designed to keep an air fluid barrier to prevent sewer gas escape. Since the water level is actually only a few inches deep it is not difficult for rodents and snakes to maneuver past the pipe bend. They can thus travel from the via the municipal sewer system to a toilet in a home without any physical barrier other than a few inches of water. A variety of rodents, dangerous spiders, and snakes, including tree snakes and pythons, have travelled into people's homes through this route, and human injury from rodent, spider, and snake bites have occurred when using the bathroom.

The device used to clear a drain and toilet sewer line is also known as a snake, because of the way it can maneuver itself through the system. Since the sewer system is open access pipes throughout its length the rodent, spider, and snake visitors have appeared in luxury homes as well as public facilities. In New York, stories of alligators in the sewers have been popularized since the 1930's, but they are probably just urban legends. In Paris a crocodile was found in the city's sewers in the 1980's under Pont Neuf. In spite of the theoretical possibilities of a sewer population of alligators and crocodiles there is no record of an animal of this size being able to get round a 'U' or S bend and arriving in a toilet. It is extremely rare to be at risk, but you just might want to have a look before you make yourself too comfortable on a toilet!

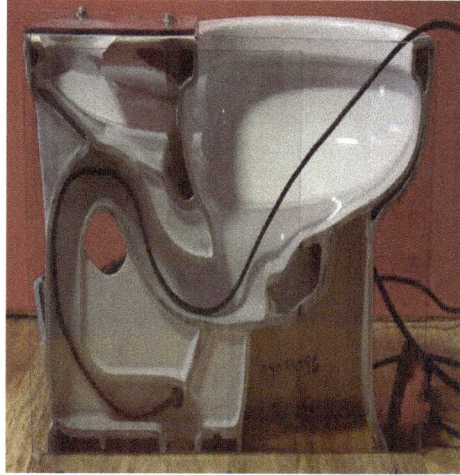

Two kinds of toilet snake. The one that arrives unannounced from the sewer system, and the plumber device to clear clogged drains and sewer lines.

Trypsin, Trypsinogen

A number of pancreatic enzymes are critical for the digestion and absorption of nutrients, including carbohydrates, lipids, and proteins. If the pancreas has been injured, such as by repeated bouts of pancreatitis, cystic fibrosis, or other conditions, deficiency of enzymes can lead to malabsorption and maldigestion. When lipids are malabsorbed a type of diarrhea with large amounts of undigested fat called steatorrhea can occur. Intestinal gas in the presence of excess undigested fat has a strong and offensive odor. Trypsinogen, Trypsin, Chymotrypsin, Pepsinogen, and Pepsin are just a few of the proteolytic enzymes produced in the pancreas which digest proteins to allow their absorption as individual or short chains of amino acids.

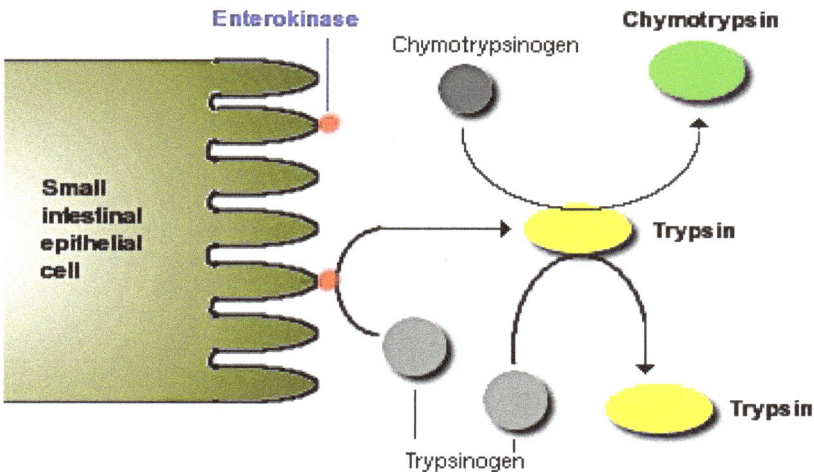

AirVeda: Ancient & New Medical Wisdom

The precursor enzyme, known as a zymogen, trypsinogen is produced in the pancreas. The hormone cholecystokinin (CCK) stimulates the pancreas to secrete it via the pancreatic duct into the duodenum, where it is activated to trypsin by another enzyme enteropeptidase. Trypsin cleaves peptide chains releasing the amino acids lysine and arginine for absorption by the small intestine.

Underground Miners (see Atmospheric Pressure and Ideal Gas Laws)

Underground mining has significant occupational hazards. Some mines are subjected to pressurization to prevent the seepage of ground water into the mine. In other instances, the mining activity may expose pockets of toxic gasses that can lead to injury or death. For those engaged in spelunking, the exploring of caves, descending to depths within the earth have hazards similar to mining related to atmospheric pressure changes. An understanding of the effects and dangers of changes in atmospheric pressure is critical to mine and cave exploration safety. Please see the entries on atmospheric pressure and ideal gas laws for further details.

Vagina (see Fart, Vagina)

Valsalva Maneuver

The Valsalva maneuver is performed by attempted exhalation against a closed airway. This can usually be done by closing the mouth, pinching the nose and nostrils, and attempting to exhale. The maneuver is often used subconsciously when straining on the toilet or with heavy lifting. It is also the technique most commonly used to voluntarily release intestinal gas as a fart. The technique is named after Antonio Maria Valsalva a seventeenth century physician and anatomist from Bologna whose principal scientific interest was the human ear.

www.myweightlifting.com/image-files/valsalva-maneuver.

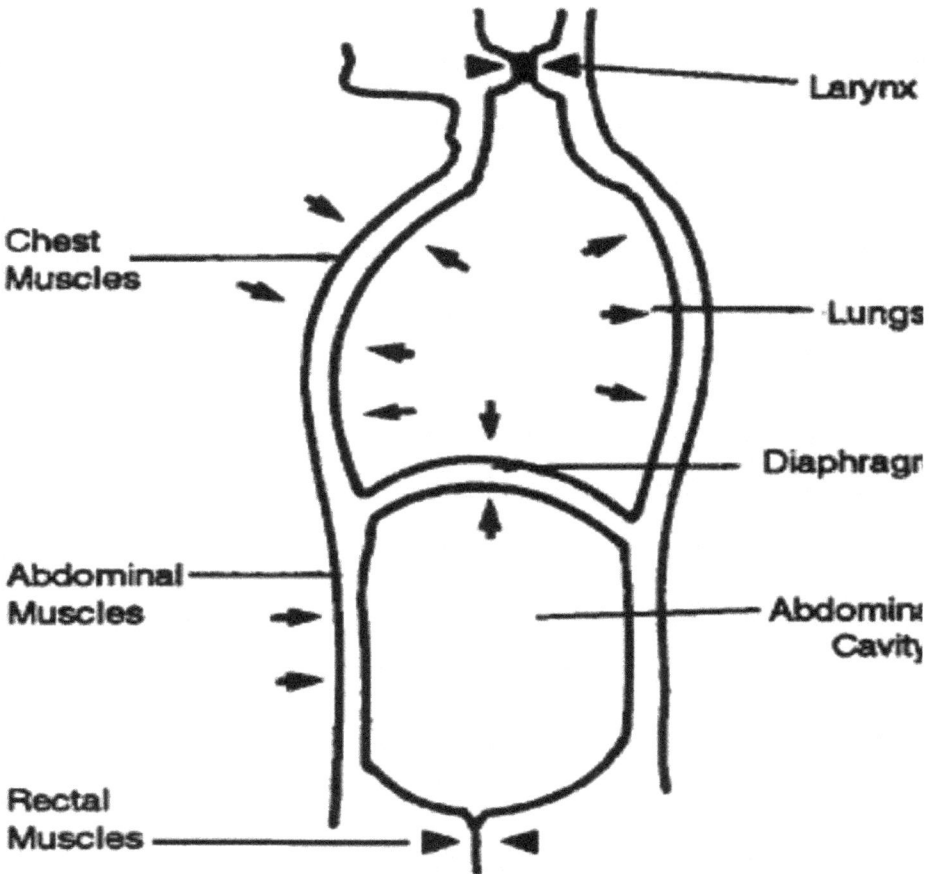

A VALSALVA MANEUVER
www.valsalva.org/vman.

The maneuver can be used in medical examination as well as to equalize pressures in the sinus and ear canal with a change in atmospheric pressure such as with scuba diving or air travel. With air travel, but not with diving, swallowing, chewing gum, and yawning may also be helpful in equalizing pressure. Failure to equalize pressures can lead to ear pain and possibly eardrum perforation.

Villi

The villi are the long finger like projections of the gut mucosal lining, which dramatically increases the surface area for digestion and absorption. The villi are in continuous motion and are a major contributor to intestinal stirring and mixing. In spite of the relatively long length of the small intestine, its absorptive capacity would not be sufficient to maintain nutrition for an organism the size of a human without modifications to increase its surface area.

The deep circular folds of the mucosa and submucosa known as plica circulares or plica, in conjunction with the fingerlike extensions of the mucosa called villi and the microscopic projections of the mucosal cell plasma membranes called microvilli, dramatically increase the surface area. The surface area of the human small intestine thus available for digestive processes, enzymatic activity, and absorption exceeds that of a championship tennis court.

Using electron microscopy, super magnified view of surface of microvilli reveal enhanced surface area. Each villus has thousands of microvilli, as demonstrated on this scanning Transmission electron microscope image of a thin section cut through a human jejunum microfilament.
images.fineartamerica.com

*Air*Veda: Ancient & New Medical Wisdom

Virus (see Microbiome, Pathogen)

Whoopee Cushion

A whoopee cushion is a device used as a practical joke which mimics the sound of flatulence when compressed. It is commonly placed on a chair or cushion so that the sound is generated when someone sits on it. It is typically constructed as a rubber bladder, which is inflated with air. A vibrating exit flap creates an audible fart like sound that is generated when sat upon. The modern commercially successful version was developed in the 1920's by the JEM Rubber Co. of Toronto, Canada. A more discrete alternate remote controlled version that can be hidden under a chair electronically generates prerecorded fart sounds.

Elagabalus, Marcus Aurelius Antoninus Augustus, (c. 203 AD–222 AD) was Roman Emperor from 218 to 222. According to the findings of archeologist Warwick Ball the Roman Emperor Elagabalus played practical jokes on his guests. At dinner parties he would place whoopee cushion like devices under their seats from which fart like sounds would emanate. He showed a disregard for Roman traditions and taboos, insulted the Roman Senate, the common people, and his own protectors the Praetorian Guard. It is therefore not terribly surprising that he was assassinated at the age of eighteen.

Yoga

Yoga is a physical, mental, and spiritual practice that comprises many different schools and approaches. It has often been associated with the practice of Hinduism, Buddhism, Jainism, and other belief systems that originated in the East. The origins of yoga are not clearly defined but were thought to arise in pre-Vedic Indian traditions. The first documents ascribed to yoga are found in the Buddhist Nikayas and the Yoga Sutras of Patanjali recorded around 400 AD. Recognizing its role in general health and wellness, it is no longer an exclusive religious practice but has become increasingly adopted into the mainstream. Of course any general physical activity is beneficial as it increases bowel motility, yet there are a number of specific yoga postures that may provide additional benefit from compression and release of intra-abdominal pressure. The yoga breathing techniques are also found to stimulate the vagus nerve and the autonomic nervous system. Perhaps surprisingly, stimulation of the vagus nerve by FDA approved neurostimulators has been found to be effective in treatment of depression and mood disorders. There is growing evidence that the gut-brain-microbiome axis is powerfully influenced by such vagal nerve stimulation, and yoga breathing techniques may have a similar effect.

A yogi seated in a garden, North Indian or Deccani miniature painting, c. 1620-40
www.columbia.edu/itc Public Domain

Yoga originally had been a religious practice and over thousands of years has become incorporated into secular wellness programs as well. Its effect on natural bodily functions, including intestinal gas were well recognized even in ancient times. Yogic masters and Brahmins in India practiced goze (flatus, eructation, belch) as a means of concentration in ridding the flesh of all evil. Yoga may provide benefit for some individuals with irritable bowel syndrome, especially poses that exercise the lower abdomen. It may also stimulate the passage of intestinal gas. In fact, there is a specific yoga posture designed to aid in the release of intestinal gas. It is not unusual for participants in a yoga class to experience the auditory or olfactory consequences of someone else's, or their own, successful assumption of the yoga gas release pose.

ADHO MUKHA SHVANASANA

- HELPS WITH ARTHRITIS OF THE SHOULDER JOINTS
- PROMOTES A RUSH OF BLOOD TO THE HEAD
- STRENGTHENS THE ANKLES
- RELIEVES PAIN IN HEELS
- HELPS DIGESTION
- RELIEVES FATIGUE

CONTRAINDICATIONS: HIGH PRESSURE; INJURIES TO THE WRIST; HEADACHE; LAST TRIMESTER OF PREGNANCY

Shutterstock/StarikovaVeronika

Yoga helped to achieve the suppression of consciousness and reaching towards enlightenment through union with the Supreme Being (Nirvana). Belching & forcing wind from the buttocks the yogi would chant: "Glory to those keen ebullitions which escape above & below!" (Allen Edwardes: *The Jewel in the Lotus*). Among certain Brahmins, a spiritual blessing was required after each bite of food: He takes a little rice soaked in melted butter and puts it into his mouth, saying: "Glory to the wind which dwells in the chest!' At the second mouthful, "Glory to the wind which dwells in the face!" At the third, "Glory to the wind which dwells in the throat!" At the fourth, "Glory to the wind which dwells in the whole body!" At the fifth, "Glory to those noisy ebullitions which escape above and below!" Any general physical activity is beneficial as it increases bowel motility, yet there are a number of yoga postures that may provide additional benefit from compression and release of intra-abdominal pressure.

The Wind Relieving Pose (Pavanamuktasana) is particularly effective. (Sanskrit: Pavana wind, mukta relieve , Asana Posture) Technique: Lie on your back, arms by your side and feet together. Inhale and as you exhale bend your right knee and flex your right leg bringing the right thigh up pressing on the abdomen. Inhale again and as you exhale lift your head and chest up off the floor and touch your chin to your right knee. Hold this position for several more cycles of inspiration and expiration. Then relax and after a rest repeat the sets with the opposite side. After a second period of rest and relaxation repeat the exercises using both legs at the same time. Avoid practicing the Wind Relieving Pose (Pavanamuktasana) if you have high blood pressure, heart problems, excess acidity reflux or GERD, hernia, slipped disc, neck or back problems, are pregnant, or if you feel any ill effects from the exercise. Other yoga positions and moves that may be helpful include Balasana (Child's Pose) supported, Paschimottanasana (Seated Forward Bend), Supta Baddha Konasana (Reclining Bound Angle Pose) supported, Janu Sirsasana (Head of the Knee Pose) supported, and Jathara Parivartanasana (Revolved Abdomen Pose).

ARDHA MATSIENDRASANA

- STRENGTHENS THE DEEP MUSCLES OF THE SPINE
- INCREASES JOINT MOBILITY OF THE PELVIS
- INCREASES THE MOBILITY OF THE SPINE
- INCREASES BLOOD FLOW TO THE SPINE
- A BENEFICIAL EFFECT ON THE LIVER, INTESTINES, STOMACH, PANCREAS, SPLEEN, REPRODUCTIVE SYSTEM, URINARY SYSTEM, THE KIDNEYS

CONTRAINDICATIONS: HIGH OR LOW PRESSURE; PREGNANCY; ACUTE BOWEL LUMBAR SPINE; RECENT INJURY KNEES AND SPINE

Shutterstock/StarikovaVeronika

Sthala Basti, also called Vata Basti, Air Basti, Air Enema, is an advanced Hatha yoga technique that is best learned from an expert teacher. There are a number of different approaches and techniques but mastery of anal sphincter control is a challenging practice. Once you master this technique you may not become as famous as Le Pétomane of the Moulin Rouge but you will certainly be able to entertain your soon to be former friends.

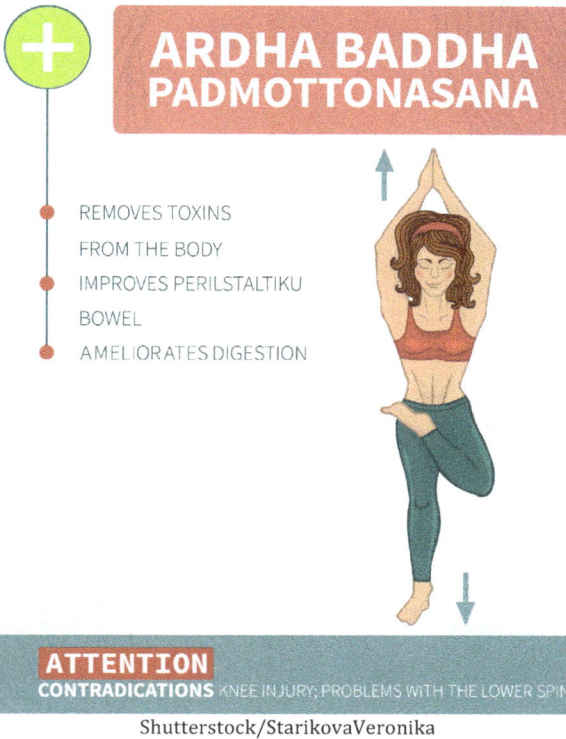

ARDHA BADDHA PADMOTTONASANA

- REMOVES TOXINS FROM THE BODY
- IMPROVES PERILSTALTIKU BOWEL
- AMELIORATES DIGESTION

ATTENTION
CONTRADICATIONS KNEE INJURY; PROBLEMS WITH THE LOWER SPINE

Shutterstock/StarikovaVeronika

Sthala Basti starting from Paschimottanasana technique. Sit with your legs stretched out in front of you and then bend forward halfway. You do not however fully place your upper body on your legs but only bend forward halfway. Perform Uddiyana Bandha by exhaling completely then taking a false inhalation while holding the breath. This flattens and pulls in the abdomen under the rib cage as if the chest was suctioning it in. The process is repeated many times followed by relaxation of the anal sphincter muscles to allow air to be drawn in with the uddiyanna Bandha maneuver. The air suctioned in is released as flatus.

Sthala Basti in lying position technique. Lying on the back bend the knees up towards the chest and raise the buttocks. Practice developing control of the anal sphincter muscles by contraction and relaxation of the sphincter. When the sphincter is relaxed air suctioned into the colon is released as flatulence.

Sthala Basti in Utkatasana technique. Sit in Utkatasana, also called the chair or lightning bolt pose, by squatting while standing with the knees bent ninety degrees backwards to thighs. The back and upright arms form a forward facing ninety-degree angle from the thighs. If necessary until sphincter control is mastered a hollow tube like bamboo or a catheter is placed in the anus and Uddiyama Bandha is performed. Air is sucked into the colon and released as flatus.

441

+ **UTTANASANA**

STIMULATES THE KIDNEYS
AND LIVER
LOOSENS THE PELVIS AND
THE CALF MUSCLES
STRETCHES THE BACK
OF THE THIGHS
PULLS THE SPINE
IMPROVES DIGESTION

ATTENTION HIGH AND LOW BLOOD PRESSURE;
CONTRADICTIONS CIRCULATORY DISORDERS OF THE HEAD

Shutterstock/StarikovaVeronika

Yoga is often associated with the Indian medical system of Ayurveda. The word agni is Sanskrit term for 'fire'. Sanskrit is in the Indo-European family of languages as is Latin, English, Greek and others. The Sanskrit word 'agni' is the equivalent of the Latin 'ignis', which is the root of the English word ignite often used as descriptive action to start a fire. Agni is a central concept in Ayurveda, as it represents the fire energy equivalent produced by the metabolic process of digestion. It allows the breakdown, absorption, and assimilation of food nutrients while eliminating waste and toxins, known as the Ayurveda term 'ama', from the body. The accumulation of ama results in the slow but progressive deterioration of the body which ultimately leads to ill health and disease.

Agni also refers more broadly to our ability to process and digest all aspects of life, including food, experiences, memories, and sensory impressions. It transforms the physical matter of food into the useable forms of energy the cells of the body require. *Jathar-agni* determines the production of hydrochloric acid in the stomach, while *Bhuta-agni* determines the production of bile in the liver. *Kloma-agni* determines the production of the pancreatic enzymes, while *Jatru-agni* regulates the thyroid gland. *Dhatu-agni* is the agni at the level of tissue and cellular metabolism. The Ayurvedic concept of agni beliefs continues to an even subtler level of *Indrya-agni,* described as the door of perception, which transforms external information into internal knowledge. In Ayurveda a stronger agni allows for a stronger and clearer body and mind. The nature and quality of the various *agnis* depend on the individual's blend of the three doshas: vata, pitta, and kapha. In individuals with a predominance of the vata and kapha doshas the agni tends to be weak resulting in a digestive system that is cold, irregular, and sluggish. This is believed to contribute to signs and symptoms of constipation, malabsorption, and excess intestinal gas. In pittas the fires of agni is excessive and can result in heartburn, acid reflux, colitis, and other burning symptoms.

Culinary herbs and spices are used in Ayurveda to enhance the level of agni between and during meals. The meals should be balanced and provide a sampling of each of the tastes, sweet, sour, astringent, bitter, salty, and pungent. One popular Ayurvedic practice is to consume a small piece of fresh ginger with a few drops of lemon juice prior to eating a meal. This allows a slow and progressive awakening of the fire of digestive Agni. Other aromatic spices that aid in digestion include black pepper, cayenne pepper, cardamon, and liquorice. They are believed to aid in the cooking and predigestion of foods. The spices also stimulate the secretions of saliva and digestive enzymes which reduces the work load of the Agni and results in less fatigue after eating. By assisting digestion the Herb's and spices reduce gas and ama. When digestion is incomplete, fermentation takes place and it is this process which produces gas and ama which can contribute to gastrointestinal signs and symptoms. Fennel is a common herb offered in Indian restaurants as a carminative. The seeds are chewed, the juice swallowed, and the pulp spit out. It relaxes the lower esophageal sphincter to allow swallowed air to be released and may reduce gas, discomfort, and fatigue. Hing is also used in Ayurveda cooking to assist weak agni and digestion. It is a resinous sap from the asafetida plant and, when combined with other aromatic and carminative herbs in the Ayurveduc remedy hingavashtak, it is believed to promote the deeper assimilation of nutrients.

Ojas is the Ayurveduc term for the vital nectar of life. To achieve optimal health it is important to eliminate ama and focus on the production of Ojas, the Sanskrit term meaning 'vigor'. Ojas is the pure and subtle essence that has been extracted from food that has been completely and properly digested. It circulates throughout the body tissues and heart, sustaining the physical body, providing clarity to the mind, and nurturing emotional balance. A diet of pure easily digested foods, described in Ayurveda as 'Sattvic', promotes the creation and flow of Ojas. Sattvic foods include organic milk, almonds, honey, sesame, rice, and fruits.

Some foods are difficult if not impossible for the body to convert into ojas, including meat, poultry, fish, oily foods, cheese, processed food, and items with an excess of sour or salty tastes. Freshly prepared meals produce more Ojas than foods that has been canned, frozen, or reheated. Alcohol and tobacco use reduce and eliminate ojas. Signs of Ojas includ: You feel rested upon awakening, Your skin has a healthy glow, Your tongue is clear and pink, Your body feels light, regardless of the number on the scale, You feel centered throughout the day, Your digestion is strong without bloating, You feel energized & enthusiastic, Your mind is clear, Your body has a pleasant smell, You rarely get sick. Signs of Ama include: Bad breath, Coated tongue, Dull appetite, Delicate digestion, Sluggish or irritable elimination, Generalized pain, Fatigue, Depression, Susceptibility to infections, Difficulty manifesting intentions.

Oma's is the essence of the processing of all signals our body receives, not just the foods we eat. Much as important as the quality and character of the foods, is the quality of our experience and environment. If we are in a stressful or uncomfortable environment creating ojas cannot take place because we are experiencing what are basically indigestible emotions that are distributing distressed chemical messages throughout our cells and organs. To create a nurturing atmosphere for meals it is important to pay attention to all of the senses — taste, sound, sight, touch, and smell. Here are a few suggestions to enhance the production if ojas

- Eat in a comfortable environment and atmosphere
- Do not eat when you are upset.
- Sit down comfortably to enjoy your meal.
- Do not multitask while you are eating, do not eat while reading, watching television, or while on a computer or mobile device.
- Only eat when you are hungry.
- Dine at a moderate pace. Chew your food well and with enjoyment of the taste, texture, and aroma. Don't gulp down your food or eat too slowly.
- Moderate the quantity of raw foods, which are harder to digest than cooked ones.
- Include all six tastes (sweet, sour, astringent, bitter, salty, and pungent) with each meal.
- Drink water to maintain adequate hydration
- Use spices and herbs that assist the digestive process
- Enjoy pure Sattvic foods they are easily digestible, including organic milk, almonds, honey, sesame, rice, and fruits.

Zymogen

A zymogen is an enzyme precursor, which can be converted to the active form of the enzyme with the appropriate stimulus or conditions. The protein digesting enzyme zymogens pepsinogen and trypsinogen are converted to their respective active enzymes pepsin and trypsin in the presence of gastric hydrochloric acid. Other zymogens require another specific enzyme to initiate the activation process. Such restricted activation makes perfect sense to avoid the destructive properties of the enzymes being prematurely activated, where their protein digesting properties can otherwise damage the organs in which they are produced. The dangerous condition of pancreatitis can arise when acid enters the pancreatic duct and activates the zymogens to the active enzyme which then inflame and destroy pancreatic tissue as a form of autodigestion.

The enzyme is specific for a substrate such as proteins, carbohydrates, or lipids. They can be restricted to a unique substrate such as the individual carbohydrates lactose, fructose, sucrose, etc. If a zymogen or its active enzyme is defective or present in inadequate quantities the consequences are dependent on the importance of the enzyme. Some digestive enzymes are critical for the health and welfare of the individual. Fortunately, most of the digestive enzymes are available commercially and can be taken orally if needed. Other enzymes play critical roles in various cells and tissues and their absence can lead to specific conditions and diseases. Many are needed in internal organs and tissues, and delivery is much more challenging than simply taking an oral supplement.

Shutterstock/joshya

Afterword

Medicine and the life sciences are undergoing dramatic advances in knowledge and understanding. We are at the threshold of a revolutionary understanding of genomics and the microbiome, with the analogy being made that this is the equivalent of the discovery of an enormous unexplored continent. Actually this analogy is inadequate, it is more as if an entire parallel universe has been identified. This discovery is partly due to advances in technology which allow deeper exploration of the universe around us, including peering more deeply into the previously invisible microscopic and molecular worlds. Another contributing advance is the enhanced ability to communicate, a critical aspect of the collaboration that most often results in scientific breakthroughs. It is ironic and tragic that many of the lifesaving advances in science and medicine such as immunization, antibiotics, and effective therapeutics were delayed for hundreds of years, resulting in the deaths of millions, because of lapses in communication, usually because of language barriers.

Humans on Earth use six thousand five hundred different languages and 46 different alphabets. Approximately four hundred of these languages belong to the Indo-European family, which includes Greek, Latin, English, Sanskrit and many languages spoken in Europe, Iran, and the Indian subcontinent. Although they only account for seven percent of all languages, they are spoken by three billion people, nearly half the world's population. In spite of the rich tapestry of world culture, the communication challenges have contributed to a fragmented world community, hostilities, and a barrier to societal, scientific, and human achievements. The English language is the richest language on the planet with over one million words using its twenty-six-character alphabet. Although English has become the dominant language in medicine and science, computers have advanced translation capabilities to become virtually universal and instantaneous. Imagine the world with one universal language and only one alphabet. Now imagine that the alphabet consists of only four main characters or letters. Welcome to the universal world of genomics, where all life forms on the planet communicate and understand this single language.

Although, for better or for worse, we consider ourselves closer relatives to the other humans on the planet than all other life forms, we actually share a deeper level of a common communication language with all living creatures on the planet. This is the language of the universal genetic code, consisting of a limited alphabet of characters that can be counted on one hand. The sequence of the acid bases, adenine, guanine, cytosine, and thymine, encodes the genetic information within genes on the double helix of deoxyribonucleic acid. The single helix of ribonucleic acid uses the nucleic acid uracil in place of thymine. The Swiss scientist Friedrich Miescher (1844-1895) discovered nucleic acids in 1869, and later proposed their possible role in heredity. Nobel Laureate Erwin Schrödinger (1887-1961) further developed the theory that heredity must be transmitted by a chemical structure found in the nucleus with a provocative publication entitled *What is Life?* Francis Crick (1916-2004) and James Watson (1928-) identified the double helix structure of DNA based on the groundbreaking work of Rosalyn Franklin who tragically died at a young age before the Nobel Prize was awarded for the discovery.

The theory of evolution posits that all life on earth originated with a single organism, and mutations that proved beneficial for survival and reproduction eventually led to further advancement of life forms. Mutations that were not beneficial and that did not contribute to survival of the fittest were removed from the gene pool with the demise and eventual extinction of the disadvantaged species. As expected with this theory, one can trace the progress of evolution over eons and the course of present day and extinct life forms that inhabited the planet. The oldest evolutionary life forms have a genetic fingerprint of genes that have remained vital for enhanced survival, and are virtually universal in spite of otherwise significant genetic diversity. If we accept our anthropomorphic notion that humans are the highest evolutionary life form, it can be humbling that we share approximately one third of our entire genome with the most primitive of microscopic life, bacteria and Archaea. Perhaps just as humbling is that our nearest genetic relative the chimpanzee shares just under ninety-nine percent of the human genome.

One of the most startling of the scientific advances of the last generation is actually a reassessment of the consensus one hundred years ago that Charles Darwin (1809-1882) was correct in genetic inheritance, and his contemporary Jean-Baptiste Lamarck (1744-1829) was wrong in proposing that genetics can be influenced by the environment. It appears that actually they were both right dependent on different circumstances. The original belief that mapping the human genome would unlock the secrets of human health and disease was disproven with the discovery of a new field called epigenetics. This rapidly evolving science has demonstrated that the environment and external factors can determine the activity or restriction of genes. Not only the environment, but also other genes can have potent and consequential epigenetic properties. It is no longer just the human genome that is key to human health and disease, but it is also the environment and the genes and epigenetic activity of all of the nonhuman genes we are constantly exposed to.

Humans have approximately twenty-three thousand genes of which between thirty percent to ninety-eight point five percent are already shared with and interchangeable with other organisms on the planet. The trillions of organisms representing thousands of different species that live within the human microbiome, the majority within the gut microbiome, represent an exposure pool of over one million nonhuman genes. Because all genes, no matter the origin, speak a universally understood language, the instructions from a nonhuman source are not necessarily recognized by the host as being of alien origin. Of particular importance is that the universal communication has distinct advantages for the human host, and indeed its survival is dependent on these gene supplements from the microbiome.

*Air*Veda: Ancient & New Medical Wisdom

Although pathogenic organism occurs, and can contribute to disease and mortality, the vast majority of the microbiome are commensal organisms which enhance human health and longevity. There is growing evidence that most human disease is related to a disruption of the normal healthy microbiome. Ironically, the lifesaving development of antibiotics appears to be a contributor to the disruption of the healthy microbiome, a condition called dysbiosis. Not only has antibiotic usage become profligate, but its common incorporation into the animal food supply as a growth enhancer has led to its widespread dissemination into the environment, food, water supply.

It is clear that the human microbiome, especially the gut microbiome, is dependent on the host diet. The presence of fiber in the diet is critical for microbiome health, as it is a main source of microbial nutrition, and is thus referred to as a prebiotic. Dietary changes, above and beyond prebiotics and probiotics, can lead to major changes in the microbiome, and thus human health and disease. A previously underappreciated implication of the universal communication of nonhuman genes and the human host is that humans are exposed to additional millions of genes in the diet. All food sources have their own genomes and whether plant or animal, Archaea or bacteria, virus or prion, parasite or protist, a gene of any origin can be understood by the human host, and if acted upon can change the host. The diet can play a critical, and direct role in human health and disease, both through manipulation of the microbiome as well as directly from food based genomic information.

The gut-brain axis has been known for a long time with its origins in the concept of gut instincts and gut feelings. The discovery of the extremely well developed enteric nervous system gave rise to the concept that the gut is actually a secondary or primitive brain. Surprisingly the major neurotransmitter serotonin, most often thought of in association with depression, is found to be unevenly distributed in the human body, only five percent is in the brain, ninety-five percent is in the gut. The neurotransmitter dopamine is found in equal fifty percent proportions in both the brain and the gut. The condition of Parkinson disease associated with dopamine deficiency is now believed to originate in the gut, and after many years or decades eventually affect the brain. The ability of microbes to affect the brain has been known since their discovery, especially with the recognition that infections of the brain can lead to severe symptoms, such as seen with syphilis, rabies, encephalitis, etc. The role of parasites, such as the extremely common cat protist parasite *Toxoplasma gondii* is just becoming more recognized. With the enormous domesticated cat population around the world, it is not surprising that humans may become infected directly by contact with cats and their droppings, or by ingesting undercooked foods that contain the cysts. The number of people infected because of their proximity to cats is numbered in the billions.

Although many people are impressed with cats use of a litter box and their reputation for cleanliness, the feral outdoor cat population more than compensates by leaving contaminated droppings everywhere. As far as an outdoor cat is concerned, a children's playground sandbox is just an oversized kitty litter box. When a pregnant human is exposed to Toxoplasma catastrophic and tragic infection of the fetus is all too common. It had previously been believed that only a minority of infections with Toxoplasma led to symptoms of the disease state known as toxoplasmosis. Growing evidence highlights the importance of the parasite in modulating the brain and behavior. There is growing evidence that *Toxoplasma gondii* may contribute, or perhaps even be the single causative agent in specific individuals, of mental health disorders such as depression, schizophrenia, mood disorders, hostility, psychosis, risk taking behavior and other conditions.

NEGLECTED PARASITIC INFECTION:
Toxoplasmosis

Toxoplasmosis is the **2nd leadin** **cause of death** from foodborn illness in the United States.

The effect of hormones on mood and mental function has likewise been long recognized. The ability of food, drink, tobacco, alcohol, psychoactive mushrooms and seafood, herbs, etc. to effect human mood and behavior has long been apparent. The concept of psychopharmacology was originally based on plant isolated and derived pharmaceuticals and chemicals. The most recent scientific advances suggest that depression, anxiety, Parkinson, Alzheimer, and perhaps even autism and multiple sclerosis may have gut origins related to the microbiome. Probiotics that may be beneficial in therapy for these conditions are now being classified as potential pscychobiotics. Manipulation of the microbiome is a potential approach to managing obesity and diabetes mellitus. Fecal microbiota transplants in animal models shows a reversal of obesity and mood disorders. Investigation of its utility in humans is ongoing for these conditions, after already been proven effective in managing dysbiosis due to the life threatening colitis caused by the antibiotic resistant organism *Clostridia difficile*.

*Air*Veda: Ancient & New Medical Wisdom

The gut-brain-microbiome-diet axis is just beginning to be fully explored and holds great promise for major advances in human health and longevity. The golden age of discovery is not in the past, but hopefully in the present and the near future. Unfortunately, medicine and the life sciences have a long history of missteps and false hopes, especially when commerce has an opportunity for financial gain. The burgeoning industry of probiotics has already exceeded forty billion dollars of revenue each year, in spite of the lack of the lack of knowledge about the optional microbiome. It is more than likely that the optimal microbiome will have to be tailored and individualized for each person based on genomics, environmental exposure, diet, and other yet to be identified variables.

The other important message to remember about the microbiome is that it is not one organism, but a community of hundreds if not thousands of distinct species that together create the optimal microbial environment. The probiotics offered in the marketplace today offer only a single or several species. The results of supplements of a single or a few species of microbes may be beneficial to a limited number of individuals who may offer well-meaning testimonials. It is just as likely that a limited number of others will have adverse reactions, and the majority will probably not notice a change one way or the other. When it comes to the probiotic marketplace it is not regulated by the Food and Drug Administration (FDA), and even if it were, that would not be a meaningful assurance of either safety or benefit. Until there is scientific validation, hopefully that will be generated over the next few years, it would be prudent to use probiotics that occur naturally in foods that have been consumed for generations. Yogurt, kefir, sauerkraut, pickles, kimchi, etc. are safer and much less expensive.

The personalized and precision medicine that is on the horizon will be a major advance. The previous concept of population based medicine based on the statistical average patient has been a poor substitute for recognizing the unique needs and requirements of the individual. Everything from selection of therapy, dosage, risks of side effects, diet, exercise, probiotics, etc. will be based on the genomics and physiology of the individual. Further advances will undoubtedly make even this most current concept outdated and obsolete. The greater the knowledge base, the more we can define effective and beneficial approaches. Although the books in this series will with time be superseded by future writings, the knowledge contained provides our current understanding and wisdom. It is the author's hope that they have provided practical and useful information in an enlightening and entertaining manner, yet encouraged an open mind that future advances may either validate or disprove and replace current concepts. With future advances all but certain, it is important to seek competent professional advice on health matters, and not rely on books and readings. It is also prudent to remember a witticism from Mark Twain (1835-1910): "Be careful about reading health books. You may die of a misprint!" With that caveat, the reader is encouraged to peruse the author's other offerings that will hopefully likewise be found to be intriguing, informative, and entertaining.

To 'Air' is Human: Everything You Ever Wanted to Know About Intestinal Gas
cover everything you ever wanted to know about the burp, belch, bloat, fart, and
digestive topics but were either too afraid or too embarrassed to ask. Intestinal
gas has been produced and released by virtually every human who has ever lived,
yet very few people have been provided with the knowledge that can offer
comfort and relief. These volumes are overflowing with practical information,
fascinating facts, surprising trivia, and tasteful humorous insight about this
universal phenomenon. The following companion volumes may also be of
interest.

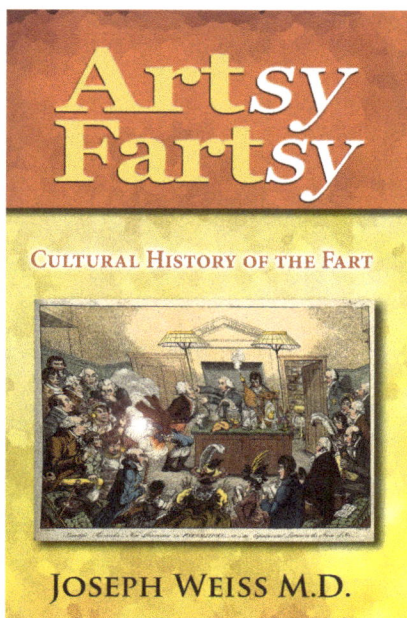

Artsy Fartsy, Cultural History of the Fart is a fascinating and factually correct
review of the common fart through human culture and history. The cough, sneeze,
hiccup, stomach rumble, burp, belch, and other bodily sounds simply cannot
compete with the notoriety of the fart. Whether encountered live and in person or
through the medium of literature, television, film, art, or music it may leave a
powerful and lingering memory. The intent of the book is to demonstrate that the
ubiquitous fart has a more illustrious story to share than just lowbrow humor.
The societal standards and cultural acceptance of this normal physiologic event
have evolved over the years, and it is currently popular as a point of humor even
in sophisticated circles.

The history of the fart in culture and society is a seldom told but fascinating tale.
The very same fart that has triggered wars and the deaths of thousands of
innocents (see entry on Josephus Flavius) has also led to the laughter and
entertainment of millions worldwide (see entry on Joseph Pujol and Cinematic
Arts). Even today the response to a fart can reach from the extremes of triggering

violence to inducing spasms of uncontrollable laughter. This volume is a chronological survey of some of the high and low points in the cultural history of this ubiquitous but inherently controversial activity. Rather than an exhaustive and long-winded discourse, this volume is meant to introduce the reader to the colorful and extremely varied response to the fart over the course of human history.

The Scoop on Poop, Flush with Knowledge is the equally unique volume that continues the series in a scatological vein. Digestion, genomics, gut-brain-microbiome-diet axis, and poop are just some of the important topics covered that profoundly impact human health and wellness. It provides a wealth of knowledge on the rarely told but engrossing subject of the digestive residue of the gastrointestinal tract. From potentially life-saving information to the bizarre and obscure, the book completely covers a subject many people mistakenly consider a simple waste. It is much more complex than that, and this book uncovers and airs its mysteries! The wealth of valuable information and trivia in these volumes can sustain a long social conversation, or cut it short abruptly!

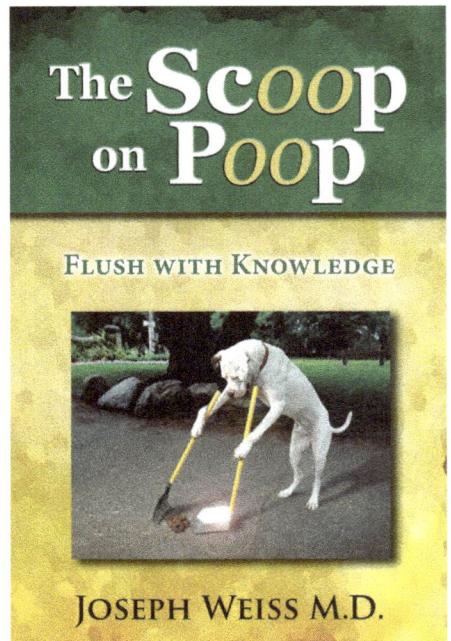

How Do You Doo? Everybody Pees & Poops! A delightfully informative, entertaining, and colorfully illustrated volume with valuable practical insights on toilet training. Tasteful color photographs of animals answering the call of nature allows the child to understand that everybody does it! Additional informative relevant content to entertain the adult while the child is 'on the potty' is included.

The Quest for Immortality, Advances in Vitality & Longevity provides an informative and enlightening overview of the remarkable advances in science and medicine that are dramatically enhancing human health and lifespan. The volume is written in clear, understandable, and engaging language with striking colorful illustrations. From groundbreaking nanotechnology to genomics and stem cells, the secrets of vitality and longevity are being uncovered along with more traditional advances and practical insights into disease prevention and health enhancement.

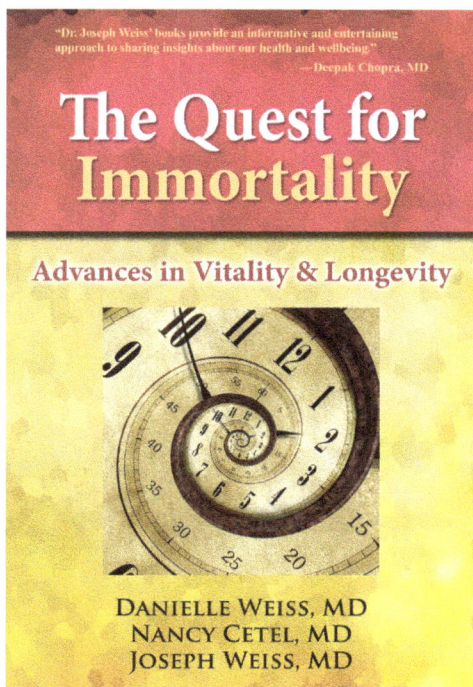

An even more comprehensive yet entertaining series are the extensive volumes of ***Digestive Health & Disease, an Illustrated Encyclopedia of Everything You Ever Wanted to Know About Digestion & Nutrition***. These volumes are a uniquely informative, entertaining, and lavishly illustrated compendium of alimentary knowledge and eccentricities. It covers everything you ever wanted to know about digestion and nutrition in health and disease. Volumes One through Five are available on Amazon.com. Organized as a reader friendly encyclopedia, the volumes cover over two thousand five hundred subject topics. Each volume may be utilized as an independent fully contained resource for the subjects it covers. The extensive size and scope of the series allows topics to be included that are rarely discussed in other books in the field and may be of great interest to the curious mind. The website www.smartaskbooks.com has a complete list of books and programs.

Index

Small Bowel (see Small Intestine)
Small Intestine (see Digestion, Gastrointestinal Tract, Duodenum, Jejunum, Ileum)
x, 42, 43, 47, 48, 54, 90, 91, 92, 93, 96, 103, 121, 134, 147-149, 249, 251,
256, 258, 259, 263, 265, 266, 268-277, 279-283, 291, 309, 313-320, 323,
329, 344, 346, 347, 384, 387-389, 421-424, 427, 431, 433
Small Intestine Bacterial Overgrowth 90-91, 282, 309, 312, 330, 346-347
Smell (see Fart, Smell) 18, 58, 87, 113, 141, 170, 173, 176, 186, 193, 197, 202-210,
214, 221, 225, 230, 236, 250, 256, 306, 310, 382, 385, 411, 417, 420, 421,
430
Smoking (see Carminative, Aerophagia, Tobacco) 26-27, 135, 136, 163, 166, 186,
210, 230, 261, 263, 292, 308, 322, 327, 328, 349, 444
Snake 435-436
Sneeze (see Diffusion, Sternutation) 112, 173-175, 192, 210, 217, 218, 446
Sodium Bicarbonate xv, 96-97, 132-134, 147, 148, 167, 170, 186, 187, 230, 231,
249, 259-261, 272, 273, 377, 385-387, 424, 425
Soft Drinks (see Aerophagia, Carbonation) 31-35, 61-67, 113, 125-131, 131-134,
161-164
Soluble Fiber 246-250
Speed (see Fart Speed) 148, 169, 170, 173-176, 187, 214, 216-218, 231, 249
Spelunking (see Atmospheric Pressure) 85, 424-425, 432
Sphincter, Anal 40, 54-56, 107, 108, 213, 217, 250, 269, 380, 392, 393, 417, 438
Sphincter, Lower Esophageal 25, 103, 134-137, 147, 159, 161, 164-166, 261-263,
291-294, 308, 326-329, 412, 427
Spontaneous Human Combustion (see Fart, Flammable) 185-186, 214
Sprue (see Gluten Sensitive Enteropathy) 137, 254, 280-283, 307, 330
Stachyose 47, 94, 143, 169, 254, 307
Sternutation (see Sneeze) 112, 173-175, 192, 210, 217, 218, 446
Stinkbug 200-201
Stomach (see Digestion, Gastrointestinal Tract) viii, x, 31, 42, 43, 80, 83, 84, 89,
92, 93, 96, 100, 101, 103-105, 111, 125, 132, 133, 135, 136, 138, 145, 147,
148, 149, 151, 159, 161, 163-165, 167, 187-192, 194, 231, 248, 249, 259-
261, 263, 271-272, 284,285, 291-294, 308, 316, 319, 323, 327, 329, 334, 344,
376, 377, 380, 383, 387, 388, 411, 418, 419, 421-423, 425-426, 446
Stomach (Gastric) Acid 96, 132, 133, 147, 148, 164, 165, 167, 187, 231, 249, 259-
261, 263-272, 276-278, 292-294, 308, 327, 377, 383, 387, 425-426
Stool (Feces, Excrement) 40, 43, 55, 65, 70-74, 99, 107, 108, 150, 174, 183, 196,
206, 210, 218, 221, 225, 227, 230, 233-246, 284, 286, 289, 297, 306, 310,
332, 365, 385, 410, 413, 417, 443, 446, 447
Sucrase 48, 117, 121, 256, 426-428
Sucrose 31, 47, 116-120, 125, 158, 254, 256-258, 330, 381, 426-428, 440
Sucrose Intolerance 427-428
Sugars (see Carbohydrate, Glucose, Sucrose, Fructose, Lactose) 29, 31, 48, 49, 98,
116-121, 124, 125, 131, 140, 146, 162, 163, 249, 251, 265, 269, 280, 290,
309, 313, 329, 341, 357, 376, 383, 385, 387, 392, 397, 423, 431, 440
Surface Area (see Activated Charcoal, Digestion, & Gastrointestinal Tract) 17-18,
20, 130, 137, 146, 148, 205, 274, 354, 402, 4122, 433, 434

*Air*Veda: Ancient & New Medical Wisdom

www.ingramcontent.com/pod-product-compliance
Lightning Source LLC
Chambersburg PA
CBHW051242020426
42333CB00025B/3017